AF449368

Anne Grethe Jurik (Ed.)

# Imaging of the Sternocostoclavicular Region

Anne Grethe Jurik (Ed.)

# Imaging of the Sternocostoclavicular Region

With 101 Figures and 1 Table

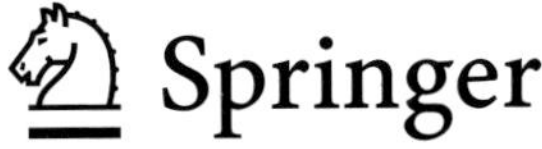
Springer

**Anne Grethe Jurik, MD, DMSc**
Associate Professor, Consultant and Director of Research,
Department of Radiology
Aarhus University Hospital
Noerrebrogade 44
DK-8000 Aarhus C
Denmark
E-mail: jurik@dadlnet.dk

ISBN 10 3-540-33147-6   Springer Berlin Heidelberg New York
ISBN 13 978-3-540-33147-6   Springer Berlin Heidelberg New York
Library of Congress Control Number: 2006929195



Springer is a part of Springer Science + Business Media
springer.com
©Springer-Verlag Berlin Heidelberg 2007



Editor: Dr. Ute Heilmann, Heidelberg
Deskeditor: Meike Stoeck, Heidelberg
Coverdesign: Frido Steinen-Broo, eStudio Calamar, Spain
Production & Typesetting: LE-TEX Jelonek, Schmidt & Vöckler GbR ,Leipzig
Printed on acid-freepaper   21/3100/YL – 5 4 3 2 1 0

# Preface

The sternocostoclavicular region often presents diagnostic challenges for both the clinician and the radiologist. It is commonly involved in rheumatologic disorders, sometimes with pain referred to areas distant from the joints. This potentially can lead to delayed diagnosis. In addition, the region is difficult to visualise by conventional radiography implying the need for more demanding examinations to confirm the disorder. As a result the region has generally not achieved the attention it merits by radiologists.

The purpose of this book is to give a survey of sternocostoclavicular disorders and their imaging based on the literature and the authors' experience.

ANNE GRETHE JURIK
AARHUS, DENMARK

# Contents

## V   CLINICAL PROBLEMS

# List of Contributors

**Yasuaki Arai, MD, PhD**
Divisions of Diagnostic Radiology and Nuclear Medicine, National Cancer Centre Hospital, 104-0045 Tokyo, Japan

**Richard M. Blaquiere, MD**
Department of Radiology, Southampton General Hospital, Tremona Road, Southampton, SO16 6YD, UK

**Hirokazu Chuman, MD**
Division of Orthopedics, National Cancer Centre Hospital, Tokyo, Japan

**Giuseppe Guglielmi, MD**
Professor, Department of Radiology, Scientific Institute Hospital "Casa Sollievo della Sofferenza", Viale Cappuccini 1, 71013 San Giovanni Rotondo, Italy

**Stephen P. Harden, MD**
Department of Radiology, Southampton General Hospital, Tremona Road, Southampton, SO16 6YD, UK

**Anne Grethe Jurik, MD**
Department of Radiology,
Aarhus University Hospital, Noerrebrogade 44, DK-8000 Aarhus C, Denmark

**Tetsuo Maeda, MD**
Divisions of Diagnostic Radiology and Nuclear Medicine, National Cancer Centre Hospital, 104-0045 Tokyo, Japan

**Mototaka Miyake, MD**
Divisions of Diagnostic Radiology and Nuclear Medicine, National Cancer Centre Hospital, 104-0045 Tokyo, Japan

**Mariano Scaglione, MD**
Emergency and Trauma CT Section, Department of Radiology, Cardarelli Hospital, Via A. Cardarelli 9, 80131, Naples, Italy

**Flemming Brandt Soerensen, MD, DMSc**
Professor, Department of Pathology, Aarhus University Hospital, Noerrebrogade 44, DK-8000 Aarhus C, Denmark

**Ukihide Tateishi, MD, PhD**
Divisions of Diagnostic Radiology and Nuclear Medicine, National Cancer Centre Hospital, 104-0045 Tokyo, Japan

**Michele Tonerini, MD**
Department of Emergency Radiology, S. Chiara Hospital, Via Bonanno Pisano, 56100 Pisa, Italy

**Umio Yamaguchi, MD**
Division of Orthopedics, National Cancer Centre Hospital, Tokyo, Japan

# Abbreviations

| | | | |
|---|---|---|---|
| **AS** | Ankylosing spondylitis | **RA** | Rheumatoid arthritis |
| **CRMO** | Chronic recurrent multifocal osteomyelitis | **ReA** | Reactive arthritis |
| **CRP** | C-reactive protein | **SAPHO** | Synovitis, acne, pustulosis, hyperostosis and osteitis |
| **CT** | Computed tomography | **SCC** | Sternocostoclavicular |
| **CVC** | Central venous catheter | **SCCH** | Sternocostoclavicular hyperostosis |
| **ESR** | Erythrocyte sedimentation rate | **SCJ** | Sternoclavicular joint |
| **FDG** | $^{18}$F-fluorodeoxyglucose | **SCoJ** | Sternocostal joint |
| **FOV** | Field of view | **SpA** | Spondylarthropathy |
| **Gd** | Gadolinium | **SPECT** | Single-photon emission computed tomography |
| **ISCCO** | Intersternocostoclavicular ossification | **STIR** | Short-tau inversion recovery (MR sequence) |
| **MPR** | Multiplanar reconstruction | **T1 FS** | T1-weighted fat suppressed (MR sequence) |
| **MRI** | Magnetic resonance imaging | | |
| **MSCT** | Multislice computed tomography | **T2 FS** | T2-weighted fat suppressed (MR sequence) |
| **MSJ** | Manubriosternal joint | | |
| **OA** | Osteoarthritis | **VIP** | Volume intensity projection (CT projection) |
| **PAO** | Pustulotic arthro-osteitis | | |
| **PET** | Positron emission tomography | | |
| **PPP** | Pustulosis palmoplantaris | | |

# I

# DEVELOPMENT OF THE STERNOCOSTOCLAVICULAR REGION

# 1 Bones, Cartilages and Joints

ANNE GRETHE JURIK

## Contents



## 1.1 Introduction

The sternocostoclavicular (SCC) region represents the anterior part of the chest wall. It consists of the sternum, the adjacent articulating first to seventh costal cartilages, the sternoclavicular joint, the medial part of the clavicles and the surrounding soft tissue. The normal anatomy and development of the region has gained attention, partly because it can be used for determination of age and gender.

This chapter includes a summary of the normal fetal and postnatal development of the SCC region until the skeleton is fully developed.

## 1.2 Sternum, Including Manubriosternal Joint

In the embryo the sternum develops from two cartilaginous plates (sternal bands), one on either side of the midline, which normally fuse during the 2nd month of fetal life (Fig. 1.1) [14]. During the 9th week, the two sternal bands are completely fused in the midline, and the sternum is uniformly cartilaginous and resembles the

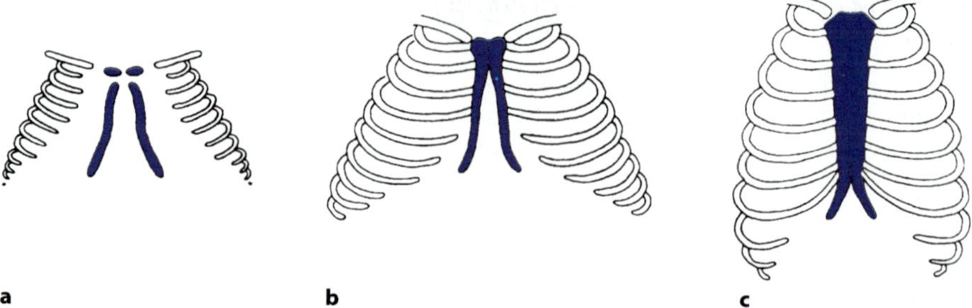

**Fig. 1.1** Cartilaginous sternal development. The sternal cartilaginous primordia in embryos of 6 **a**, 8 **b** and 9 weeks **c** of age

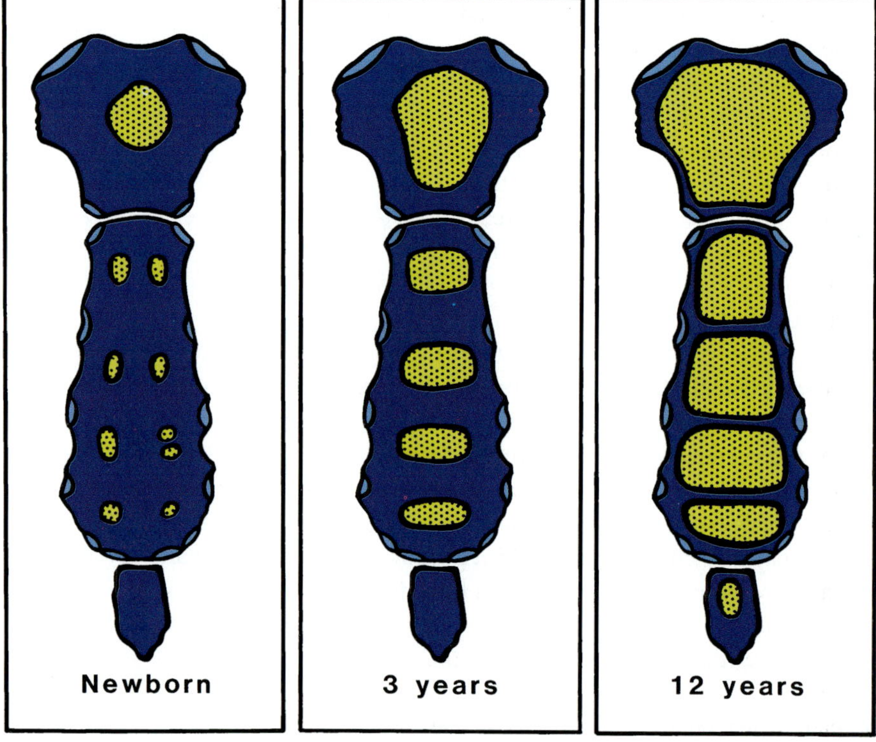



**Fig. 1.2** Development of sternal ossification. The ossification of the individual sternebrae starts during the 5th to 6th month of gestation. There are ossified nuclei in the manubrium sterni and the first to fourth sternebrae at birth, but they may vary in number and configuration. The ossification centres gradually expand and fuse across the midline

mature sternum in shape. Sternal segmentation occurs shortly afterwards. Deposition of bone (ossific centres) in the cartilaginous sternebrae begins to appear in this cartilage in the 5th to 6th fetal months [1, 9, 15]. The first centre is that of the manubrium, followed by the nucleus of the second, third and fourth pieces during the interval before birth (Fig. 1.2). There is a wide variability in the number and configuration of the ossification centres of the developing sternum. Ossification of the manubrium commonly starts from a single centre, but sometimes there are two centres located cranially, and occasionally multiple centres [9, 13]. Some or all of the sternebrae develop from paired or even multiple ossification centres [9]. The lower segment(s) and the xiphoid process ossify postnatally, and the more or less final pattern of sternal ossification centres is not found until several years after birth [9, 13]. The wide variation of sternal development in the embryo seems to preclude its use for satisfactory gestational age estimation; it is clearly less valuable than other morphological criteria already available [9, 15].

The postnatal development and maturation of the sternum also vary [13]. The ossified nuclei in childhood may vary considerably in size and shape depending on age. Expansion of individual ossification centres progresses within the peripheral part of the cartilaginous sternal anlage in consistence with the biology of endochondral ossification of hyaline cartilage [13]. The gradual expansion of ossification centres results in decreasing areas of cartilage between the ossified nuclei in the manubrium and sternal body (Fig. 1.2). Bifid ossification within a segment usually coalesces prior to adjoining adjacent sternebrae (Fig. 1.3) [13]. In most individuals there is fusion across the midline of the manubrium and the upper sternal nuclei before the age of 6 years [16], but the horizontal segmentation of the body usually persist until about puberty and will on radiographs appear as distinct bones (segments) separated by a narrow strip of cartilage (Fig. 1.4). The segments usually start to fuse at the age of 11–16 years. The fusion of sternebrae proceeds in a caudal-to-cranial direction, and thus is reciprocal to the appearance of the ossification (Fig. 1.5). Union of adjacent sternebrae is usually initiated through a central osseous bridge (Fig. 1.6), which progresses to achieve synostosis. There is a wide age variation in the development of fusion [5]. In a huge postmortem study commencement or partial fusion of the third and fourth sternebrae had already occurred in a majority of specimen in the 0- to 5-year-old age group. Although the earliest complete fusion of these segments was in the 6- to 10-year-old group, complete fusion in all subjects was first seen at 15–17 years of age. In both sexes the earliest complete fusion between the second and third sternebrae was observed in 11- to 14-year-olds and was present in all men over 25 years and all women over 30 years. Thus a complete fusion of all sternebrae may imply an age greater than 25 years in men and greater than 30 years in women [5].

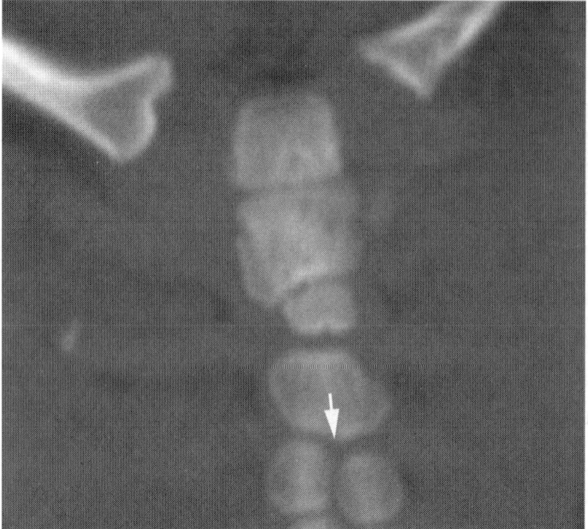

Fig. 1.3 Sternum in a 5-year-old boy. Coronal CT reconstruction shows fusion across the midline corresponding to the first sternal segment but not at the lower segments (*arrow*). The nuclei of the manubrium have not yet fused

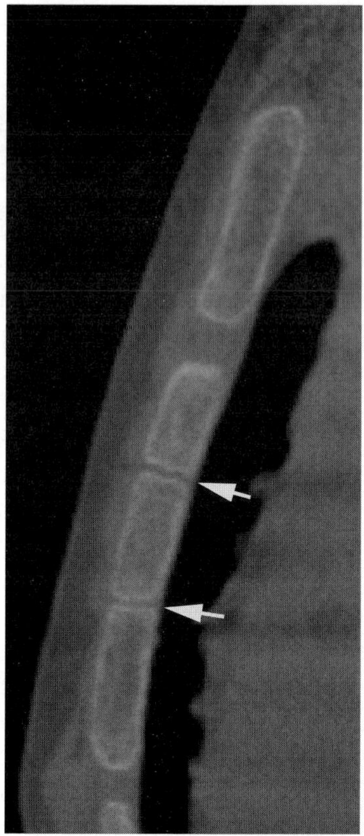

Fig. 1.4 Sternum in an 11-year-old boy. Sagittal reconstruction shows the persistence of cartilage between the ossified nuclei of the sternal body (*arrows*)

The "joints" between the sternal segments and between the body and the xiphoid process are synchondroses, composed of hyaline cartilage until they are obliterated by fusion of adjacent bony segments [7, 12]. The manubrium usually remains as a separate bone throughout life [7]. In the chondrified plate between the manubrium and the upper body segment a thin layer remains hyaline in nature, but an intervening zone becomes fibrocartilaginous before birth [13], together forming the amphiarthrodial manubriosternal joint (MSJ). The centre of the fibrocartilaginous plate may be modified either by a slit-like cavity lined by synovia, as in the pubic symphysis, or by the presence of a core of pulpy soft tissue, as in the intervertebral disc.

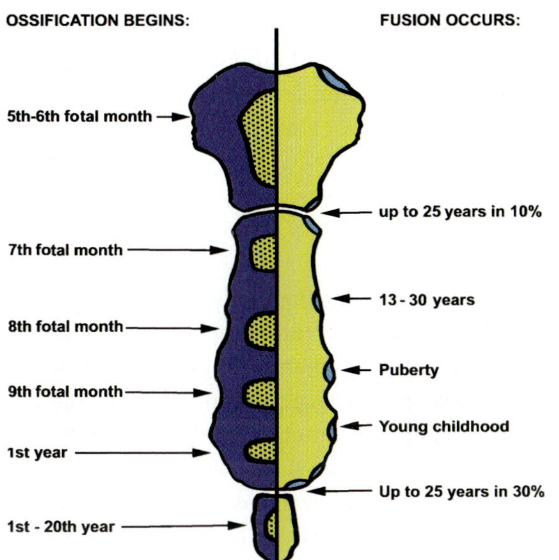



**Fig. 1.5** Development of sternal fusion. Ages at which ossification begins and fusion occurs are indicated

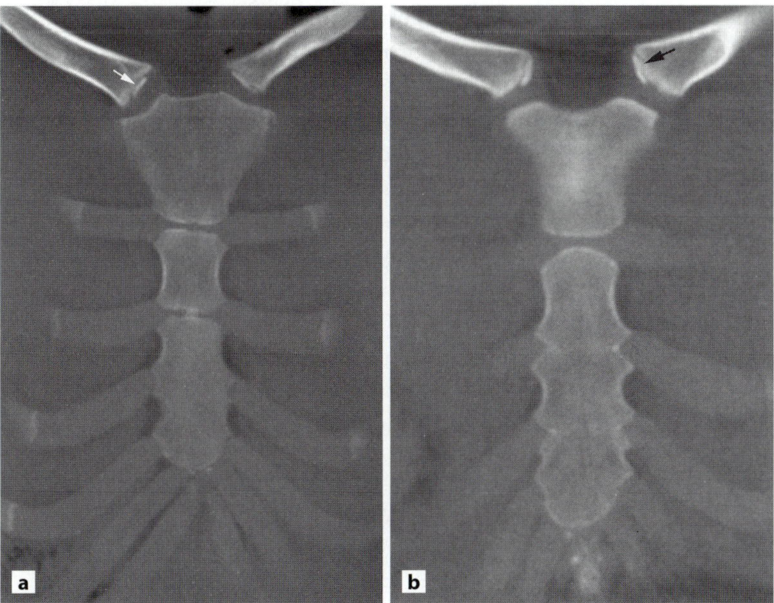



**Fig. 1.6** Normal SCC region at the age of 17 years. Coronal CT reconstruction of male (**a**) and female (**b**) previously healthy crime victims. There is persistence of segmentation between the two upper sternal segments in the boy with a little bridging ossification indicating a start of the fusion process. Secondary ossification centres are seen at the sternal end of the clavicles in both cases (*arrows*)

The xiphoid process remains connected to the most caudal sternal segments via a common zone of hyaline cartilage that ossifies in adulthood [13]. The xiphoid process often articulates with the inferior angle of the seventh ribs [13].

## 1.3
## Clavicle

The clavicle is the only long bone that develops almost entirely by a process of intramembranous ossification, with a direct transition from mesenchyme to ossified bone without the intermediate step of cartilage formation [3, 4]. In the embryo the clavicle is formed by two membranous primary centres appearing in the 6th week and fusing approximately 1 week later. The junction of the two centres of ossification is situated between the lateral and middle thirds of the clavicle, which does not correspond to the site of congenital pseudoarthrosis [10]. Subsequently hyaline cartilage develops at both ends of the clavicle. These two centres contribute to the growth in length of the clavicle, the medial cartilaginous mass more than the lateral, whereas the primary membranous derivate centres contribute little to the growth in length. The clavicles begin to ossify at a fetal age of about 5 months. The development of endochondral bone formation at the ossification centres in the ends of the clavicle in combination with their spatial orientation lead to the characteristic clavicular shape. Endochondral ossification occurs only in the sternal and acromial ends with subsequent membranous appositional ossification [11].

Postnatally the clavicles undergo their most active growth during the first 5 years, mainly by diaphyseal membranous ossification. This may explain the exuberant callus formation often seen in clavicular fractures in childhood [11]. Secondary ossification centres usually appear at the sternal end of the clavicle between 16 and 18 years of age (Fig. 1.6) [6]. They are among the last ones in the body to complete ossification. Osseous fusion usually starts at 20–22 years of age with complete fusion occurring at the age of 25–27 years [6, 8]. These features can therefore be used to determine age in early adulthood, when the epiphyseal plates of tubular bones are closed (Chapter 2).

## 1.4
## Joints and Costal Cartilages

Early in the embryo the clavicle is connected with the sternal anlage without any visible border, but an interzone develops in the 2nd fetal month as the primordium of the sternoclavicular articulation and the disc [1]. The sternoclavicular and the temporomandibular joints are very similar morphologically throughout the growth period with an intra-articular fibrocartilaginous disc [2]. The cartilage on the clavicular head and the mandibular condyle are similar at each age during growth [2], making it possible to achieve material for mandibular osteocartilaginous transplantation from the clavicle.

The costal cartilages are hyaline and initially coalesce with the cartilage of the sternal primordium. The primordium of the first rib continues into the sternum without any border. During development, the second to seventh sternocostal junctions are provided with interzones of fibrocartilage and the presence of synovial sternocostal joint cavities has been recognised shortly after birth although not at all levels [13]. The costal cartilages are laterally connected to the ribs by a junction showing similarity with the growth plate of a long bone epiphysis [2].

## 1.5
## Conclusions

The development of the SCC region varies. A single pattern of development does not occur and morphological variants are very common, but seem not to be fundamental for successful growth.

The wide variation in fetal sternal development precludes its use for satisfactory gestational age estimation, being less valuable than other morphological criteria already available. However, knowledge about fetal development does greatly assist in understanding the prepubertal and postpubertal sternal patterns, and the development of normal variants. Postnatally the development of the sternum and especially the clavicle can be used in the determination of age.

## References


1.  Doskocil M (1993) Contribution to the study of the development and ossification of human sternum. Funct Dev Morphol 3:251–257
2.  Ellis E III, Carlson DS (1986) Histologic comparison of the costochondral, sternoclavicular, and temporomandibular joints during growth in *Macaca mulatta*. J Oral Maxillofac Surg 44:312–321
3.  Gardner E (1968) The embryology of the clavicle. Clin Orthop Relat Res 58:9–16
4.  Gardner E, Gray DJ (1953) Prenatal development of the human shoulder and acromioclavicular joints. Am J Anat 92:219–276
5.  Jit I, Kaur H (1989) Time of fusion of the human sternebrae with one another in northwest India. Am J Phys Anthropol 80:195–202

6.  Jit I, Kulkarni M (1976) Times of appearance and fusion of epiphysis at the medial end of the clavicle. Indian J Med Res 64:773–782
7.  Johnston T, Whillis J (1975) Gray's Anatomy. Anatomy of the Human Body. Lea & Febiger, Philadelphia
8.  Kreitner KF, Schweden FJ, Riepert T, Nafe B, Thelen M (1998) Bone age determination based on the study of the medial extremity of the clavicle. Eur Radiol 8:1116–1122
9.  McCormick WF, Nichols MM (1981) Formation and maturation of the human sternum. I. Fetal period. Am J Forensic Med Pathol 2:323–328
10. Ogata S, Uhthoff HK (1990) The early development and ossification of the human clavicle: an embryologic study. Acta Orthop Scand 61:330–334
11. Ogden JA, Conlogue GJ, Bronson ML (1979) Radiology of postnatal skeletal development. III. The clavicle. Skeletal Radiol 4:196–203
12. Ogden JA, Conlogue GJ, Bronson ML, Jensen PS (1979) Radiology of postnatal skeletal development. II. The manubrium and sternum. Skeletal Radiol 4:189–195
13. O'Neal ML, Dwornik JJ, Ganey TM, Ogden JA (1998) Postnatal development of the human sternum. J Pediatr Orthop 18:398–405
14. Sadler TW (2000) Embryology of the sternum. Chest Surg Clin N Am 10:237–244
15. Zalel Y, Lipitz S, Soriano D, Achiron R (1999) The development of the fetal sternum: a cross-sectional sonographic study. Ultrasound Obstet Gynecol 13:187–190
16. Zimmer EA (1939) Archiv und Atlas der normalen und pathologischen Anatomie in typischen Röntgenbilden. Das Brustbein und seine Gelenke: Normale und krankhafte Befunde, dargestellt zum Teil mittels neuer röntgenologischer Methoden. Thieme, Leipzig

# II

# NORMAL ANATOMY AND VARIANTS

# 2  Bones and Cartilages

**ANNE GRETHE JURIK**

## Contents



## 2.1
## Introduction

The anatomical structures of the sternocostoclavicular (SCC) region are the sternum, the first to seventh sternocostal joints with adjacent costal cartilages, the sternoclavicular joint and the medial part of the clavicles, and the surrounding soft tissue structures, including ligaments and muscles (Fig. 2.1). The normal anatomy of the SCC region has gained great attention, partly because the region plays a major role in forensic medicine for determination of age and gender. Unfortunately, the anatomy of the region varies considerably. This is partly due to a wide variety of developmental variants [14, 31, 39] and the nearly constant strain due to movement of the joints during respiration.

The region is anatomically somewhat special by containing several amphiarthrodial joints, characterised by the connection of contiguous bony surfaces by cartilage. There are two forms of amphiarthrodial joint, a symphysis and a synchondrosis. In a symphysis the bony ends are connected by fibrocartilage as in the manubriosternal joint (MSJ). A synchondrosis is a joint where the bones are united by temporary hyaline cartilage, for example the growth plate of long tubular

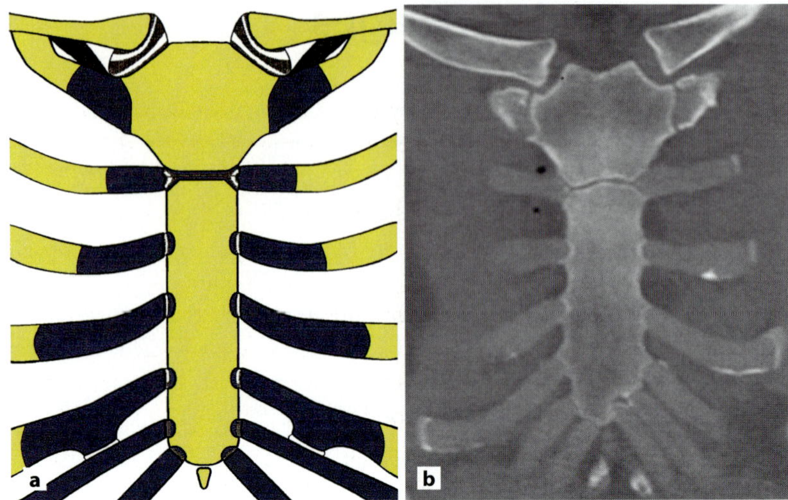

**Fig. 2.1** The sternocostoclavicular region displayed on **a** a drawing and **b** a coronal MSCT reconstruction of a 45-year-old previously healthy male crime victim. The region consists of the sternum, the adjacent articulating first to seventh costal cartilages, the medial part of the clavicles and the surrounding soft tissue structures. The CT image displayed slight slit-like calcifications corresponding to the cartilages, which are a typical male pattern

bones. The junctions between sternal segments during development are synchondroses and the first sternocostal joint is anatomically built as a synchondrosis.

There are numerous normal variants in the SCC region, which have been excellently reviewed in textbooks [14, 31], and they should not be mistaken for disease [6, 38]. This chapter includes a summary of the normal findings and the most common developmental variants. Developmental malformations influencing life are dealt with in Chapter 10.

## 2.2
## Sternum, Including Manubriosternal Joint

In most healthy individuals the sternum consist of two bones, the manubrium sterni and the sternal body, held together by the MSJ. The xiphoid process occurs as an appendix caudally.

## 2.2.1
## Sternal Bones

The sternal bones are composed of highly vascular cancellous tissue covered by a thin layer of compact bone that is thickest in the manubrium (Fig. 2.2) [23]. The shape and size of the bones generally vary considerably. On transaxial views the sternal bones can be ovoid or rectangular [8]. Some sex differences have been observed, including a significantly larger manubriosternal length in men than in women [34].

Sternal developmental variants are numerous and include persistent horizontal segmentation, sternal foramina, asymmetric bones, accessory ossification centres, etc. They may not be interpreted as disease. The same applies to variants regarding ossification of sternal segments in childhood [27].

*Persistent horizontal segmentation* of the sternal body is a well known variant. In a study of 580 non-rheumatologic patients 8 had persistence of a joint between the first and second sternal segments. Five of them had a normal MSJ, whereas 3 had osseous fusion of the MSJ [33] and their sternal segmentation can be regarded

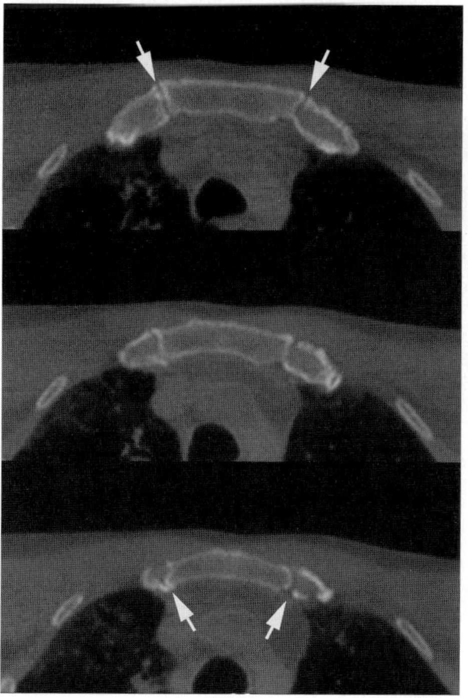

**Fig. 2.2** Axial CT slices of the manubrium of a 45-year-old previously healthy man also shown in Fig. 2.1. Note the cleft-like separation between the bone and the partly mineralised first costal cartilages (*arrows*)

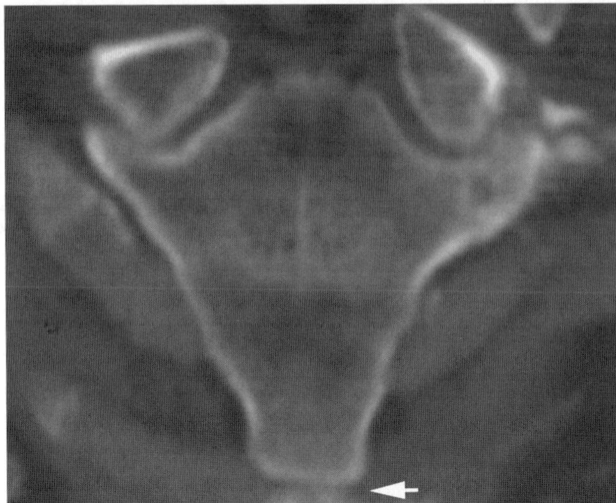

**Fig 2.3** Displaced MSJ in a 27-year-old woman presenting with swelling of the sternoclavicular joints. CT, coronal MPR shows a normal variant with lack of the first costal cartilage on the right side, ankylosis of the MSJ and instead persistence of a joint in the region of the third costal cartilage (*arrow*). Plain radiograph and tomography are shown in Fig. 5.1

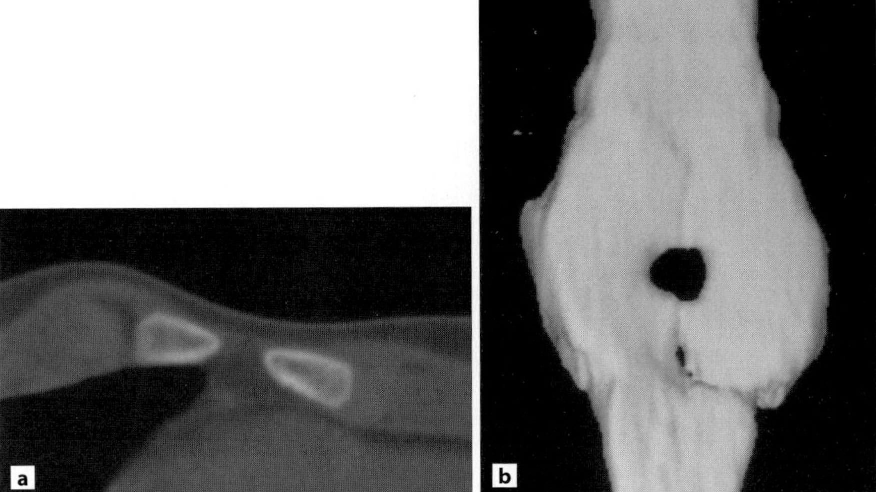

**Fig. 2.4** Sternal foramen, CT in a 17-year-old girl. **a** Axial slice. **b** Frontal 3D reconstruction showing a well-delineated osseous defect in the sternal bone

as a displaced MSJ. A hot spot in the sternal body at scintigraphy may be due to this variant [3]. An atypical location of the MSJ can occur together with other developmental variants such as hypogenesis or agenesis of the first costal cartilage (Fig. 2.3).

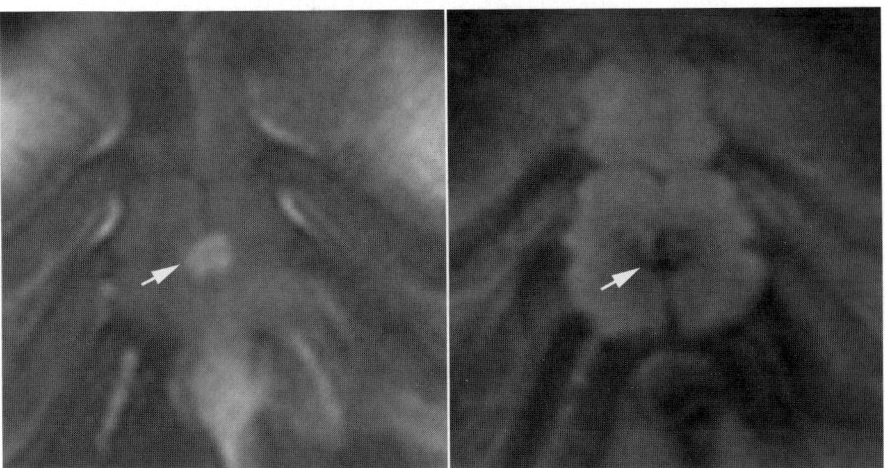

**Fig. 2.5** Sternal foramina. MRI, T1 (*left*) and STIR (*right*) of an 18-year-old girl showing persistence of an oval foramen in the lower part of the sternum (*arrows*). There is still persistence of non-fused cartilages around the foramen supporting the hypothesis that it is due to lack of cartilage coalesce. There are no high signal vessels on the STIR

*Sternal foramina* are congenital bony defects in the sternum usually occurring as a solitary oval defect in the lower third of the sternal body (Fig. 2.4), but can occur occasionally in the manubrium [5]. The incidence has been reported to be about 7%, being present in children as young as 8 years as well as in persons of advanced age [5, 19]. Their aetiology is unknown, but they may be due to incomplete fusion of multiple ossification centres (Fig. 2.5) or a passage for great vessels through the sternum. A sternal foramen is not associated with symptoms and is usually not seen at conventional radiography, but can be an incidental finding at CT or MRI performed for other reasons [38]. They should not be misinterpreted as acquired lesions such as gunshot wounds and bone destruction by tumour or infection [5, 7]. Awareness of the anomaly is important in acupuncture to avoid heart damage [7].

*Accessory ossification centres* can occur incidentally. They are usually located adjacent to the manubrium in the form of ossa suprasternale or ossiculum parasternale [14, 31]. However, extra ossification can also be part of skeletal dysplasia such as diastrophic dysplasia (Chapter 10) [26].

The blood supply to the sternum and the surrounding joints comes from the internal thoracic artery (previously named internal mammary artery) [11, 32], which has to be taken into account when suspecting infection or aseptic necrosis.

## 2.2.2
## Manubriosternal Joint

The MSJ is formed by two bony surfaces covered with hyaline cartilage and separated by a disc of fibrocartilage (Fig. 2.6) [11], just as the symphysis pubis. The fibrocartilaginous disc is anchored to the ventral and dorsal surface of the sternum by ligaments. In about 30% of individuals, a synovial-lined cavity develops in the disc area, probably preceded by partial or complete absorption of the fibrocartilaginous disc [11]. The MSJ may have different orientation in the coronal plane, but is frequently parallel [39] (Fig. 2.7). In the lateral plane the surfaces are mostly convex, but occasionally slightly concave [28]. The articular margins can be irregular due to unequal growth of the ossification centres during development [39]. Small defects in the articular surfaces may also occur. They are considered analogous to Schmorl's nodes in vertebral bodies having clear-cut margins that distinguish them from the ragged erosion with subchondral sclerosis seen in seronegative arthritis.

Degenerative changes of the MSJ often occur in old age (Fig. 2.8) and consist of narrowing of the MSJ and osteophyte formation, sometimes with bridging osteophytes, but the joint margins usually remain smooth [31].

The normal appearance of the MSJ at radiography or CT varies with age. In young individuals the MSJ usually has slightly undulating well-defined bony margins [16]. In older persons bone appositions at the margins are common [16]. Erosion-like changes may occur in 12% (12 of 95) of individuals, and have together with reactive sclerosis and/or ankylosis been observed in 28% of non-rheumatic individuals [18]. The observed erosion is probably related to osteoarthritis or to herniation of the intra-articular disc [15].

Osteoarthritis of the MSJ demanding therapy is rare, but when occurring pre-operative CT images with three-dimensional (3D) reconstruction can be used to measure the dimension of the material to be used at arthrodesis [1].

Fusion of the MSJ (Fig. 2.9) occurs in 6–10% of adults without rheumatologic disorders [2, 33, 39]. It is apparently more common in women than in men and

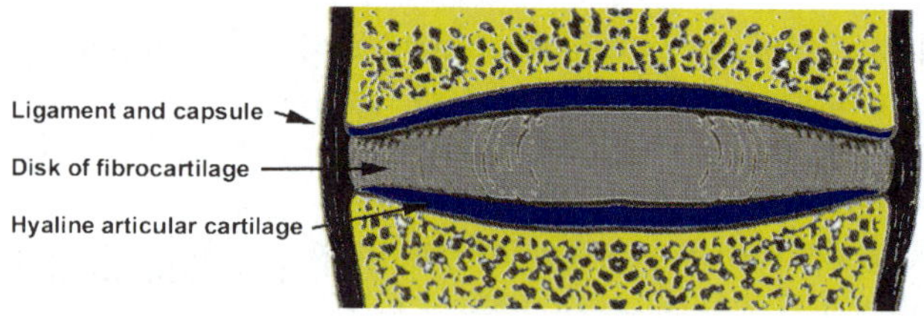


**Fig. 2.6** Drawing showing the anatomical structure of the amphiarthrodial MSJ consisting of bony ends covered by hyaline cartilage with an intervening plate of fibrocartilage

is not related to aging [37]. In a large series of necropsy material (606 bodies), the mean incidence of fusion was 14%, but there were two peak incidences for MSJ fusion, one at the age of 30–40 years and one at 70–80 years. The latter peak seems related to thoracolumbar disc degeneration [4]. The large amount of com-

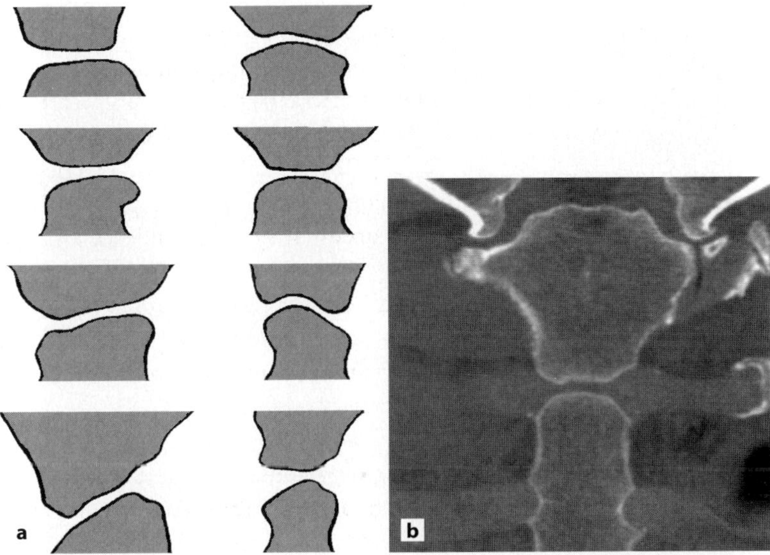

**Fig. 2.7 a** Different types of MSJ orientation in the coronal plan according to Zimmer [39]. **b** The most frequently occurring parallel appearance in a 41-year-old woman

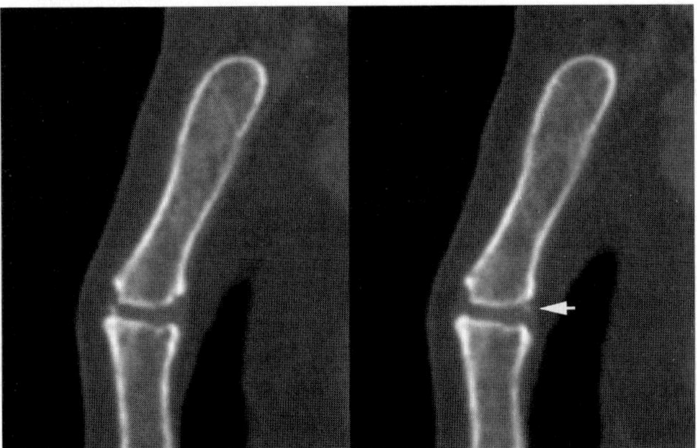

**Fig. 2.8** Slight degenerative changes in a 73-year-old man. Sagittal CT reconstructions showing small osteophytes and calcification in the disc area (*arrow*)

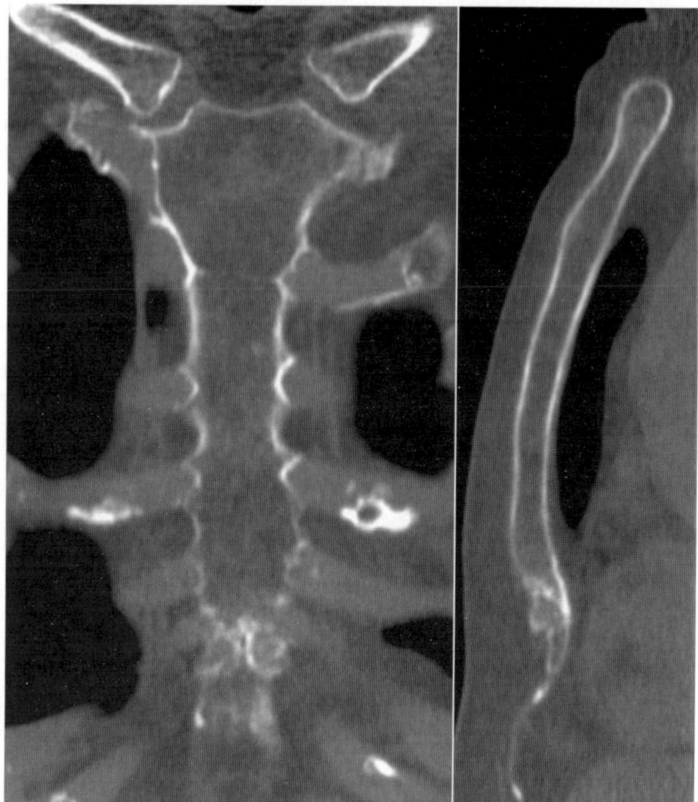

**Fig. 2.9** Fusion of the MSJ in a 60-year-old woman without SCC complaints. Coronal (*left*) and sagittal (*right*) CT reconstruction shows homogeneous osseous structure throughout the bone

bined material (2,787 individuals) analysed by Ashley in 1954 and including previously published material also disclose two peaks, the incidence of fusion being 9.3% in 30- to 39-year-olds, 11.5% in 40- to 49-year-olds, 10.6% in 50- to 59-year-olds and 60- to 69-year-olds, but 12.7% in 70- to 79-year-olds and 7.9% at age 80–89 years [2].

Persons with osseous fusion of the MSJ have probably failed to develop a fibro-cartilaginous lamina between the manubrium and the sternal body in the embryo. The joint will then be a synchondrosis comparable to the growth plate of long tubular bones, which inevitably undergo fusion [2]. In accordance with this, MSJ fusion may be accompanied by a persistent segmentation between the two upper sternal segments (Fig. 2.3) [12, 33]. The presence of a homogeneous osseous structure across the "joint" in non-inflammatory fusion (Fig. 2.9) is in accordance with this (Chapter 12). The osseous structure at ankylosis secondary to inflammation is often irregular and may be accompanied by hyperostosis. It is, however, possible that degenerative changes, including osteoarthritis and diffuse idiopathic skeletal hyperostosis (DISH), can also be the cause of MSJ fusion.

### 2.2.3
### Xiphoid Process

The xiphoid process varies considerably in size and shape among normal persons [14, 31]. Variants are frequent, but significant anomalies consisting of agenesis or abnormal location seem rare (Chapter 10).

### 2.3
### Clavicle

The clavicles occupy the ventral position of the shoulder girdle and extend from the acromial processes to the upper border of the manubrium sterni. They serve as the only osseous connection between the shoulder girdle and the trunk [22] and have a superficial location at the base of the neck (making them vulnerable to trauma). The clavicles are unique bones in several aspects. Only mammals using their forelimbs for catching have them to enable lateral movement of the limbs. Their shape is optimised for the function. The clavicle is double-curved, like the letter "S", of which the sternal two thirds are anterior convex, while the acromial one third is anteriorly concave. Each clavicle articulates with the sternum and first rib medially and with the acromion laterally. The clavicle consists of cancellous tissue enveloped by a compact layer, which is thicker in the intermediate part than at the medial and lateral part of the bone. The clavicle contains only a little red marrow. The blood supply is comparatively poor which probably accounts for the low incidence of metastatic tumours and haematogenous bacterial infections.

The clavicle is the site of many developmental variants and acquired lesions, the latter most commonly resulting from trauma. The unique anatomy may imply that lesions normally exhibiting benign radiological features in other bones may have a more aggressive appearance. Several factors can contribute to this: the unusual shape of the bone with its irregular ridges and rough cortical surface, the variable thickness of its cortex and the unique embryological development.

Clavicular developmental variants include rhomboid fossae, accessory ossicles, asymmetric closure of the growth plate, etc. [14, 31, 39]. An irregular excavation

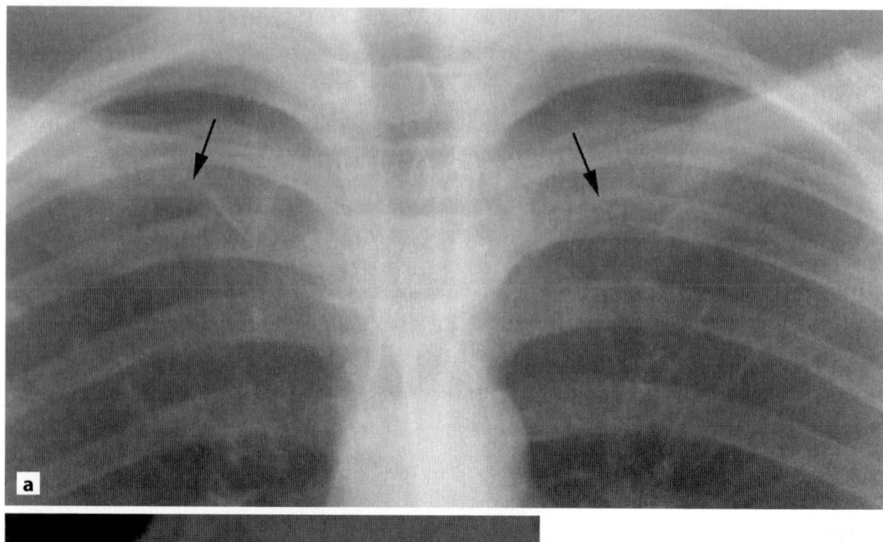

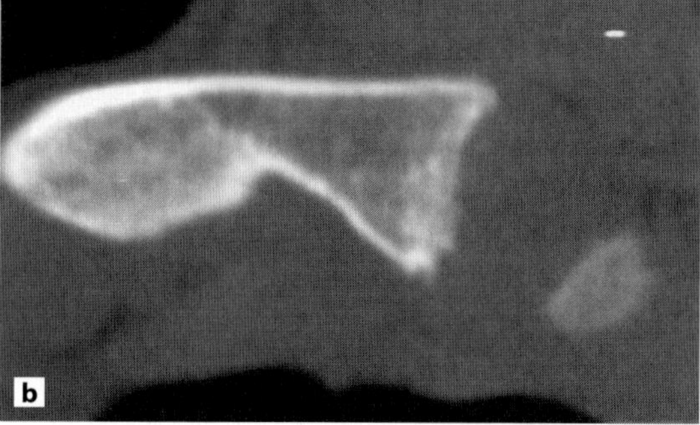

**Fig. 2.10** Rhomboid fossa in a 14-year-old boy. **a** At chest radiography there is irregular excavation of the inferior part of both clavicles (*arrows*) most pronounced on the right side. **b** Semicoronal CT reconstruction of the right clavicle displays a regular cortical bone surface corresponding to the indentation and thus no signs indicating infectious or malignant destruction

of the inferior part of the clavicle, named *rhomboid fossa*, is a frequent normal variant occurring both in children and adults (Fig. 2.10) [10]. Bilateral rhomboid fossae were found to be present in 44% of male and 54% of female children below 18 years of age and unilaterally in 16.5% of male and 20.8% of female children [10]. The incidence is nearly similar in adulthood, where bilateral fossae occurred in 59% of men and 54% of women, and unilateral fossae in 13% of men and 17% of women. Unilateral fossae occurred significantly more frequently on the right than on the left side. Factors responsible for creating a deep fossa unilaterally are not understood, but it is not found in newborns [10].

## 2.4
## Cartilages and Their Articulation

The costal cartilages consist of hyaline cartilage extending from the ribs anteriorly to the sternum and are part of the thoracic cage (Fig. 2.11). There are numerous developmental variants of costal cartilages mainly related to rib variants [14, 31, 39].

### 2.4.1
### Costal Cartilages

In young persons the cartilages are purely hyaline, but calcification within the cartilage occurs as a normal aging phenomenon. Detectable calcification is rare before the age of 15 years (Fig. 1.6) [20], but at least a trace of ossification has been found present in all cadavers over the age of 25 years and may be seen at radiography after the age of 30 years [25]. However, calcification occurring in young adults is usually slight (Fig. 2.11). Moderate calcification is rare below 40 years of age, but common above 60 years, and marked calcification rarely occurs before the age of 50 years (Fig. 2.12).

At radiography the calcification is usually first detectable in the first costal cartilage (Fig. 2.12), but in autopsy studies has been found earlier adjacent to the sternal border in the sixth, seventh and eighth cartilages, which may appear at CT (Fig. 2.11) [20]. The calcification is usually more or less symmetrical [39]. There are no convincing sex differences in the pattern of costal cartilage calcification of the first rib. There is often a slit-like cleft between an ossified first costal cartilage and the sternum (Fig. 2.2), sometimes with formation of osteophytes between the cartilage and the bone, and a homogeneous fusion is rare. Corresponding to the other cartilages there is a somewhat different appearance in women and men. The cartilage calcification of women is typically irregular, speckled and centrally located, whereas it is more peripheral at the margin of the cartilage (sheath-like calcification) in men (Figs. 2.1 and 2.11) [21]. This difference may be due to different degenerative changes in the cartilage depending on the vascularisation, different mechanical factors, hormones, etc.

In the development of a roentgenographic method to determine age, race and gender of cadaver material, an absolutely distinctive pattern of ossification of the costal cartilages in older women was identified [35]. Spherical or globular foci of calcification occurring in the subperichondrial location in the central portion of the cartilage were a feature unique to elderly women. In a large sample of autopsy material it was found only in postmenopausal women over the age of 50 years, and especially after 60 years [35]. Not encountered in men, this distinctive sex and age pattern was found in about one third of the adult female autopsy population.

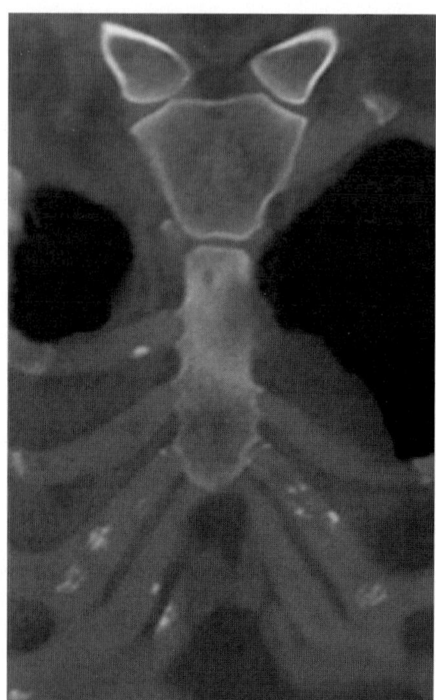

Fig. 2.11 Central costal cartilage calcification in a 40-year-old woman (previously healthy crime victim); coronal CT reconstruction

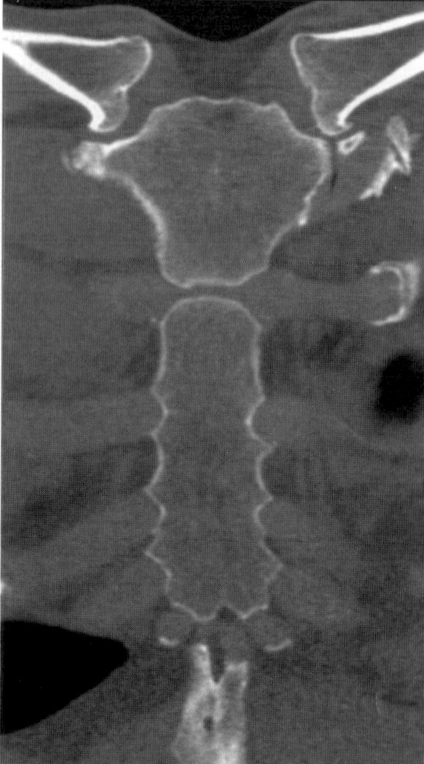

Fig. 2.12 Normal sternocostal joints. Coronal CT reconstruction in a 41-year-old woman

At the costochondral junctions the lateral end of each costal cartilage is held together with the rib by the periosteum [11]. They are important sites of muscle tensions due to muscle origin and insertion on both sides of the junction.

## 2.4.2
## Sternocostal Joints

The anatomy of the sternocostal joints (SCoJs) is rather variable. The first SCoJ is a synchondrosis in which the costal cartilage and the sternal bone are united directly by hyaline cartilage [9, 11, 24, 29, 36]. The second to fourth SCoJs are usually diarthrodial with small synovial-lined cavities and joint facets consisting of fibro-cartilage with underlying hyaline cartilage [9, 36]. The fifth to seventh SCoJs may be similarly diarthrodial, but sometimes the synovial membrane is absent, and the joints are built like a synchondrosis or symphysis [9, 11, 29, 36]. The second SCoJ contains a fibrocartilaginous intra-articular sternocostal ligament that is attached to the fibrocartilage of the MSJ and to the joint facet on the costal cartilage [9]. It divides the joint into two cavities in about 50% of individuals. A similar ligament occurs occasionally at the third SCoJ, but is rare at the fourth to seventh SCoJs [9]. The articular capsule of the second to seventh joints is reinforced by a ventral and dorsal sternocostal ligament.

In young persons the joint facets are smooth without subchondral sclerosis or peripheral osteophytes (Figs. 1.6 and 2.12). After middle age the articular surfaces of the second to seventh SCoJs lose their polish, become roughened and the synovial membrane apparently disappears. In old age the joint cavities are often obliterated [11] and the cartilage of most of the ribs becomes continuous with the sternum [11].

The SCoJs are not visible at conventional radiography, but can be evaluated by conventional tomography [13] or better by multislice CT (Figs. 1.6 and 2.12). The normal appearance at imaging varies considerably due to differences in the sternal development and the influence of ageing. There can be osteoarthritis-like changes at the first SCoJ with osteophyte formation sometimes appearing as a pseudoar-throsis.

## 2.5
## Age Determination

Age estimations of living individuals are increasingly important in criminal matters. If doubts arise regarding the age of a person suspected of a criminal offence, forensic age estimation is prompted by the need to ascertain whether the person concerned has reached the age of criminal responsibility and whether general criminal law in force for older juveniles or adults is to be applied. In such cases age estimates are usually based on a general physical examination, X-ray examination of the hand and odontological examination, including an Orthopantomogram.

The development of the peripheral skeleton is completed before the age of 18 years. The eruption and calcification the third molars, which is fundamental for dental age estimation is usually completed by the age of 19 or 20 years and cannot be used to ascertain whether a person has attained the forensically relevant age of 21 years. If it has to be determined, it may be necessary to perform an X-ray examination or CT of the medial clavicular epiphyseal region [30] or better

MRI to avoid irradiation. Based on the analysis of Kreitner et al. (1998) [17] the finding of a complete union of the medial clavicular epiphysis implies an age of 22 years or above. Age determination based on the development of the medial part of the clavicle can also be important for identifying human remains whose age is estimated to be under 30 years [17]. Information about age in childhood, adolescence and young adulthood can be gained based on the development of the medial clavicular epiphysis, closure of the adjacent growth plates and fusion of sternal segments [17].

Sternal length and the pattern of costal cartilage calcification can also contribute to the determination of gender and age [17, 34].


## 2.6
## Conclusions

The normal anatomy of the bones and cartilages in the SCC region vary considerably and there are numerous normal variants that should not be interpreted as signs of disease. Bone age estimation based on the study of the development of the medial clavicular epiphysis may be a useful tool in forensic age identification in living individuals, especially if the age of the subject is about the end of the second or the beginning of the third decade of life.


## References


1. Al Dahiri A, Pallister I (2006) Arthrodesis for osteoarthritis of the manubriosternal joint. Eur J Cardiothorac Surg 29:119–121
2. Ashley GT (1954) The morphological and pathological significance of synostosis at the manubrio-sternal joint. Thorax 9:159–166
3. Baas J, Eijsvogel M, Dijkstra P (1988) Persistent sternum synchondroses on bone scintigraphy. Eur J Nucl Med 13:572–573
4. Cameron HU, Fornasier VL (1974) The manubriosternal joint: an anatomico-radiological survey. Thorax 29:472–474
5. Cooper PD, Stewart JH, McCormick WF (1988) Development and morphology of the sternal foramen. Am J Forensic Med Pathol 9:342–347
6. Donnelly LF, Frush DP, Foss JN, O'Hara SM, Bisset GS III (1999) Anterior chest wall: frequency of anatomic variations in children. Radiology 212:837–840
7. Fokin AA (2000) Cleft sternum and sternal foramen. Chest Surg Clin N Am 10:261–276
8. Goodman LR, Teplick SK, Kay H (1983) Computed tomography of the normal sternum. Am J Roentgenol 141:219–223

9. Gray DJ, Gardner ED (1943) The human sternochondral joints. Anat Rec 87:235–253

10. Jit I, Kaur H (1986) Rhomboid fossa in the clavicles of North Indians. Am J Phys Anthropol 70:97–103

11. Johnston T, Whillis J (1975) Gray's Anatomy. Anatomy of the Human Body. In: Lea & Febiger P (ed)

12. Jurik AG, Graudal H (1987) Monarthritis of the manubriosternal joint. A follow-up study. Rheumatol Int 7:235–241

13. Jurik AG, Graudal H (1988) Sternocostal joint swelling: clinical Tietze's syndrome. Report of sixteen cases and review of the literature. Scand J Rheumatol 17:33–42

14. Keats T (1996) Atlas of normal roentgen variants that may simulate disease. Mosby, St. Louis

15. Kormano M (1970) A microradiographic and histological study of the manubrio-sternal joint in rheumatoid arthritis. Acta Rheumatol Scand 16:47–59

16. Kormano M, Karvonen J, Lassus A (1975) Psoriatic lesion of the sternal synchondrosis. Acta Radiol Diagn (Stockh) 16:463–468

17. Kreitner KF, Schweden FJ, Riepert T, Nafe B, Thelen M (1998) Bone age determination based on the study of the medial extremity of the clavicle. Eur Radiol 8:1116–1122

18. Laitinen H, Saksanen S, Suoranta H (1970) Involvement of the manubrio-sternal articulation in rheumatoid arthritis. Acta Rheum Scand 16:40–46

19. McCormick WF (1981) Sternal foramina in man. Am J Forensic Med Pathol 2:249–252

20. McCormick WF, Stewart JH (1983) Ossification patterns of costal cartilages as an indicator of sex. Arch Pathol Lab Med 107:206–210

21. Navani S, Shah JR, Levy PS (1970) Determination of sex by costal cartilage calcification. Am J Roentgenol Radium Ther Nucl Med 108:771–774

22. Ogden JA, Conlogue GJ, Bronson ML (1979) Radiology of postnatal skeletal development. III. The clavicle. Skeletal Radiol 4:196–203

23. Ogden JA, Conlogue GJ, Bronson ML, Jensen PS (1979) Radiology of postnatal skeletal development. II. The manubrium and sternum. Skeletal Radiol 4:189–195

24. O'Neal ML, Dwornik JJ, Ganey TM, Ogden JA (1998) Postnatal development of the human sternum. J Pediatr Orthop 18:398–405

25. Ontell FK, Moore EH, Shepard JA, Shelton DK (1997) The costal cartilages in health and disease. Radiographics 17:571–577

26. Remes VM, Helenius IJ, Marttinen EJ (2001) Manubrium sterni in patients with diastrophic dysplasia: radiological analysis of 50 patients. Pediatr Radiol 31:555–558

27. Rush WJ, Donnelly LF, Brody AS, Anton CG, Poe SA (2002) "Missing" sternal ossification center: potential mimicker of disease in young children. Radiology 224:120–123

28. Savill DL (1951) The manubrio-sternal joint in ankylosing spondylitis. J Bone Joint Surg Br 33:56–64

29. Schils JP, Resnick D, Haghighi P, Trudell D, Sartoris DJ (1989) Sternocostal joints. Anatomic, radiographic and pathologic features in adult cadavers. Invest Radiol 24:596–603

30. Schmeling A, Olze A, Reisinger W, Rosing FW, Geserick G (2003) Forensic age diagnostics of living individuals in criminal proceedings. Homo 54:162–169

31. Schmidt H, Freyschmidt J (1993) Kohler/Zimmer. Borderlands of normal and early pathologic findings in skeletal radiography. Thieme Medical, New York

32. Sick H, Ring P (1976) Vascularization of the sternoclavicular articulation (author's transl). Arch Anat Histol Embryol 59:71–78

33. Solovay J, Gardner C (1951) Involvement of the manubriosternal joint in Marie-Strümpell disease. Am J Roentgenol 65:749–759

34. Stewart JH, McCormick WF (1983) The gender predictive value of sternal length. Am J Forensic Med Pathol 4:217–220

35. Stewart JH, McCormick WF (1984) A sex- and age-limited ossification pattern in human costal cartilages. Am J Clin Pathol 81:765–769

36. Taddei A, Sick H (1983) Contribution to the study of the anterior joints of the thorax. Arch Anat Histol Embryol 66:3–54

37. Trotter M (1934) Synostosis between manubrium and body of the sternum in whites and negroes. Am J Phys Anthrop 18:439–442

38. Yekeler E, Tunaci M, Tunaci A, Dursun M, Acunas G (2006) Frequency of sternal variations and anomalies evaluated by MDCT. Am J Roentgenol 186:956–960

39. Zimmer EA (1939) Archiv und Atlas der normalen und pathologischen Anatomie in typischen Röntgenbilden. Das Brustbein und seine Gelenke: Normale und krankhafte Befunde, dargestellt zum Teil mittels neuer röntgenologischer Methoden. Thieme, Leipzig

# 3   Sternoclavicular Joints

ANNE GRETHE JURIK
AND FLEMMING BRANDT SOERENSEN

## Contents



## 3.1 Introduction

The normal anatomy of the sternoclavicular joints varies due to many developmental variations, age and different normal signs caused by a rather constant load on the joints. They are the only synovial joints between the upper extremity and the axial skeleton. They accompany movement of the arms and move slightly during respiration, which contributes to continuous strain.

## 3.2 Macroscopic Anatomy

The sternoclavicular joint is formed by the articulation of the medial end of the clavicle with the clavicular notch of the manubrium sterni and the adjacent cartilage of the first rib. The articular surfaces of the sternum and the clavicle are incongruent. Only a relatively small area of the medial clavicle is in contact with the manubrium sterni, but the joint contains a fibrocartilaginous intra-articular disc that fills the space between the apposing articular surfaces (Fig. 3.1). The disc is strongly attached to the superior margin of the clavicular articular surface and to the first costal cartilage inferiorly and attached to the interior of the capsule (Fig. 3.1). The disc is an important buffer between the joint surfaces acting as a check-rein against medial displacement of the clavicle. In 97% of individuals this disc divides the joint into two compartments or a double gliding joint [5].

Owing to the discrepancy in size between the two articular surfaces, the stability of the sternoclavicular joint depends on surrounding ligaments in addition to the disc. The fibrous articular capsule surrounding the articulation is reinforced by the anterior and posterior sternoclavicular ligaments and the interclavicular ligament (Fig. 3.1). The joint is further stabilised by the costoclavicular ligament,

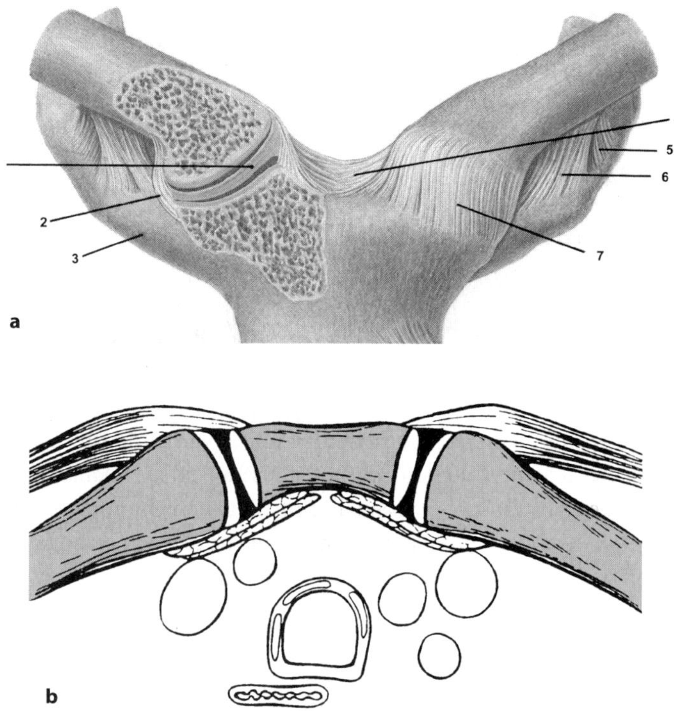

Fig. 3.1 Sternoclavicular joints. **a** Anterior aspect of the joints. The right joint is cut in the coronal plane. *1* Intra-articular disc, *2* articular capsule, *3* costal cartilage, *4* interclavicular ligament, *5* costoclavicular ligament, posterior fibres, *6* costoclavicular ligament, anterior fibres, *7* anterior sternoclavicular ligament. **b** Superior aspect of the sternoclavicular joint demonstrating the incongruence of the joint facets and intra-articular disc attached to the capsule anteriorly and posteriorly

which extends from the inferior surface of the medial end of the clavicle to the first rib and the adjacent costal cartilage [2, 11]. It is a short, flat, strong, rhomboid-shaped ligament with an anterior and posterior sheet separated by a bursa [2]. It nearly always merges with the sternoclavicular joint capsule [2]. The costoclavicular ligament resists forces that attempt to displace the medial clavicle anteriorly, posteriorly or medially and stabilises the joint by acting as a fulcrum with motion occurring around the axis through this ligament [10]. Ossification of this ligament does not occur in persons without rheumatologic disorders [9, 11]. The presence of stabilising surrounding ligaments implies that the costoclavicular region contains many areas with insertion of fibrous tissue into bones, usually named entheses [3], which can be involved in inflammatory disorders (enthesopathy).

The blood supply to the sternoclavicular joints comes from the internal thoracic artery, and this has to be taken into account when suspecting infection or aseptic necrosis.

## 3.3
## Microscopic Anatomy

The sternoclavicular joint is a true diarthrodial synovial-lined joint. It has been described to differ from other diarthroses, except the temporomandibular joints, by containing fibrocartilaginous and not hyaline articular cartilage when fully developed [4, 7, 8, 11]. The cartilage has been reported placed directly on the bone and fixed by a network of fibrous fibres penetrating into the bone [8], making the junction between cartilage and bone anatomically somewhat similar to entheses [3]. However, examination of three necropsy specimens (a 23-year-old male, and two 47- and 49-year-old female crime victims) performed at our institution revealed that, for their age and sex, the cartilage is hyaline, but with intermingling fibrous fibres at the peripheral part corresponding to the attachment of the intra-articular disc, the capsule and the surrounding ligaments (Fig. 3.2a). These areas therefore gain an appearance similar to fibrocartilage. At the age of 47–49 years there was also dispersed fibrous fibres in the superficial part of the cartilage centrally, but with underlying hyaline cartilage (Fig. 3.2b). At the age of 23 years the cartilage was also hyaline superficially (Fig. 3.2c). Our finding of hyaline cartilage in adults is in accordance with the reported presence of hyaline cartilage in childhood and adolescence [4, 8]. The reported appearance simulating conversion to fibrocartilage in adulthood may be explained by more prominent intermingling ligamentous structures and probably also to the frequent occurrence of degenerative changes [6]. Irrespective of the type of cartilage, the articular cartilage of adults has been reported to be thicker on the clavicle than on the manubrium sterni [8, 11].

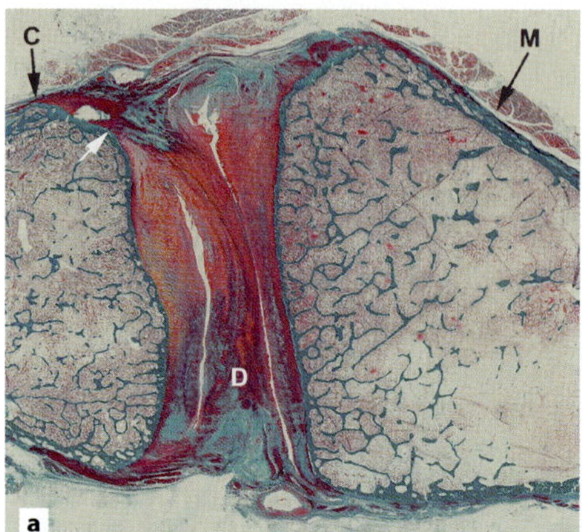

**Fig. 3.2a** Microscopic appearance of the sternoclavicular joint. Semiaxial 10-µm-thick methyl methacrylate-embedded section though the joint of a 47-year-old woman stained with Goldner–trichrome. The intra-articular disc is seen to divide the joint into two compartments, being attached to the capsule anteriorly and posteriorly and also to the clavicle by a strong ligamentous structure (*white arrow*).

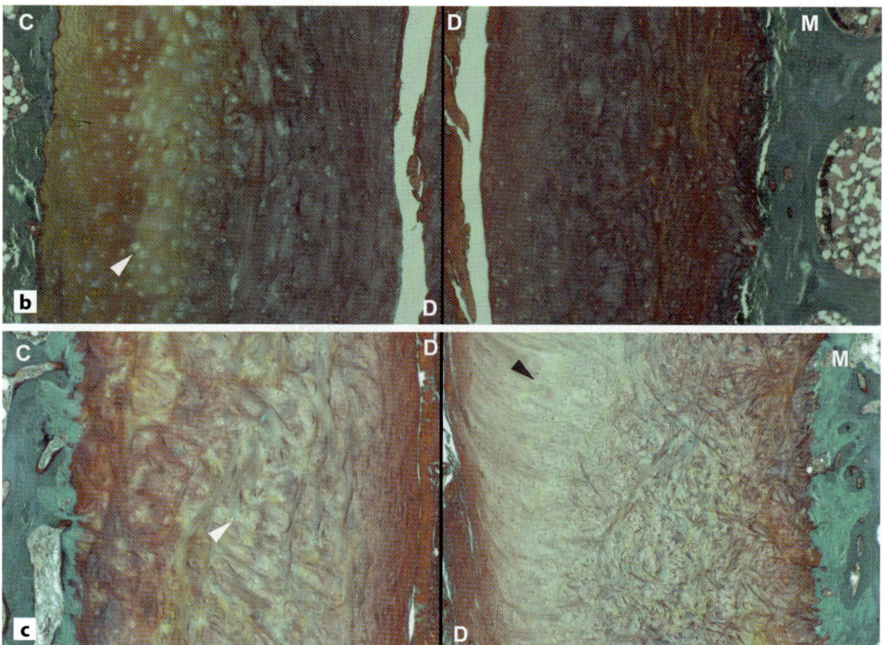

**Fig. 3.2b,c** Microscopic appearance of the sternoclavicular joint. **b** Magnified views of the clavicular (*left*) and the sternal cartilage (*right*) in Fig. 3.2a show the existence of hyaline cartilage beneath a layer of cartilage intermingled with fibrous structures, most obvious in the clavicular cartilage (*white arrowhead*). **c** Joint from a 23-year-old man (stained similarly). Magnified histological sections of the clavicular (*left*) and the sternal cartilage (*right*) show hyaline cartilage superficially, especially on the sternal side (*black arrowhead*). At the clavicular side there were some fibrous structures surrounding cartilage cells (*white arrowhead*). *C* Clavicle, *M* manubrium sterni, *D* intra-articular disc

## 3.4
## Appearance at Imaging

The normal sternoclavicular joints are difficult to visualise by conventional radiography due to overprojecting structures. Computed tomography eliminates this problem and can visualise the osseous structures clearly, especially when using multislice CT (MSCT) with secondary reconstructions. The increasing use of MSCT with routine multiplanar reconstructions has revealed a wide variable appearance, for example seen at chest CT for other disorders. This is due to a frequent occurrence of degenerative changes. Advanced osteoarthritis is infrequent before the age of 40 years, but occurs in almost all persons older than 70 years [6]. Osteoarthritis often includes calcification of the first costal cartilage (Fig. 3.3). MSCT is

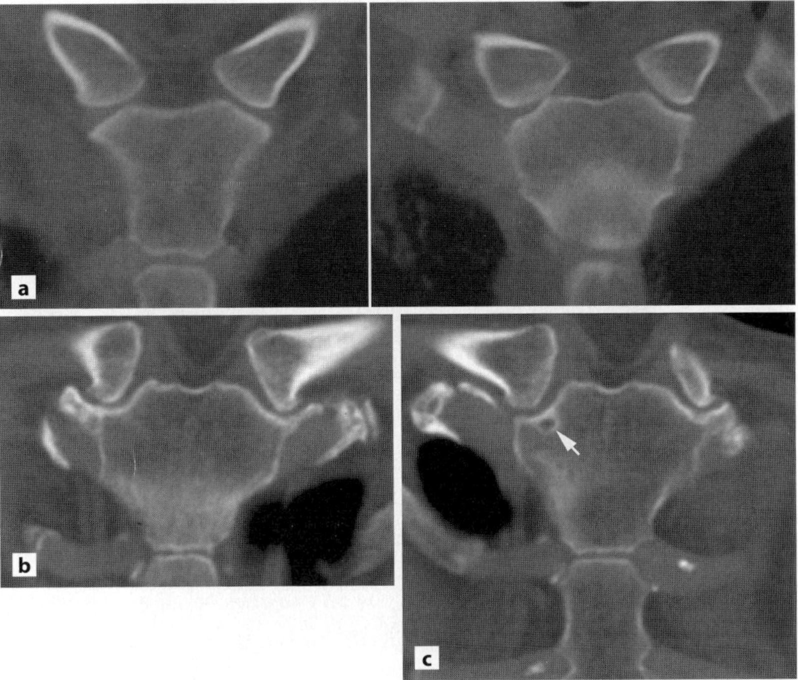

**Fig. 3.3** Computed tomography appearance of normal sternoclavicular joints. **a** Coronal MSCT reconstructions of a 40-year-old woman without signs of degenerative changes. **b** In a 47-year-old woman there is slight joint space narrowing inferiorly with small clavicular osteophytes and also calcification of the first costal cartilage. **c** A 57-year-old woman who in addition to joint space alteration had a subchondral cyst (*arrow*) in the manubrium. **d** see Page 34

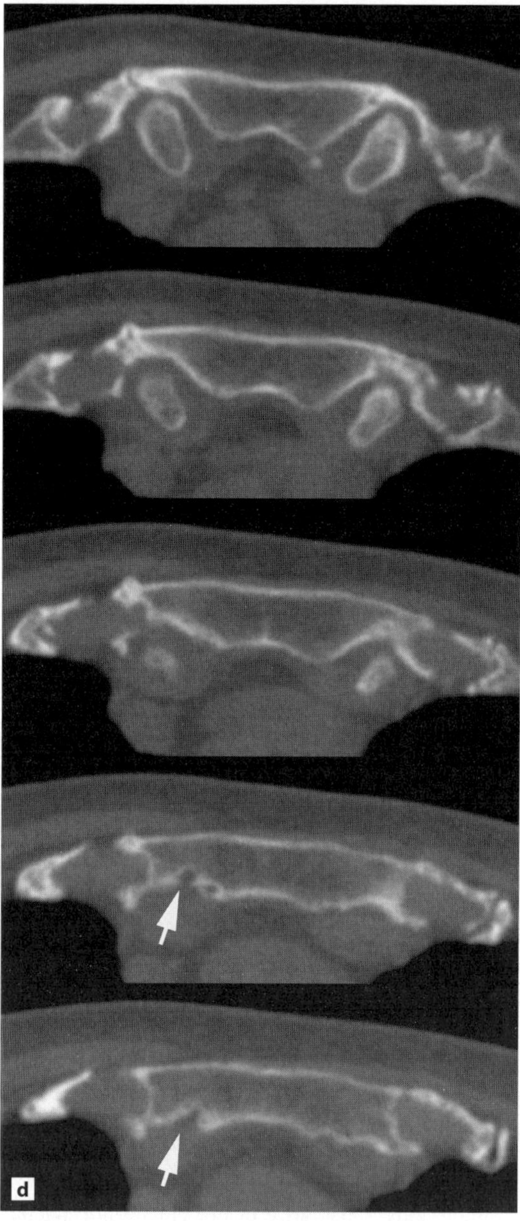

**Fig. 3.3** (*continued*) Computed tomography appearance of normal sternoclavicular joints. **d** Supplementary axial slices show that the cystic appearance may be due to cortical indentations (*arrows*)

an excellent method for delineating calcified structures, but soft tissue structures can only be visualised to the extent possible by X-ray attenuation.

Magnetic resonance imaging (MRI) allows detailed imaging of the normal soft tissue structures of the sternoclavicular joint (Chapter 7). This has been documented by MRI of non-moving specimens [1]. The normal anatomical structures can usually be delineated at clinical MRI when performed appropriately and not influenced by the occasional problems with movement artefacts. On axial images the anterior and posterior part of the capsule, and the anterior and posterior sternoclavicular ligament are delineated, in addition to the anterior and posterior attachment of the disc, and the costoclavicular and interclavicular ligaments. Coronal images are superior for displaying the articular surface of the medial end of the clavicle and the manubrium in addition to the disc. The costoclavicular ligament is also well delineated, but differentiation between the anterior and posterior portion is not possible. The thickness of the costoclavicular ligament is best delineated on sagittal images, but the two fascicles of this ligament and the bursa between them are seldom seen. The extent of the anterior and posterior sternoclavicular ligaments and the attachment of the intra-articular disc to the capsule anteriorly and posteriorly is also delineated by this slice orientation [1].

## 3.5
## Conclusions

The anatomy of the sternoclavicular joint is rather complex being composed of incongruent joint facets with an intervening intra-articular disc and with many surrounding ligaments and entheses, which may be involved in seronegative arthritis. The joint cartilage is basically hyaline, but with intermingled fibrous fibres which contribute to an appearance simulating fibrocartilage. This may partly be due to a frequent occurrence of degenerative changes.

## References


1. Brossmann J, Stabler A, Preidler KW, Trudell D, Resnick D (1996) Sternoclavicular joint: MR imaging—anatomic correlation. Radiology 198:193–198
2. Cave AJ (1961) The nature and morphology of the costoclavicular ligament. J Anat 95:170–179
3. Cooper RR, Misol S (1970) Tendon and ligament insertion. A light and electron microscopic study. J Bone Joint Surg Am 52:1–20
4. DePalma AF (1957) Degenerative changes in the sternoclavicular and acromioclavicular joints in the various decades. Thomas, Springfield, Illinois.

5. DePalma AF (1959) The role of the disks of the sternoclavicular and the acromioclavicular joints. Clin Orthop 13:222–233
6. Hagemann R, Ruttner JR (1979) [Arthrosis of the sternoclavicular joint.] Z Rheumatol 38:27–38
7. Klein MA, Miro PA, Spreitzer AM, Carrera GF (1995) MR imaging of the normal sternoclavicular joint: spectrum of findings. Am J Roentgenol 165:391–393
8. Langen P (1934) Untersuchungen über Altersveränderungen und Abnutzungserscheinungen am Sternoclaviculargelenk. Virchows Arch Pathol Anat 293:381–408
9. Lucet L, Le Loët X, Ménard JF, Mejjad O, Louvel JP, Janvresse A, Daragon A (1996) Computed tomography of the normal sternoclavicular joint. Skeletal Radiol 25:237–241
10. Milch H (1952) The rhomboid ligament in surgery of the sternoclavicular joint. J Int Coll Surg 17:41–51
11. Sutro CJ (1974) The sternoclavicular joint and attached structures (costoclavicular ligament). Bull Hosp Joint Dis 35:168–201

# BIOMECHANICS OF THE STERNOCOSTOCLAVICULAR REGION

# 4 Biomechanics of Joints and Cartilages

ANNE GRETHE JURIK

**Contents**



## 4.1
## Introduction

The sternocostoclavicular (SCC) region is part of the chest wall (Fig. 4.1) and thereby contributes to respiratory movements. In addition, the sternoclavicular joints are the only synovial joints between the upper extremity and the trunk.

## 4.2
## Sternoclavicular Joints

The sternoclavicular joint is a non-weight-bearing joint, but one of the most frequently used joints in the trunk. It accompanies every movement of the arm, and functions like a ball-and-socket joint permitting motion in all planes [2, 3]. With movement of the arm its movements consist of a cone of 60 degrees with the tip in the middle of the clavicular head. Movement in the sternoclavicular joint contributes to shoulder abduction and flexion via elevation of the lateral end and rotation of the clavicle. In the first 90 degrees of abduction, the clavicle raises approximately 30 degrees. With abduction beyond 90 degrees, the clavicle rotates about its

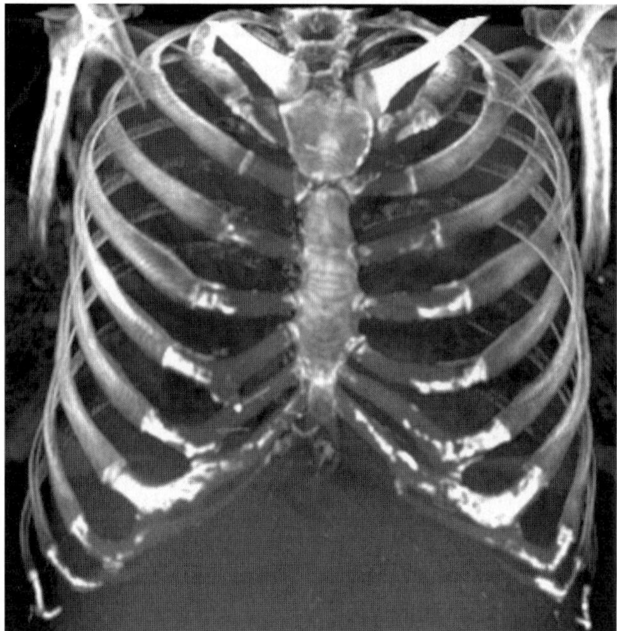

Fig. 4.1 Computed tomography, 3D reconstruction of the thoracic cage in a 58-year-old woman shows the intimate relation of the SCC region and the rest of the thoracic cage

longitudinal axis. Due to the crankshaft shape of the clavicle, this rotation elevates the lateral end, but also implies rotation at the sternoclavicular joint. Moreover, the sternoclavicular joint moves slightly during respiration contributing to continuous strain, although to a lesser degree. It seems there is always some strain on the joint especially in the upright position, and it is apparently only relaxed in the supine position. This may explain the frequent occurrence of degenerative changes (Fig. 3.3) (Chapter 15) [4, 5].

## 4.3
## Manubriosternal Joint

The manubriosternal joint (MSJ) is located between the manubrium sterni and the sternal body. It is slightly moveable and contributes to the mobility of the SCC region; it thus has a function during respiration. During inspiration, the ribs move upward and forward to expand the thoracic cavity. The first rib is much shorter than the succeeding ribs. Therefore, the upward and forward excursion of its anterior end is lesser, and the adjacent manubrium sterni is only slightly raised forward. The greater excursion, especially in the forward direction, imposed upon the rest of the sternum by the longer ribs causes a bending at the MSJ. An opposite

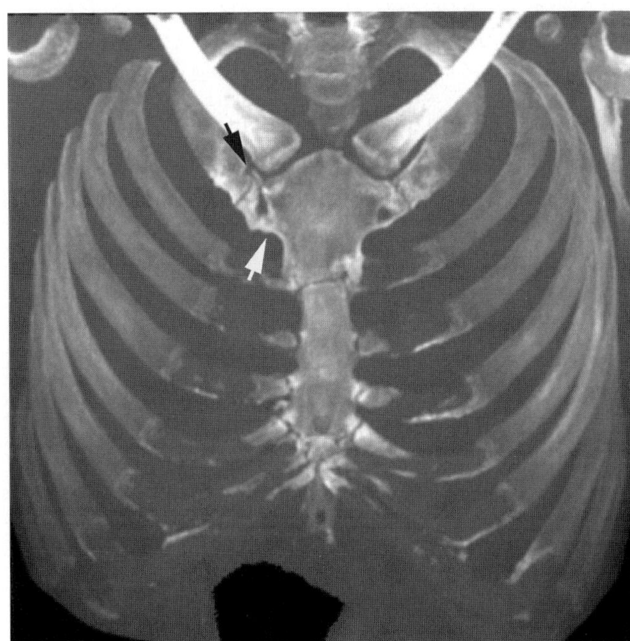

**Fig. 4.2** Computed tomography, 3D reconstruction of the SCC region in a 63-year-old man. There is pronounced calcification of the first costal cartilages with a cleft-like space and osteophytes on the right side (*arrows*). There are also degenerative changes at other sternocostal joints most pronounced corresponding to the left-sided second and fourth to seventh joints

movement occurs during expiration [1]. The forces thus imposed on the joint may cause degenerative changes (Fig. 2.8).

## 4.4
## Sternocostal Joints

The first costal cartilages and sternocostal joints have a special function. The cartilages are originally united directly to the sternal bone forming synchondrotic first sternocostal joints. However, mineralisation occurs early in these cartilages, but often a non-calcified cleavage will persist between the cartilages and the sternum. During each respiration the torsion of the cartilages is made possible by these joint-like cleavages. Due to a nearly continuous strain imposed on the region osteoarthritis-like changes can occur with osteophyte formation, sometimes appearing as a pseudoarthrosis (Fig. 4.2).

The second sternocostal joints are intimately related to the MSJ and adjacent cartilages and contribute to the extension during inspiration [1]. Similarly, the third to the seventh sternocostal joints will move during respiration, and the strain thereby imposed on the joints may cause degenerative changes in addition to calcification of the adjacent costal cartilages (Fig. 4.2).

## 4.5
## Conclusions

The sternoclavicular, manubriosternal and sternocostal joints are important for the biomechanics of the chest during respiration. This implies a nearly constant strain on the joints, which may result in degenerative changes. In addition, the sternoclavicular joints accompany every movement of the arms being the only joints between the trunk and the upper extremities.

## References


1.  Asley GT (1954) The morphological and pathological significance of synostosis at the manubrio-sternal joint. Thorax 9:159–166
2.  DePalma AF (1957) Degenerative changes in the sternoclavicular and acromioclavicular joints in the various decades. Thomas, Springfield, Illinois
3.  DePalma AF (1963) Surgical anatomy of acromioclavicular and sternoclavicular joints. Surg Clin North Am 43:1541–1550
4.  Hagemann R, Ruttner JR (1979) [Arthrosis of the sternoclavicular joint.] Z Rheumatol 38:27–38
5.  Langen P (1934) Untersuchungen über Altersveränderungen und Abnutzungserscheinungen am Sternoclaviculargelenk. Virchows Arch Pathol Anat 293:381–408

# IV IMAGING TECHNIQUES AND PROCEDURES

# 5  Conventional Radiography and Tomography

ANNE GRETHE JURIK

**Contents**



## 5.1
## Conventional Radiography

The sternocostoclavicular (SCC) region, consisting of the sternum and the sternoclavicular and sternocostal joints, may be difficult to assess with routine radiographic techniques. On a *frontal radiograph* overlaying spine, ribs, mediastinal structures, lung and/or soft tissue of the chest wall often obscure minor joint and bone details. However, the presence of manifest osseous hyperostosis and sclerosis in the SCC region may be detected by frontal radiography, and even at chest radiography, but a clear delineation of osteoarticular changes demands elimination of superimposed structures (Fig. 5.1). *Oblique radiographic views* of the sternoclavicular joints allow visualisation of the sternal and clavicular contours, but fine articular and osseous details are invisible due to the superimposed structures. Several special views of the sternoclavicular region have been invented in an attempt to eliminate this problem [1, 3, 6]. The success has, however, been limited, partly because such views often are difficult to obtain and interpret.

A *lateral radiograph* of the sternum can visualise the anterior and posterior cortex, and the manubriosternal joint (MSJ) may be adequately visualised by this view (Fig. 12.3a). Most sternal fractures are transverse and can be detected on a lateral radiograph, likewise disruption of the MSJ (Chapter 11) [8]. However, the

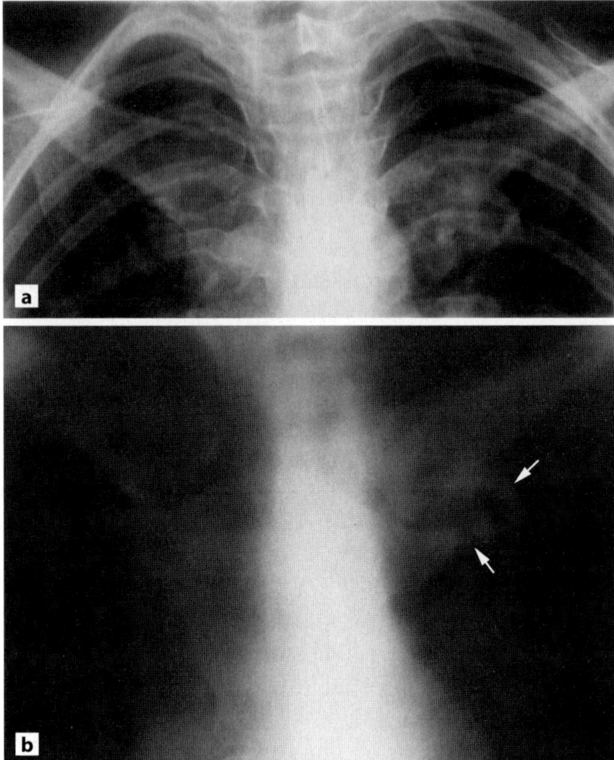

**Fig. 5.1 a** Anterior radiograph of the sternoclavicular joint in a 27-year-old woman with swelling at both joints and left-sided pain. There is narrowing of the left sternoclavicular joint with surrounding osseous proliferations. Also, at least on the right side, is a congenital variant with lack of the first rib. **b** Supplementary tomography revealed definite narrowing of the left sternoclavicular joint with osteophyte formation (*arrows*) as a sign of degenerative changes. Supplementary CT is shown in Fig. 2.3. Coronal reconstructions confirmed the presence of left-sided osteoarthritis, but also a normal variant with lack of the first costal cartilage on the right side, and ankylosis of the MSJ, corresponding to the location of the second sternocostal joints. There is instead persistence of a joint between the two upper sternal segments

sternoclavicular joints and the medial part of the clavicles are usually not visualised by lateral radiography due the considerable distance from the film and overlying shadows.

## 5.2
## Conventional Tomography

Elimination of shadows from overlaying structures can be achieved to some degree by frontal tomography depending on the technique used [2, 4, 7]. The osseous structures may not be clearly delineated by linear tomography. Multidirectional tomography improves the diagnostic quality and can detect even minor joint or bone lesions, including abnormalities of the sternocostal joints [4], but the radiation dose is relatively high. Irrespective of the tomography technique, it is time-consuming, and soft tissue structures are only shown as shadows. Computed tomography (CT) has the advantage of visualising soft tissue structures in addition to elimination of shadows from superimposed structures. CT is more convenient for the patient, less time-consuming and does not basically imply a higher radiation dose than tomography [5]. Imaging of the SCC region has therefore in most institutions been changed to CT or magnetic resonance imaging (MRI).

## 5.3
## Conclusions

Over the years there have been many attempts to visualise the SCC region by conventional radiography, but most have been unsuccessful. The osseous structures can be visualised by conventional tomography, but not to the extent obtained by CT or MRI, which in addition visualise the surrounding soft tissue structures. The conventional radiographic methods have therefore been substituted by cross-sectional imaging in most departments.

## References


1.   Abel MS (1979) Symmetrical anteroposterior projections of the sternoclavicular joints with motion studies. Radiology 132:757–759
2.   Hermann G, Rothenberg RR, Spiera H (1983) The value of tomography in diagnosing infection of the sternoclavicular joint. Mt Sinai J Med 50:52–55
3.   Hobbs DW (1968) Sternoclavicular joint: a new axial radiographic view. Radiology 90:801
4.   Jurik AG (1992) Seronegative anterior chest wall syndromes. A study of the findings and course at radiography. Acta Radiol Suppl 381:1–42
5.   Jurik AG, Jensen LC, Hansen J (1996) Radiation dose by spiral CT and conventional tomography of the sternoclavicular joints and the manubrium sterni. Skeletal Radiol 25:467–470

6.  Kattan KR (1973) Modified view for use in roentgen examination of the sternoclavicular joints. Radiology 108:8
7.  Morag B, Shahin N (1975) The value of tomography of the sterno-clavicular region. Clin Radiol 26:57–62
8.  von Garrel T, Ince A, Junge A, Schnabel M, Bahrs C (2004) The sternal fracture: radiographic analysis of 200 fractures with special reference to concomitant injuries. J Trauma 57:837–844

# 6 Computed Tomography

ANNE GRETHE JURIK

**Contents**



## 6.1 Introduction

Computed tomography (CT) is today available in all advanced radiological departments. It is generally accepted that the diagnostic information obtained by CT is better than by conventional tomography [14]. CT can provide excellent visualisation of osseous structures. In addition to eliminating superimposed structures it visualises soft tissue structures to the extent possible by X-ray attenuation [7, 13, 22]. Moreover, CT is less time-consuming, more comfortable for the patient and the radiation dose can be decreased compared to conventional tomography [15]. CT is thus preferable compared to conventional tomography with regard to osteoarticular lesions.

This chapter encompasses the technical aspects and the normal CT appearance of the sternocostoclavicular (SCC) region. The chapter also deals with indications for CT, offering advice to determine the role of CT in the imaging of the SCC region.

## 6.2
## Technical Aspects

The technical level of the CT scanners available may differ due to a constant evolution of CT technique. The recent development of sub-second multislice CT (MSCT) with up to 64 detector rows is, in particular, diagnostically important [5]. The acquisition of isotropic or nearly isotropic image voxels improves the quality of secondary reconstructions, which is important in the evaluation of the SCC region. Also, the acquisition can be obtained in less than 10 s thereby omitting problems of breath holding. Irrespective of the technique used, the radiation dose always has to be taken into consideration. It is important to be aware that high-contrast osseous structures provide adequate image quality at a relative low mAs value [15]. The dose can therefore be reduced compared to conventional tomography by single-slice helical CT [15]. MSCT can also be optimised to achieve diagnostic quality of osteoarticular structures using a relatively low radiation dose [12].

The optimal slice thickness at MSCT depends on the scanner, but is usually ≤ 1 mm to gain isotropic voxels and optimal secondary reconstructions. For serial or single-slice helical CT it should be ≤ 3 mm to achieve a good visualisation of osteoarticular structures (Fig. 6.1). Irrespective of the technique a *bone reconstruction algorithm* should be used for clear delineation of osseous structures.

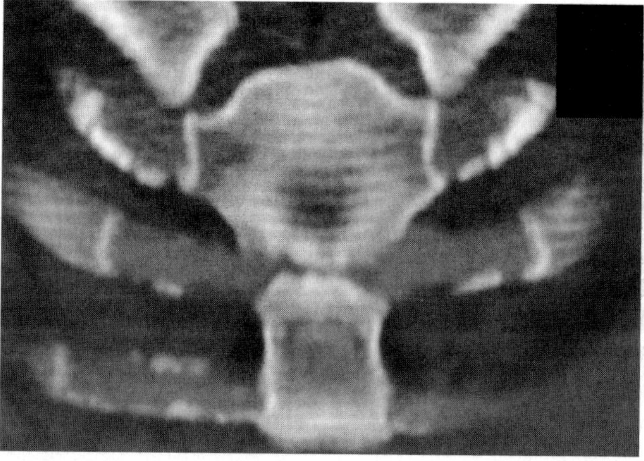

**Fig. 6.1** Single-slice helical CT, coronal reconstruction performed based on slices obtained with a thickness of 3 mm without overlap in a 23-year-old woman with clinical signs of MSJ arthritis. There is erosion of the MSJ joint facets, but there are irregular osseous contours due to technical factors, most importantly the universal streaky blurring due to the slice thickness

The field of view (FOV) should be adjusted to fit the SCC region. Decreasing the FOV increases the image resolution. Additional image reconstruction with a larger FOV may be necessary when suspecting abnormalities in other areas.

Due to the joint orientation changes of the sternoclavicular, the sternocostal and especially the manubriosternal joint (MSJ) may be difficult to evaluate on axial CT slices. Secondary *multiplanar reconstructions* (MPR) are often needed, and their diagnostic quality depends upon the acquired axial slices. The use of serial CT may imply irregularities of the osseous contours. This can also be the case for single-slice helical CT (Fig. 6.1) unless the image acquisition or reconstruction is performed with overlap. MSCT makes it possible to obtain MPR images with a high resolution (Fig. 6.2). Coronal and sagittal reconstructions should be performed routinely in the evaluation of the SCC region, but supplementary imaging planes such as oblique and curved MPR can be advantageous. With curved reconstructions, taking into account the sternal angulation at the MSJ, both the sternoclavicular joints and the MSJ can be delineated on a few reconstructed slices (Fig. 6.2). In addition to MPR images other postprocessing techniques may provide additional information. Most important are three-dimensional (3D) surface rendering and maximum intensity projection with variable thickness or volume intensity projection (VIP) (Fig. 6.2).

For delineating soft tissue abnormalities, for example as part of infection or tumour, it is often necessary to perform postcontrast scanning. It provides information about tissue vascularisation, which is important in the diagnosis of abscesses or tumours [24]. Visualisation of minor vessels always demands contrast enhancement [9].

## 6.3
## Normal Computed Tomography Appearance of the Sternocostoclavicular Region

It is important to know the normal appearance at CT to be able to diagnose disorders of the SCC region. Some variation may be seen for the normal sternoclavicular joints partly due to the occurrence of degenerative changes and costal cartilage calcification with age (Fig. 3.3). In a study of 60 non-rheumatic individuals, 20–80 years old, using serial 1.2-mm CT slices with gab of 2.5 mm, the most frequent finding was ossification of the first costal cartilage. It occurred in 88% of individuals followed in frequency by subchondral clavicular erosion (27%) or subchondral cyst (15%), uneven clavicular surface (23%) and meniscal ossification (15%). Importantly sternal hyperostosis, sternal condensation and ossification of the costoclavicular ligament never occurred in these non-rheumatic individuals [18].

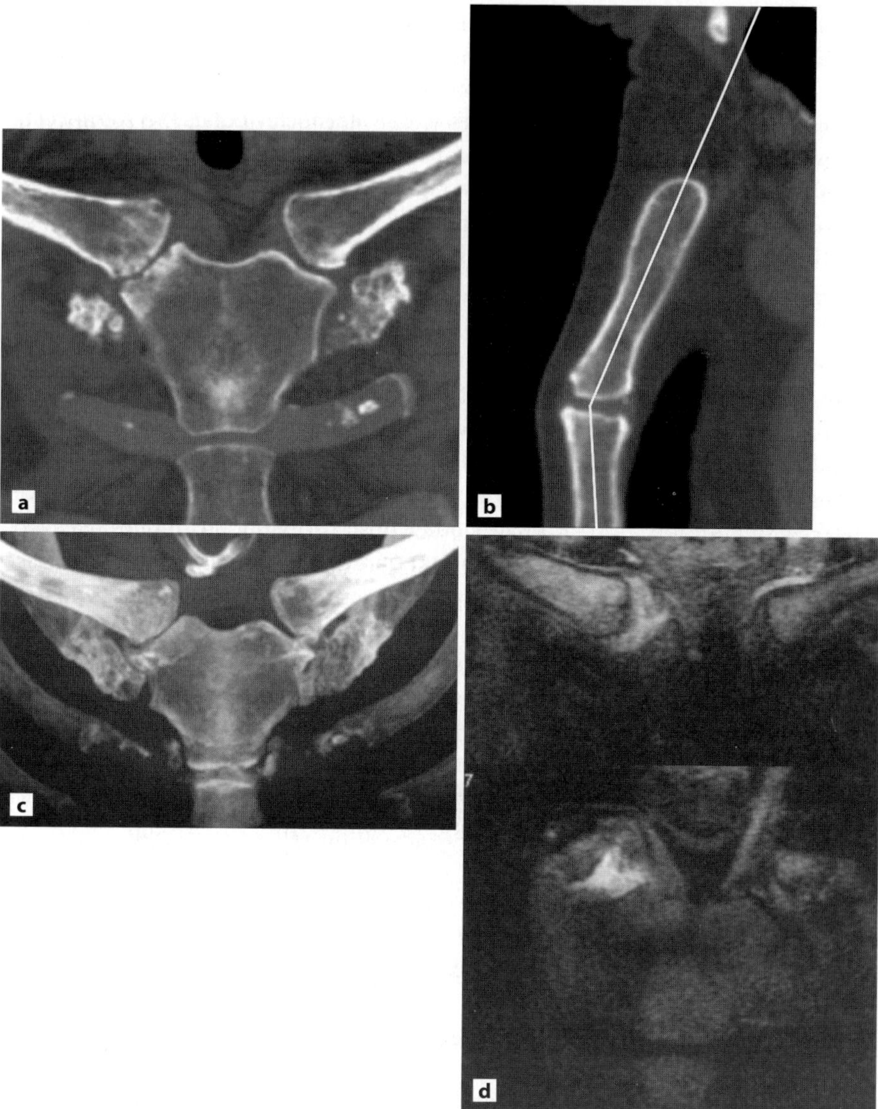

**Fig. 6.2** Multislice CT. **a** Coronal reconstruction based on slices obtained with a collimation of 64 × 0.67 mm in a 73-year-old man with joint space narrowing and erosion of the right sternoclavicular joint due to septic arthritis. **b** Sagittal view with the reconstruction line used to achieve **a**. **c** Anterior VIP image clearly delineates the calcified structures, including the extent of costal cartilage calcification. Narrowing of the right sternoclavicular joint space is also seen, but the minor changes detectable by MPR are not delineated. **d** MRI, coronal STIR shows signs of activity in the form of increased signal intensity, especially corresponding to the joint cavity

In accordance with this, a blind analysis of persons with and without inflammatory disorders revealed cysts or erosion associated with hyperostosis or osseous sclerosis only in patients with inflammatory disorders, whereas signs of degenerative lesions (osteophytes, subchondral sclerosis, uneven joint surfaces) occurred in both groups [17].

The normal CT appearance of the sternum was studied in 35 patients using 10-mm serial slices obtained for chest CT [11]. At these axial views the sternal bones were found to vary in shape and contour, the bones being ovoid to rectangular. The cortical margins of the manubrium were often blurred and irregular, especially caudally, which could simulate disease (Fig. 6.3a). Also irregular mottled calcifications and indistinct margins at the MSJ and xiphoid process could simulate bony lesions [11]. Using thin slices dedicated for visualisation of the SCC region and a bone reconstruction algorithm, the osseous contours are well defined (Fig. 6.3b).

Studies of the appearance of osseous structures of the SCC region at MSCT have not been published, although the technique has been used for vascular imaging in the region [16]. Based on forensic examination of crime victims performed in our department the appearance at axial MSCT is in accordance with the description at serial CT. The ovoid appearance of the sternal body occurred between the sternocostal joints whereas the shape mostly was rectangular at the level of joints. MSCT data offer the possibility for immediate visualisation in other reconstruction planes and the use of additional reconstruction techniques (Fig. 6.2).

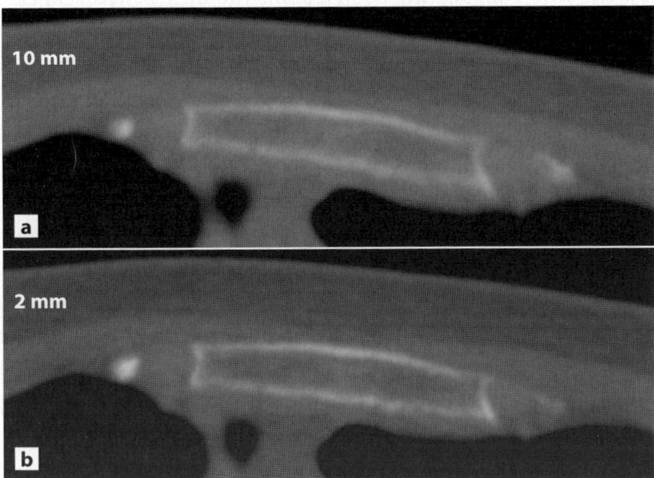


**Fig. 6.3** Axial CT slices of a normal sternal bone. **a** Ten-millimetre slice of the manubrium sterni showing irregular osseous contour posteriorly. **b** Two-millimetre slices in the same region show well-defined osseous contours

The normal CT appearance of the sternocostal joints varies considerably due to a wide range of normal variation and a frequent occurrence of degenerative changes with age. In young persons the joint facets are smooth and well defined without localised subchondral osseous changes (Fig. 1.6). With age the occurrence of osteophytes, subchondral osseous condensation and cartilage calcification may cause quite variable appearances (Figs. 2.9 and 4.2).


## 6.4
## Indications for Computed Tomography

Computed tomography is of great value in the evaluation of *trauma* patients (Chapter 11) [10]. It can visualise subtle, complex or unusual fractures [3] and joint malalignment. In addition CT can visualise the frequent concomitant thoracic or spinal injuries if the FOV is adjusted for viewing the whole thoracic cage (Chapter 11) [26].

The osteoarticular changes in *inflammatory* and *degenerative disorders* are well visualised by CT [23]. Serial CT has been shown to be superior to linear tomography in the detection of erosion, subchondral cysts and sclerosis as part of psoriatic arthritis [4, 6, 23]. By the use of MSCT detailed information regarding minor osseous lesions and soft tissue calcification can be obtained by CT, and not always by magnetic resonance imaging (MRI). MSCT can therefore be diagnostically preferable to MRI when suspecting such lesions including meniscal calcifications. However, due to the radiation dose given by CT, MRI should always be considered as an alternative method, giving the additional advantage of a clear delineation of concomitant soft tissue structures, which may be needed diagnostically (Chapters 12, 13 and 14).

Osteoarticular alterations as part of *septic arthritis* and *osteitis* can be delineated by CT (Fig. 6.2), which is the best modality for detecting sequesters. CT can also visualise the presence of local abscess formation, especially when using postcontrast scanning [2, 8, 24]. The use of CT is especially advantageous for demonstrating intrathoracic complications such as extensive chest wall abscess or phlegmon and mediastinitis (Chapter 16) [20]. However, delineation of the extent of osseous and soft tissue inflammation can be difficult at CT, also when including postcontrast scanning. The superior modality is in this case MRI (Chapter 16) [21].

Computed tomography can be valuable for assessing *complications after sternotomy*, depicting the extent and depth of the abnormalities [25]. CT can also be used to plan *sternal operations* such as arthrodesis of the MSJ giving information about the exact thickness of the sternum [1]. MSCT angiography may be used to visualise the location of the internal thoracic vessels before a parasternal transthoracic approach [9].

*Bone tumours* or *tumour-like lesions* can usually be diagnosed at CT, but supplementary MRI is often needed for delineating the local extent of malignancies (Chapters 17 and 18).

In rare cases CT may be needed to evaluate *congenital disorders* such as pectus deformities with regard to management or exclusion of other disorders. The orientation of the ribs and costal cartilages and their relationship to the sternum can be defined by 3D surface rendering, allowing exact preoperative measurement of the thoracic cage to guide individualised operative correction (Chapter 10) [19].

Computed tomography-guided *biopsy of osteoarticular lesions* can be advantageous to secure a correct location.

## 6.5
## Conclusions

Computed tomography can clearly delineate osseous structures of the SCC region making it possible to demonstrate subtle changes. Compared to conventional tomography, it additionally demonstrates soft tissue structures to the extent possible by X-ray attenuation, but not with the tissue characterisation gained by MRI. It is important to optimise the technique for achieving high-quality diagnostic images with a radiation dose as low as reasonably achievable.

Computed tomography can be diagnostically preferable to MRI when suspecting minor osseous lesions or calcified soft tissue abnormalities such as meniscal calcifications. In some patients CT is chosen due to a shorter examination time and better patient comfort or contraindications for MRI. When suspecting soft tissue abnormalities, MRI or ultrasonography should be the first modality of choice.

The main indications for CT are traumatic lesions, inflammatory and degenerative disorders, infections, postoperative complications, bone tumours and tumour-like lesions, and in rare cases congenital disorders.

## References


1. Al Dahiri A, Pallister I (2006) Arthrodesis for osteoarthritis of the manubriosternal joint. Eur J Cardiothorac Surg 29:119–121
2. Atasoy C, Oztekin PS, Ozdemir N, Sak SD, Erden I, Akyar S (2002) CT and MRI in tuberculous sternal osteomyelitis: a case report. Clin Imaging 26:112–115
3. Ayrik C, Cakmakci H, Yanturali S, Ozsarac M, Ozucelik DN (2005) A case report of an unusual sternal fracture. Emerg Med J 22:591–593
4. Baker ME, Martinez S, Kier R, Wain S (1988) High resolution computed tomography of the cadaveric sternoclavicular joint: findings in degenerative joint disease. J Comput Tomogr 12:13–18

5.  Buckwalter KA, Rydberg J, Kopecky KK, Crow K, Yang EL (2001) Musculoskeletal imaging with multislice CT. Am J Roentgenol 176:979–986

6.  Chigira M, Shimizu T (1989) Computed tomographic appearances of sternocostoclavicular hyperostosis. Skeletal Radiol 18:347–352

7.  Destouet JM, Gilula LA, Murphy WA, Sagel SS (1981) Computed tomography of the sternoclavicular joint and sternum. Radiology 138:123–128

8.  Dhillon MS, Gupta R, Rao KS, Nagi ON (2000) Bilateral sternoclavicular joint tuberculosis. Arch Orthop Trauma Surg 120:363–365

9.  Dursun M, Yekeler E, Yilmaz S, Genchellac H, Tunaci M (2005) Mapping of internal mammary vessels by multidetector computed tomography for parasternal transthoracic intervention guidance. J Comput Assist Tomogr 29:617–620

10. Ernberg LA, Potter HG (2003) Radiographic evaluation of the acromioclavicular and sternoclavicular joints. Clin Sports Med 22:255–275

11. Goodman LR, Teplick SK, Kay H (1983) Computed tomography of the normal sternum. Am J Roentgenol 141:219–223

12. Gurung J, Khan MF, Maataoui A, Herzog C, Bux R, Bratzke H, Ackermann H, Vogl TJ (2005) Multislice CT of the pelvis: dose reduction with regard to image quality using 16-row CT. Eur Radiol 15:1898–1905

13. Hatfield MK, Gross BH, Glazer GM, Martel W (1984) Computed tomography of the sternum and its articulations. Skeletal Radiol 11:197–203

14. Jurik AG, Albrechtsen J (1994) Spiral CT with three-dimensional and multiplanar reconstruction in the diagnosis of anterior chest wall joint and bone disorders. Acta Radiol 35:468–472

15. Jurik AG, Jensen LC, Hansen J (1996) Radiation dose by spiral CT and conventional tomography of the sternoclavicular joints and the manubrium sterni. Skeletal Radiol 25:467–470

16. Kamath S, Unsworth-White J, Wells IP (2005) Pseudoaneurysm of the internal mammary artery as an unusual cause of post-sternotomy hemorrhage: the role of multislice computed tomography in the diagnosis and treatment planning. Cardiovasc Intervent Radiol 28:246–248

17. Louvel JP, Duvey A, Da Silva F, Primard E, Mejjad O, Henry J, Le Loët X (1997) Computed tomography of sternoclavicular joint lesions in spondylarthropathies. Skeletal Radiol 26:419–423

18. Lucet L, Le Loët X, Ménard JF, Mejjad O, Louvel JP, Janvresse A, Daragon A (1996) Computed tomography of the normal sternoclavicular joint. Skeletal Radiol 25:237–241

19. Pretorius ES, Haller JA, Fishman EK (1998) Spiral CT with 3D reconstruction in children requiring reoperation for failure of chest wall growth after pectus excavatum surgery. Preliminary observations. Clin Imaging 22:108–116

20. Ross JJ, Shamsuddin H (2004) Sternoclavicular septic arthritis: review of 180 cases. Medicine (Baltimore) 83:139–148

21. Shah J, Patkar D, Parikh B, Parmar H, Varma R, Patankar T, Prasad S (2000) Tuberculosis of the sternum and clavicle: imaging findings in 15 patients. Skeletal Radiol 29:447–453

22. Stark P (1987) Computed tomography of the sternum. Crit Rev Diagn Imaging 27:321–349

23. Taccari E, Spadaro A, Riccieri V, Guerrisi R, Guerrisi V, Zoppini A (1992) Sternocla-vicular joint disease in psoriatic arthritis. Ann Rheum Dis 51:372–374

24. Tecce PM, Fishman EK (1995) Spiral CT with multiplanar reconstruction in the diag-nosis of sternoclavicular osteomyelitis. Skeletal Radiol 24:275–281

25. Templeton PA, Fishman EK (1992) CT evaluation of poststernotomy complications. Am J Roentgenol 159:45–50

26. von Garrel T, Ince A, Junge A, Schnabel M, Bahrs C (2004) The sternal fracture: ra-diographic analysis of 200 fractures with special reference to concomitant injuries. J Trauma 57:837–844

# 7   Magnetic Resonance Imaging

ANNE GRETHE JURIK

**Contents**



## 7.1 Introduction

Although the use of magnetic resonance imaging (MRI) has become indispensable in the evaluation of most joints, MRI has not yet gained wide clinical acceptance in evaluation of the sternocostoclavicular (SCC) region. This may be due to the wide availability of CT, which is easy to perform, whereas MRI of the SCC region can be a technical challenge. The advantage of MRI is its multiplanar capability as well as excellent spatial and contrast resolution with a superior visualisation of soft tissue structures. MRI characterises cartilage and soft tissue better than CT and is also more sensitive to marrow oedema and replacement or fatty degeneration. The disadvantage of MRI compared to CT is the longer acquisition time, which can cause respiratory blurring.

This chapter encompasses the technical aspects and the normal MRI appearance of the SCC region. Furthermore, the chapter deals with indications for MRI, offering advice to determine the role of MRI in the imaging of the SCC region.

## 7.2
## Technical Aspects

The most important factor for obtaining high-quality MRI of the SCC region is to avoid respiratory blurring. This is ensured by appropriate patient position and surface coil. The region can be stabilised by placing the patient in prone position with a surface coil over the SCC region and by supporting the patient with cushions to secure comfort [8]. The use of a body array coil and a breath-hold technique or respiratory gating is also a possibility [1].

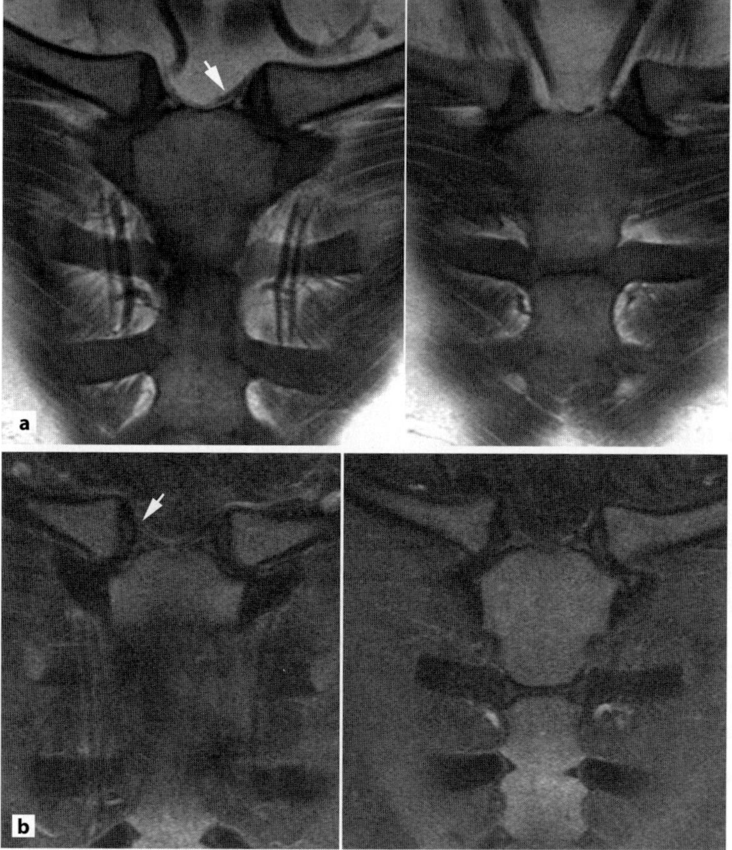

**Fig. 7.1** Normal sternum of a 33-year-old woman. **a** Coronal T1-weighted and **b** coronal STIR images. The bone marrow is relatively homogeneous, but with less fat signal than corresponding to peripheral bones indicating persistence of haematopoietic tissue. The inter-clavicular ligament (*arrow on image a*) and the intra-articular discs are well visualised on T1 images, the disc also at STIR (*arrow*)

The most appropriate sequences consist of a T1-weighted sequence and a sequence sensitive to fluid such as short-tau inversion recovery (STIR) or fat suppressed (FS) T2-weighted images (Fig. 7.1). A supplementary postcontrast T1 FS sequence may be needed to obtain information about tissue vascularisation. To avoid motion artefacts from the heart and lungs a saturation band should be placed posterior to the sternum.

The field of view (FOV) and slice thickness should be adjusted to the pathology suspected, for example a FOV of 10–12 cm for the sternoclavicular joints, a slice thickness of 3 mm, 10% gab and a matrix of 256 or preferably 512.

The slice orientation should be chosen according to the suspected pathology and its location. It is important always to obtain both coronal and axial slices. The sternal bones are often best visualised on coronal images (Fig. 7.1), preferably obtained in two planes to obtain better views of the manubrium and the sternal body, respectively, due to the angulation at the manubriosternal joint (MSJ) [1]. Axial views provide additional information, particularly about the surrounding soft tissue. A supplementary sagittal plane may be needed to clearly delineate the outer cortex and the central marrow of the manubrium and sternal body. For delineating clavicular lesions or the relation of the medial clavicle to the sternum, an oblique axial plane along the long axis of the clavicle is often advantageous. MRI of the sternoclavicular joints has to be performed in accordance with the anatomical structures involved [3]. A coronal plane is best for displaying the articular surfaces and the disc (Fig. 7.1). Also the costoclavicular ligament is well delineated by this slice orientation. Axial and sagittal images delineate the extent of the anterior and posterior sternoclavicular ligaments, the attachment of the intra-articular disc to the capsule anterior and posterior, the interclavicular ligament and the thickness of the costoclavicular ligament.

Magnetic resonance arthrography can be used to detect intra-articular abnormalities such as disc perforation and to delineate the extent of the capsule [3]. However, the method has not gained wide clinical acceptance.


## 7.3
## Normal Magnetic Resonance Imaging Appearance of the Sternocostoclavicular Region

It is important to know the normal appearance at MRI to be able to diagnose disorders of the SCC region. In a study of 119 persons cortical irregularities in normal sternoclavicular joints, erosion and destruction were not detected [8]. However, poorly defined cortical margins, non-fatty bone marrow and small amounts of fluid in the sternoclavicular joint, either alone or in combination, were identified and should not be interpreted as disease. The finding at common clinical imaging of poorly defined cortical margins in the normal sternoclavicular joint region is probably due to the curved surfaces of the joints and the slice thickness used. When performing three-dimensional (3D) volume acquisition with an effective slice thickness of less than 1 mm, the normal cortical surfaces were well defined [8].

Haematopoietic, non-fatty bone marrow occurs as a normal finding in the sternoclavicular region (Fig. 7.1). Relative to fatty marrow it appears as slightly decreased signal intensity on T1-weighted images, increased signal intensity on STIR and slightly decreased or isointense signal on T2. The bone marrow is regarded fatty if it is isointense to fat on all sequences. Persistence of haematopoietic bone marrow occurs especially in young persons. When mixed with fatty tissue the marrow signal can appear inhomogeneous (Fig. 2.5), which is predominantly seen in the sternum, but also in the clavicle [8, 17]. Conversion of the haematopoietic bone marrow in the sternum begins at the age of 6–10 years, and in the clavicle before 11 years of age. Areas of haematopoietic bone marrow often persist throughout adult life [17], although the amount decreases with age [8].

The small amounts of fluid in normal joints are particularly visible on sequences sensitive to fluid (STIR or T2 FS), but is a relatively rare finding [8].

It is possible to visualise the anatomy of the normal sternoclavicular joints in detail by MRI. In an analysis of specimens all ligaments around the sternoclavicular joint were delineated with conventional MR sequences [3]. The fibrous capsule and the ligaments had low signal intensity at all imaging sequences. The intra-articular disc was best visualised on T2-weighted images, where the low signal intensity of the disc contrasted against a high signal of the joint space and cartilage [3]. On T1 the disc displayed low-intermediate signal (Fig. 7.1) and could be difficult to differentiate from the articular surfaces except when calcified. The study showed that the costoclavicular ligament is well delineated, but differentiation between the anterior and posterior portion is not possible [3].


## 7.4
## Indications for Magnetic Resonance Imaging

If there are no contraindications for MRI, such as the presence of a pacemaker, MRI should be the modality of choice when suspecting *primary malignancies*, especially when located in the soft tissue (Fig. 7.2). The local extent and the relationship to important structures are better visualised by MRI compared to CT (Chapter 17) [1, 9, 11]. *Metastases* in the SCC region and manifestation of *myeloproliferative disorders* may be diagnosed or confirmed by MRI (Figs. 7.3 and 7.4). MRI can also be used to monitor such disorders in the SCC region, sometimes together with other

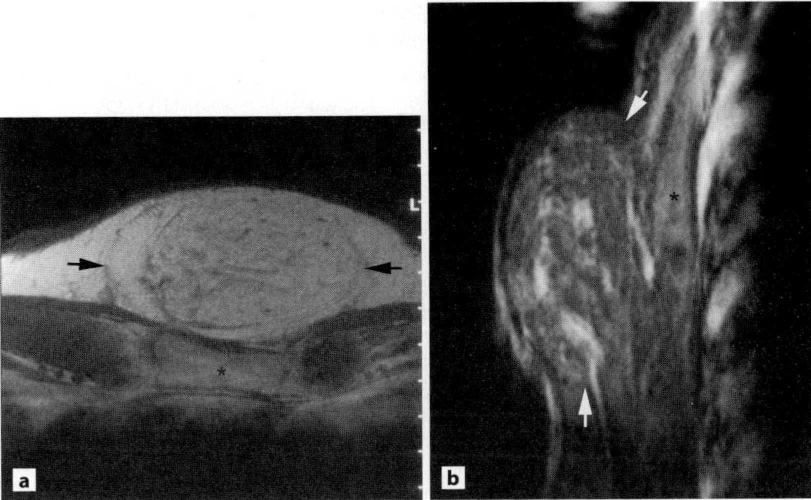

**Fig. 7.2** Liposarcoma in a 78-year-old woman. **a** Axial T1 and **b** sagittal STIR show a large soft tissue mass mainly consisting of fatty tissue, but also enhancing sarcomatous areas (*arrows*). The *asterisk* indicates the sternal bone. Biopsy confirmed the diagnosis of a highly differentiated liposarcoma

lesions using whole-body bone marrow MRI consisting of STIR and T1-weighted sequences.

Magnetic resonance imaging or CT should be obtained routinely to assess *septic arthritis* or *osteitis* in the SCC region [9, 13]. MRI has the advantage of showing the extent of osseous inflammation in addition to destructive changes also detectable by CT (Fig. 6.2d) [4]. In addition, soft tissue involvement and abscess formation are better delineated by MRI than by CT (Chapter 16) [1, 14].

Magnetic resonance imaging can be valuable for the diagnosis of *rheumatic inflammatory osteoarticular disorders*, such as rheumatoid and seronegative arthritis, and the wide spectrum of inflammatory syndromes in the SCC region, including *pustulotic arthro-osteitis* and *SAPHO* (synovitis, acne, pustulosis, hyperostosis and osteitis) [1, 6, 9, 10]. MRI is especially valuable to determine disease activity, but joint destruction and osseous alteration are also visualised. Inflammatory soft tissue lesions such as ganglion cysts originating from the sternoclavicular joint are well delineated by MRI. Such lesions can also be visualised by ultrasonography, but concomitant joint or bone lesions cannot be diagnosed or excluded with certainty by this method [7].

Magnetic resonance imaging can be used to diagnose *soft tissue injuries*, including ligamentous tears and cartilaginous injuries [2, 9]. This has been confirmed in

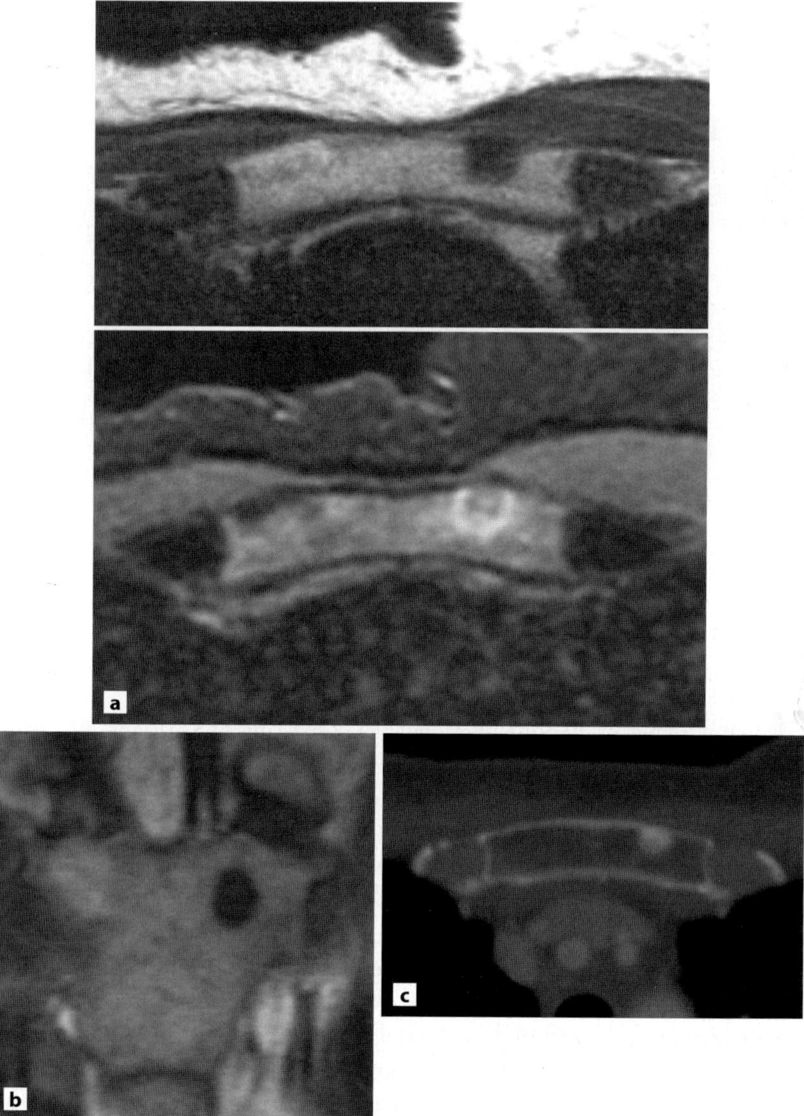

**Fig. 7.3** Sclerotic metastasis in the manubrium sterni of a 46-year-old woman with breast cancer and tracer uptake at scintigraphy corresponding to this region and in two ribs. **a** Axial T1 (*upper*) and STIR image (*lower*), and **b** coronal T1-weighted image of the manubrium show a small intramedullary process with low signal intensity centrally on both sequences, but a surrounding rim of high signal at STIR indicating metastasis and excluding the possibility of a bone island. **c** Axial CT slice from a following chest scan only shows a well-demarcated osseous condensation in addition to sclerotic metastasis in two ribs

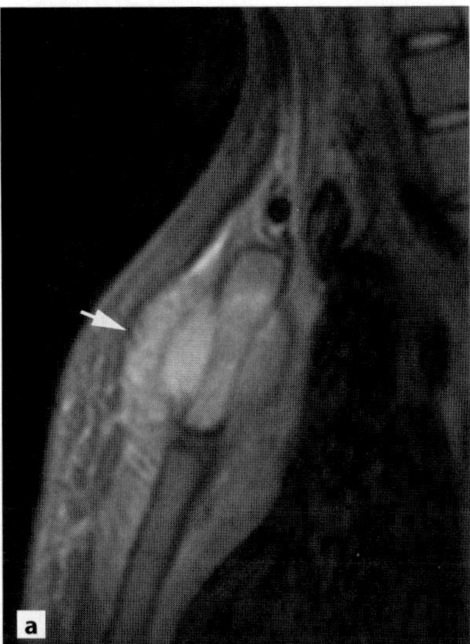

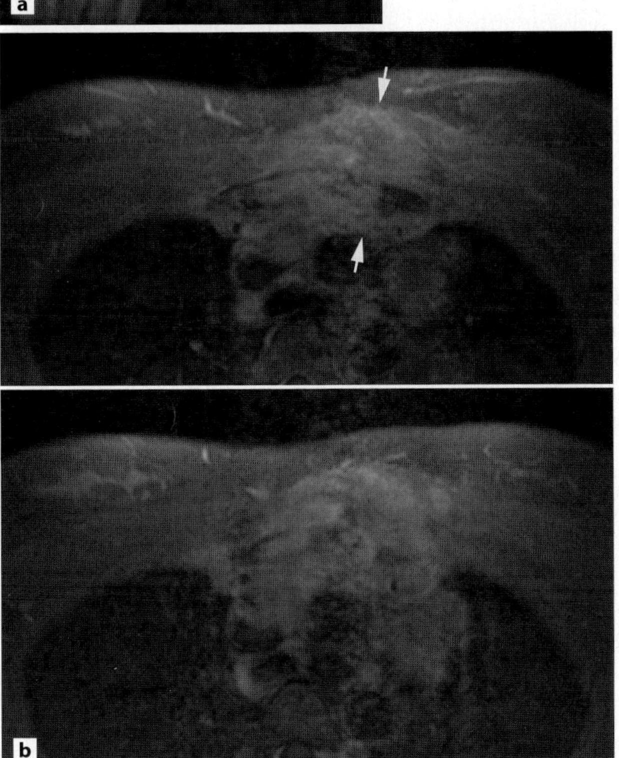

**Fig. 7.4** Malignant lymphoma in a 21-year-old woman with increasing swelling at the manubrium during 1 month. **a** Sagittal STIR and **b** postcontrast axial T1 FS show a huge tumour mass in and around the manubrium sterni with surrounding soft tissue oedema (*arrows*)

a study of 41 patients, where 80% had detectable articular disc injuries diagnosed by MRI [2]. Injuries of the anterior, posterior, interclavicular and costoclavicular ligaments occurred in 73%, 39%, 29% and 14% of patients, respectively. MRI also displayed impingement of mediastinal structures in cases of posterior clavicular subluxation. The potential occurrence of vascular injury by posterior sternoclavicular dislocations can additionally be evaluated by MR angiography [5]. Also post-traumatic dislocation of sternal segments in children can be delineated by MRI, being located either at the junction of the manubrium with the sternal body or at the junction of upper sternal segments [16]. In addition MRI can be used to assess postoperative changes in selected patients [9].

*Congenital malformation*, such as cleft sternum may be evaluated by MRI, which is especially valuable in the case of associated vascular abnormalities or other ventral developmental defects [1, 15]. In patients with pectus excavatum fast, breath-hold MRI can be very informative regarding skeletal abnormalities, chest wall motion and cardiac or diaphragmatic changes [12].

## 7.5
## Conclusions

The normal anatomical structures of the sternoclavicular region can be identified by MRI. Poorly defined cortical margins, non-fatty bone marrow and small amounts of joint fluid, either alone or combined, can be identified and should not be mistaken for pathological changes.

Magnetic resonance imaging is a sensitive method to diagnose disease. It should therefore be the first modality of choice when suspecting malignancies or infection in the SCC region. MRI often adds important diagnostic information in many other disorders such as rheumatic diseases, soft tissue injuries and congenital disorders.

## References


1. Aslam M, Rajesh A, Entwisle J, Jeyapalan K (2002) Pictorial review: MRI of the sternum and sternoclavicular joints. Br J Radiol 75:627–634
2. Benitez CL, Mintz DN, Potter HG (2004) MR imaging of the sternoclavicular joint following trauma. Clin Imaging 28:59–63
3. Brossmann J, Stabler A, Preidler KW, Trudell D, Resnick D (1996) Sternoclavicular joint: MR imaging—anatomic correlation. Radiology 198:193–198
4. Dhillon MS, Gupta R, Rao KS, Nagi ON (2000) Bilateral sternoclavicular joint tuberculosis. Arch Orthop Trauma Surg 120:363–365

5.  Ernberg LA, Potter HG (2003) Radiographic evaluation of the acromioclavicular and sternoclavicular joints. Clin Sports Med 22:255–275

6.  Ginalski JM, Landry M, Rappoport G, Chamot AM, Gerster JC (1992) MR imaging of sternocostoclavicular arthro-osteitis with palmoplantar pustulosis. Eur J Radiol 14:221–222

7.  Haber LH, Waanders NA, Thompson GH, Petersilge C, Ballock RT (2002) Sternoclavicular joint ganglion cysts in young children. J Pediatr Orthop 22:544–547

8.  Klein MA, Miro PA, Spreitzer AM, Carrera GF (1995) MR imaging of the normal sternoclavicular joint: spectrum of findings. Am J Roentgenol 165:391–393

9.  Klein MA, Spreitzer AM, Miro PA, Carrera GF (1997) MR imaging of the abnormal sternoclavicular joint: a pictorial essay. Clin Imaging 21:138–143

10.  Laiho K, Soini I, Martio J (2001) Magnetic resonance imaging findings of manubriosternal joint involvement in SAPHO syndrome. Clin Rheumatol 20:232–233

11.  Nakajo M, Ohkubo K, Nandate T, Shirahama H, Yanagi M, Anraku M, Nakajo M (2005) Primary synovial sarcoma of the sternum: computed tomography and magnetic resonance imaging findings. Radiat Med 23:208–212

12.  Raichura N, Entwisle J, Leverment J, Beardsmore CS (2001) Breath-hold MRI in evaluating patients with pectus excavatum. Br J Radiol 74:701–708

13.  Ross JJ, Shamsuddin H (2004) Sternoclavicular septic arthritis: review of 180 cases. Medicine (Baltimore) 83:139–148

14.  Shah J, Patkar D, Parikh B, Parmar H, Varma R, Patankar T, Prasad S (2000) Tuberculosis of the sternum and clavicle: imaging findings in 15 patients. Skeletal Radiol 29:447–453

15.  Tastekin A, Kantarci M, Onbas O, Ermis B, Ors R (2003) Superior sternal cleft and minor hemangiomas in a newborn. Genet Couns 14:349–352

16.  Wada A, Fujii T, Takamura K, Yanagida H, Matsuura A, Katayama A (2002) Sternal segment dislocation in children. J Pediatr Orthop 22:729–731

17.  Zawin JK, Jaramillo D (1993) Conversion of bone marrow in the humerus, sternum, and clavicle: changes with age on MR images. Radiology 188:159–164

# 8  Ultrasonography

**ANNE GRETHE JURIK**

**Contents**



## 8.1
## Introduction

The use of ultrasonography in musculoskeletal imaging has increased during recent years. This is partly due to its availability in most departments, the low cost and high patient comfort. Ultrasonography of the sternocostoclavicular (SCC) region has the advantage of showing the soft tissue structures which are not delineated by radiography. It is therefore often used as an initial examination, especially in children.

This chapter encompasses the technical aspects and the normal ultrasonography appearance of the SCC region. It also gives advice to determine the role of ultrasonography in the imaging of the SCC region.

## 8.2
## Technical Aspects

Ultrasonography can be performed with a wide variety of equipment and thereby technical possibilities. Linear or curved-linear probes with a frequency of

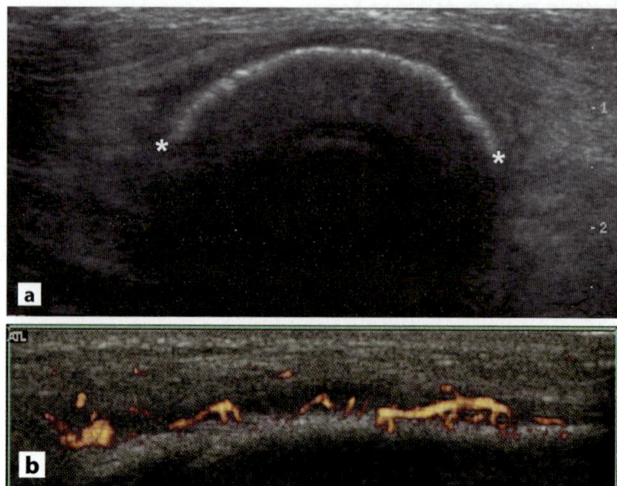

**Fig. 8.1** Chronic recurrent multifocal osteomyelitis in a 6-year-old girl presenting with a swelling at the medial part of the clavicle. **a** Conventional ultrasonography shows enlargement of the bone, but intact cortical bone (*asterisks*). There is no fluid collection in soft tissue, but it appears relatively echopenic compatible with oedema. **b** Colour Doppler shows increased vascularity in the surrounding soft tissue. Conventional radiographs and MRI are displayed in Fig. 13.1

7.5–15 MHz are most suitable for imaging the SCC region. Supplementary Doppler technique enables the assessment of tissue vascularisation via signals generated by flowing blood cells (Fig. 8.1). However, the blood flow in microvessels may be slow and difficult to detect. The administration of microbubble contrast increases the intensity of Doppler signals from the blood and can rescue or improve a non-diagnostic Doppler examination. More dedicated ultrasonography is appearing in the form of colour/power Doppler. These techniques increase the accuracy of the examination, but irrespective of the technique used, diagnostic ultrasonography is limited to visualisation of soft tissue structures and bone surfaces [10].

Ultrasound-guided biopsy or puncture of soft tissue abnormalities should be performed with dedicated guidance equipment to secure a correct location of the tissue sample.

## 8.3
## Normal Ultrasonography Appearance of the Sternocostoclavicular Region

There are few publications describing the normal ultrasonography appearance of the SCC region, mainly focusing on the cartilaginous structure [3]. The costal cartilages appear less echogenic than the adjacent muscle and are delineated by a thin echogenic anterior margin. From our clinical experience all soft tissue structures can be identified including the ligaments, capsule, cartilages and intra-articular discs anterosuperiorly, but not to the extent possible by MRI.

## 8.4
## Indications for Ultrasonography

Ultrasonography is important as an *initial diagnostic tool in children*, as the procedure is painless and easy to perform. Ultrasonography has been reported used to diagnose important congenital abnormalities such as complete cleft sternum [15], but also minor abnormalities such as superior sternal cleft [2, 11]. Ultrasonography can provide information not obtained by radiography by showing the extent of non-calcified chest wall abnormalities [9, 11]. The possibilities of evaluating the sternum in the embryo by transabdominal ultrasonography has been proved in a cross-sectional study [16], and the prenatal diagnosis of abnormalities such as cleft sternum has been described [6, 15].

Ultrasonography can be a reliable substitute for radiography in very specific circumstances such as *diagnosis of fluid collections* in the form of joint effusion, ganglion cyst and soft tissue abscesses [1, 8, 13].

Ultrasonography has also been reported to be of value in the *diagnosis of injuries* in the form of joint dislocation, stress or undisplaced fractures, such as physeal fracture of the sternal end of the clavicle in children (Chapter 11) [1, 4, 7, 8, 12, 13]. It has also been proved helpful during operation for posterior sternoclavicular joint dislocation [14].

Ultrasonography may be valuable as an initial diagnostic tool to clarify the differential *diagnosis of sternoclavicular joint lesions*. It can diagnose or exclude the presence of joint inflammation, but the cause of an inflammation is seldom detected [5].

Despite the interesting information obtained by ultrasonography, it may be mandatory to compare and prove the findings with other methods such as CT or MRI (Fig. 8.2), especially when suspecting malignancy.

Ultrasonography gives the possibility of performing guided fluid aspiration, injections or biopsy, for example of soft tissue tumours.

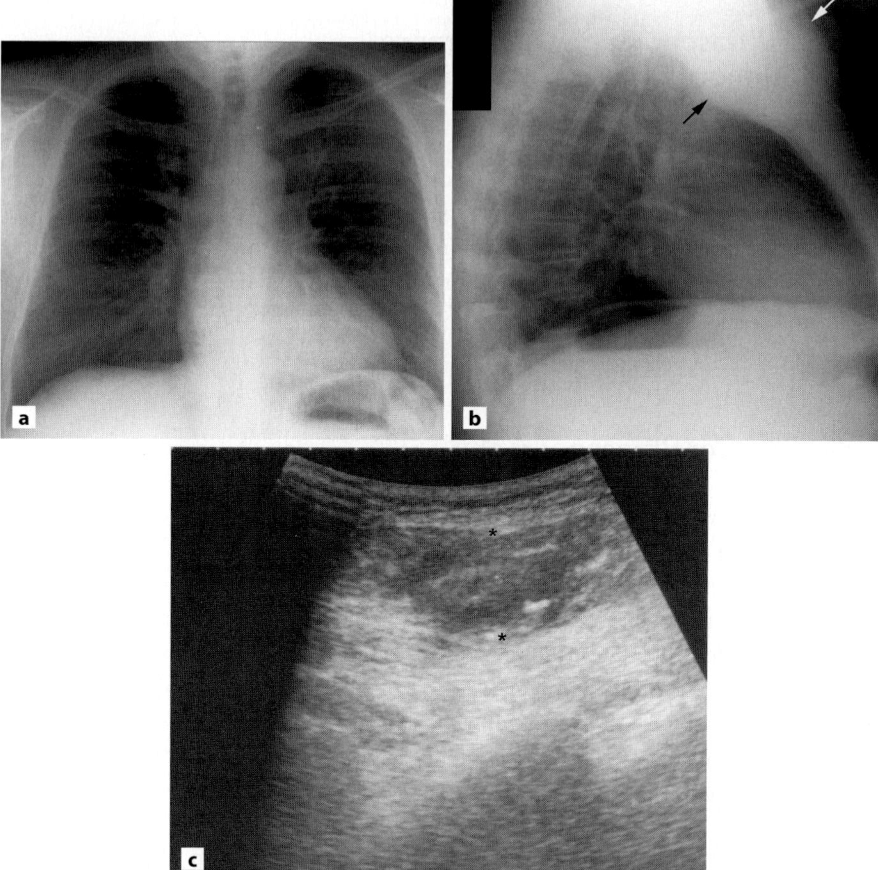

**Fig. 8.2** Septic arthritis of the sternoclavicular joint in a 48-year-old drug addict. He was admitted due to hip pain and the diagnosis of infectious hip arthritis was established. Clinical examination and chest X-ray (**a,b**) revealed a swelling in the upper sternal region (*arrows*) with blurring of the mediastinal structures on the left side. Supplementary ultrasonography (**c**) disclosed an irregular echopenic mass just inferior to the left sternoclavicular joint and superficially to the first costal cartilage (*asterisks*) and extended laterally beneath the pectoralis muscle. There was also a small intra-articular fluid collection (not shown). MRI, STIR (**d**) and T2-weighted images (**e**) semiaxial along the clavicular bone do not delineate the soft tissue involvement better than ultrasonography partly because a postcontrast sequence could not be obtained due to lack of available veins. MRI, however, displayed the extent of osseous inflammation being present in both the manubrium (M) and the clavicle (C). Also destruction of the first costal cartilage at the bottom of the infected area was detected (*arrow*)

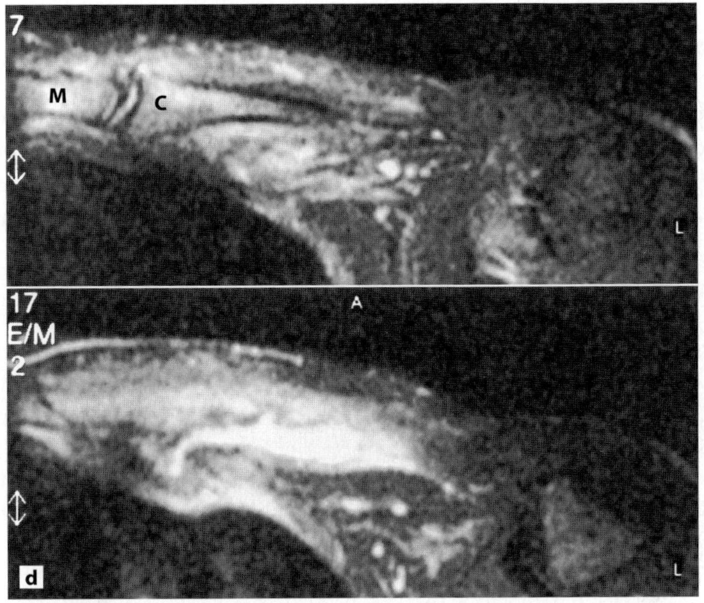
7
M
C
L
17
E/M
2
A
L
d

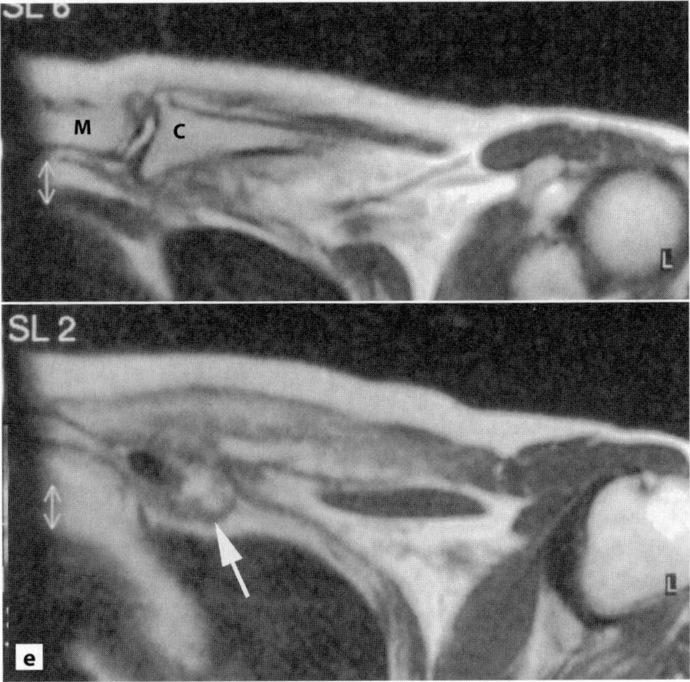
SL 6
M
C
L
SL 2
L
e

## 8.5
## Conclusions

Ultrasonography can be a reliable substitute for radiography in very specific circumstances. It is especially useful to establish or exclude disease and congenital variants in children. It can visualise soft tissue structures and diagnose fluid collections or joint effusion. Guided aspiration, injections or biopsy of soft tissue abnormalities can easily be performed.

## References


1. Boll KL, Jurik AG (1990) Sternal osteomyelitis in drug addicts. J Bone Joint Surg Br 72:328–329
2. Carles D, Pelluard F, Alberti EM, Maugey-Laulom B, Lin TY, Saura R, Roux D, Lacombe D (2005) Fetal presentation of PHACES syndrome. Am J Med Genet A 132:110
3. Choi YW, Im JG, Song CS, Lee JS (1995) Sonography of the costal cartilage: normal anatomy and preliminary clinical application. J Clin Ultrasound 23:243–250
4. Engin G, Yekeler E, Guloglu R, Acunas B, Acunas G (2000) US versus conventional radiography in the diagnosis of sternal fractures. Acta Radiol 41:296–299
5. Ernberg LA, Potter HG (2003) Radiographic evaluation of the acromioclavicular and sternoclavicular joints. Clin Sports Med 22:255–275
6. Fokin AA (2000) Cleft sternum and sternal foramen. Chest Surg Clin N Am 10:261–276
7. Griffith JF, Rainer TH, Ching AS, Law KL, Cocks RA, Metreweli C (1999) Sonography compared with radiography in revealing acute rib fracture. Am J Roentgenol 173:1603–1609
8. Haber LH, Waanders NA, Thompson GH, Petersilge C, Ballock RT (2002) Sternoclavicular joint ganglion cysts in young children. J Pediatr Orthop 22:544–547
9. Herman TE, Siegel MJ (2001) Superior congenital sternal cleft. J Perinatol 21:334–335
10. Klauser A, Demharter J, De Marchi A, Sureda D, Barile A, Masciocchi C, Faletti C, Schirmer M, Kleffel T, Bohndorf K (2005) Contrast enhanced gray-scale sonography in assessment of joint vascularity in rheumatoid arthritis: results from the IACUS study group. Eur Radiol 15:2404–2410
11. Mazzie JP, Lepore J, Price AP, Driscoll W, Bohrer S, Perlmutter S, Katz DS (2003) Superior sternal cleft associated with PHACES syndrome: postnatal sonographic findings. J Ultrasound Med 22:315–319
12. Rainer TH, Griffith JF, Lam E, Lam PK, Metreweli C (2004) Comparison of thoracic ultrasound, clinical acumen, and radiography in patients with minor chest injury. J Trauma 56:1211–1213
13. Sferopoulos NK (2003) Fracture separation of the medial clavicular epiphysis: ultrasonography findings. Arch Orthop Trauma Surg 123:367–369

14. Siddiqui AA, Turner SM (2003) Posterior sternoclavicular joint dislocation: the value of intra-operative ultrasound. Injury 34:448–453
15. Twomey EL, Moore AM, Ein S, McAuliffe F, Seaward G, Yoo SJ (2005) Prenatal ultrasonography and neonatal imaging of complete cleft sternum: a case report. Ultrasound Obstet Gynecol 25:599–601
16. Zalel Y, Lipitz S, Soriano D, Achiron R (1999) The development of the fetal sternum: a cross-sectional sonographic study. Ultrasound Obstet Gynecol 13:187–190

# 9 Radionuclide Imaging

ANNE GRETHE JURIK

**Contents**



## 9.1
## Introduction

Bone scintigraphy provides highly sensitive information about the whole skeleton in a single examination. Tracer uptake reflects increased bone turnover and vascularity, and the method is therefore very sensitive for the detection of neoplastic, infectious and inflammatory lesions [17, 19]. The specificity, however, is not impressive, as increased tracer uptake can appear in both normal and abnormal conditions. It is important to know the pitfalls, including increased uptake as a normal finding. Other forms of radionuclide imaging may be used in specific situations.

This chapter encompasses the technical aspects and the normal scintigraphic appearance of the sternocostoclavicular (SCC) region. In addition the chapter deals with the indications for bone scintigraphy and other forms of radionuclide imaging, giving advice to determine their role in the imaging of the SCC region.

## 9.2
## Technical Aspects

Conventional *bone scintigraphy* is usually performed as planar images 2–4 h after injection of [99m]technetium-methylenediphosphonate ([99m]Tc MDP) using a gamma camera. The amount of tracer uptake reflects osteoblastic activity and vascularity. Occasionally three-phase technetium bone scintigraphy can be advantageous, for example in diagnosing infection [1].

*Leukocyte scintigraphy* is performed 4–20 h after injection of [99m]Tc-hexamethyl-propyleneamine oxime (HMPAO)-labelled leukocytes. It can be performed as a planar scintigraphy, but the information will increase by additional use of *single-photon emission computed tomography* (SPECT). SPECT can provide transverse, sagittal and coronal slices, and thereby add information about the location and depth of changes.

*Positron emission tomography* (PET) is based on emission of positrons and is usually performed with [18]F-fluorodeoxyglucose (FDG). It allows sectional images of the body and provides physiological information that enables the diagnosis of disorders based on altered tissue glucose metabolism.

## 9.3
## Normal Appearance of the Sternocostoclavicular Region

When evaluating bone scintigraphy, it is important to be able to distinguish between normal variants and skeletal pathology. There are two extensive publications dealing with age-related normal scintigraphic variants in the SCC region [8, 18]. There were based on analysis of 152 (66 male and 86 female; mean age $45 \pm 19$ years) and 334 (158 male and 176 female; mean age $33 \pm 20$ years) patients, respectively, without sternal symptoms. The following variants of sternal tracer uptake were identified. A uniform pattern was most common in children ($\leq 10$–12 years). A heterogeneous uptake was frequently seen in adolescents and young adults, where a linear pattern corresponding to transverse sternal ridges may occur [8]. A heterogeneous pattern was also frequent in adults and often present as a segmented pattern in persons above the age of 60 years [18]. Predominant focal findings were a hot spot at the manubriosternal joint (MSJ) and decreased tracer uptake in the lower sternum, just above the xiphoid process. Other spots of increased tracer uptake in the sternal body also occurred, but not in subjects below 12 years of age [8, 18]. Focal hot spots may be due to normal variants such as a persistent sternal synchondrosis [2], and the occurrence of degenerative joint changes with age, for example at the sternocostal joints [8]. A well-defined area of increased uptake in the second sternocostal joint adjacent to the MSJ is usually a normal finding and not a sign of disease [4].

## 9.4
## Indications for Radionuclide Imaging

Bone scintigraphy is valuable for the staging of *neoplastic diseases* with regard to metastases. The same applies to PET, which has proved useful in assessing the extension of carcinomas, detecting tumour recurrence and monitoring responses to therapy. PET revealed more lesions than bone scintigraphy, independent of the type of tumour and the location of bone involvement [9, 13]. The combination of PET and CT (PET/CT) may have a great potential for diagnosing SCC lesions, especially malignancies (Chapters 17 and 18).

*Infectious lesions* will display increased uptake at bone scintigraphy, which is especially valuable regarding multifocal lesions (Fig. 9.1). Leukocyte scintigraphy is useful for evaluation of infection in osteoarticular areas, which will display abnormal activity at bone scintigraphy due to other abnormalities or be located to soft tissue. Leukocyte scintigraphy is a highly reliable method for early diagnosis of sternal infections after sternotomy [16].

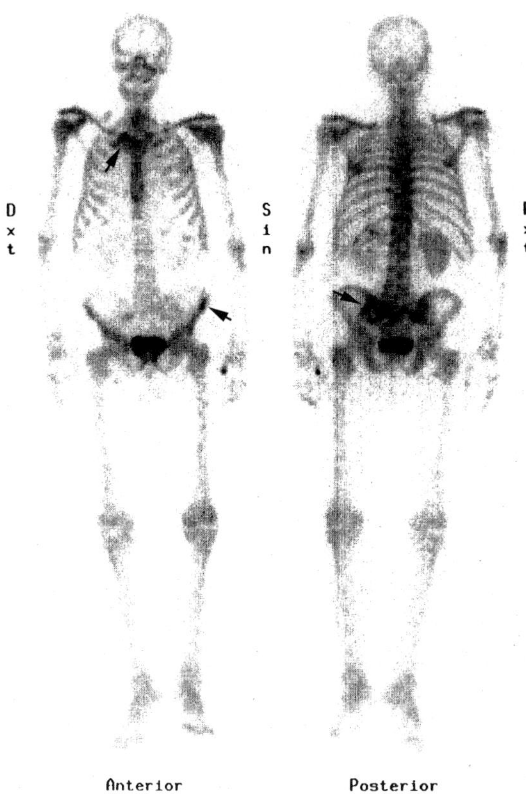


**Fig. 9.1** Septic arthritis of the right sternoclavicular joint in a 73-year-old man with diabetes mellitus and sepsis with endocarditis. Bone scintigraphy, anterior and posterior views, show increased tracer uptake corresponding to the right sternoclavicular joint, and at the left iliac bone and sacroiliac joint (*arrows*). The coexistence of septic sternoclavicular arthritis, sacroiliitis and iliac osteitis was confirmed by MRI, CT and CT-guided biopsy. CT and MRI of the SCC region is shown in Fig. 6.2

In the diagnosis of SCC lesions as part of *chronic recurrent multifocal osteomyelitis*, a rare multifocal inflammatory skeletal disorder, bone scintigraphy is valuable for identification of clinically silent lesions (Chapter 13) [12].

Bone scintigraphy may also be of diagnostic help in confirming the presence of *rheumatic inflammatory osteoarticular lesions*. The inflammatory disorders sternocostoclavicular hyperostosis (SCCH) and pustulotic arthro-osteitis (PAO) may show a characteristic "bullhead-like" tracer uptake in the SCC region with the manubrium sterni representing the upper skull and the inflamed sternoclavicular joints the horns (Fig. 9.2). The bullhead sign is a typical and highly specific scintigraphic appearance of advanced SCCH and PAO [5, 6], but may not be present in early or inactive stages of the disorders (Chapter 12). The use of FDG PET to visualise metabolically active tissue has only been reported in two cases with similar disorders [10, 15] and its value has to be evaluated further. Bone scintigraphy has been reported used to monitor the course and to assess therapeutic efficiency

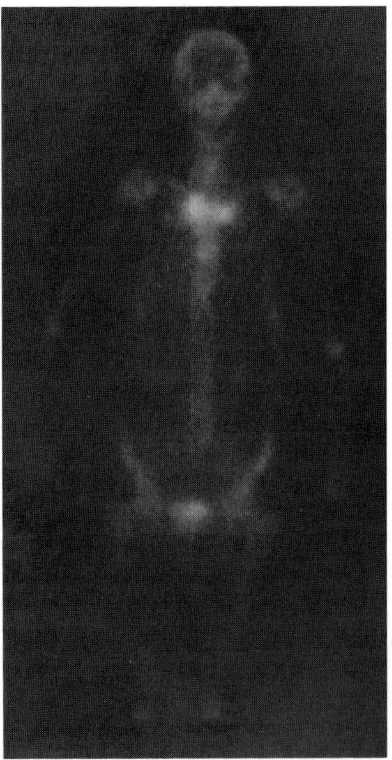

**Fig. 9.2** Pustulotic arthro-osteitis, bone scintigraphy, anterior view, in a 58-year-old woman with intermittent pain in the sternoclavicular region for 2 years accompanied by an increasing firm swelling. There is increased "bullhead-like" tracer uptake in the SCC region, most pronounced on the right side. No other foci were found. Clinical examinations revealed dermal changes compatible with pustulosis palmoplantaris

in patients with such inflammatory lesions [15]. The method can be an easy way to monitor the disease if changes are part of a multifocal disease. When limited to the SCC region it is more appropriate to monitor by MRI, as a STIR sequence will give the same information about activity as scintigraphy and will provide further pathoanatomical details. In addition, MRI is without any inherent radiation risk.

Other rheumatic disorders of the sternoclavicular joint may be difficult to visualise accurately on routine bone scintigraphy [14]. *Ankylosing spondylitis* (AS) often involves the SCC region (Chapter 12), but reports of scintigraphic SCC abnormalities have been scarce. Bone scintigraphy has mainly been used to visualise disease activity in the sacroiliac and spinal joints partly because scintigraphic activity in the SCC region may be obscured by overshadowed spinal involvement [11]. However, increased activity in the SCC region has been found to be frequent if the scan includes available views of the sternum, being present in five of six patients at the MSJ and in five at the sternoclavicular joints [3]. Awareness of the scintigraphic appearances of AS is important in order to avoid confusion with other pathology.

*Relapsing polychondritis* involving the costal cartilages may be diagnosed by scintigraphy showing increased tracer uptake in the involved cartilages [7].


## 9.5
## Conclusions

Scintigraphy is a sensitive method for detecting disorders with increased bone turnover, but is in general not specific for disorders in the SCC region except for the "bullhead-like" sign in SCCH and PAO. It is, however, valuable when suspecting multifocal disorders. Leukocyte scintigraphy can add to the diagnosis of deep infections, especially when using SPECT. PET alone or in combination with CT (PET/CT) may be valuable in the diagnosis and follow-up of malignancies and possibly other disorders.


## References


1. Atasoy C, Oztekin PS, Ozdemir N, Sak SD, Erden I, Akyar S (2002) CT and MRI in tuberculous sternal osteomyelitis: a case report. Clin Imaging 26:112–115
2. Baas J, Eijsvogel M, Dijkstra P (1988) Persistent sternum synchondroses on bone scintigraphy. Eur J Nucl Med 13:572–573
3. Collie DA, Smith GW, Merrick MV (1993) 99mTc-MDP scintigraphy in ankylosing spondylitis. Clin Radiol 48:392–397
4. Fink-Bennett DM, Shapiro EE (1984) The Angle of Louis. A potential pitfall ("Louie's Hot Spot") in bone scan interpretation. Clin Nucl Med 9:352–354

5.  Freyschmidt J, Sternberg A (1998) The bullhead sign: scintigraphic pattern of sterno-costoclavicular hyperostosis and pustulotic arthroosteitis. Eur Radiol 8:807–812

6.  Ginalski JM, Landry M, Rappoport G, Chamot AM, Gerster JC (1992) MR imaging of sternocostoclavicular arthro-osteitis with palmoplantar pustulosis. Eur J Radiol 14:221–222

7.  Imanishi Y, Mitogawa Y, Takizawa M, Konno S, Samuta H, Ohsawa A, Kawaguchi A, Fujikawa M, Sakaida H, Shinagawa T, Yamashita H (1999) Relapsing polychondritis diagnosed by Tc-99m MDP bone scintigraphy. Clin Nucl Med 24:511–513

8.  Kakhki VD, Zakavi SR (2006) Age-related normal variants of sternal uptake on bone scintigraphy. Clin Nucl Med 31:63–67

9.  Kato H, Miyazaki T, Nakajima M, Takita J, Kimura H, Faried A, Sohda M, Fukai Y, Masuda N, Fukuchi M, Manda R, Ojima H, Tsukada K, Kuwano H, Oriuchi N, Endo K (2005) Comparison between whole-body positron emission tomography and bone scintigraphy in evaluating bony metastases of esophageal carcinomas. Anticancer Res 25:4439–4444

10.  Kohlfuerst S, Igerc I, Lind P (2003) FDG PET helpful for diagnosing SAPHO syndrome. Clin Nucl Med 28:838–839

11.  Lentle BC, Russell AS, Percy JS, Jackson FI (1977) Scintigraphic findings in ankylosing spondylitis. J Nucl Med 18:524–528

12.  Mandell GA, Contreras SJ, Conard K, Harcke HT, Maas KW (1998) Bone scintigraphy in the detection of chronic recurrent multifocal osteomyelitis. J Nucl Med 39:1778–1783

13.  Nakamoto Y, Osman M, Wahl RL (2003) Prevalence and patterns of bone metastases detected with positron emission tomography using F-18 FDG. Clin Nucl Med 28:302–307

14.  Oppenheim BE, Cantez S (1977) What causes lower neck uptake in bone scans? Radiology 124:749–752

15.  Pichler R, Weiglein K, Schmekal B, Sfetsos K, Maschek W (2003) Bone scintigraphy using Tc-99m DPD and F18-FDG in a patient with SAPHO syndrome. Scand J Rheumatol 32:58–60

16.  Quirce R, Carril JM, Gutierrez-Mendiguchia C, Serrano J, Rabasa JM, Bernal JM (2002) Assessment of the diagnostic capacity of planar scintigraphy and SPECT with 99mTc-HMPAO-labelled leukocytes in superficial and deep sternal infections after median sternotomy. Nucl Med Commun 23:453–459

17.  Shanley DJ, Vassallo CJ, Buckner AB (1991) Sternoclavicular pyarthrosis demonstrated on bone scan. Correlation with CT and MRI. Clin Nucl Med 16:786–787

18.  Syed GM, Fielding HW, Collier BD (2005) Sternal uptake on bone scintigraphy: age-related variants. Nucl Med Commun 26:253–257

19.  Taccari E, Spadaro A, Riccieri V, Guerrisi R, Guerrisi V, Zoppini A (1992) Sternoclavicular joint disease in psoriatic arthritis. Ann Rheum Dis 51:372–374

CLINICAL PROBLEMS

V

# 10 Congenital and Developmental Abnormalities

ANNE GRETHE JURIK

**Contents**



## 10.1 Introduction

Congenital and developmental variants of the sternocostoclavicular (SCC) region are numerous [13, 21], but abnormalities influencing or impairing life are relatively rare. They mainly consist of deformities and fusion abnormalities.

## 10.2 Pectus Deformities

Pectus deformities are relatively common. They are often only of cosmetic importance in childhood and adolescence. However, the elasticity of costal cartilages decrease with age and pulmonary complications may occur in adults [8].

## 10.2.1
## Pathoanatomy

*Pectus excavatum* is the most common congenital deformity of the sternum, in which the sternum is displaced posteriorly with associated changes in the adjacent costal cartilages. This results in reduction of the prevertebral space. The deformity is usually classified in accordance with the clinical presentation according to Haje et al. [8, 9]. It can include the whole sternum or be localised. The opposite deformity, *pectus carinatum*, with the sternum displaced anteriorly can be superior, inferior and lateral.

The aetiology of pectus deformities is uncertain, but at least the localised form of pectus excavatum and also pectus carinatum deformities seem to be caused by growth disturbances. Lesions of the cartilaginous growth plates between the bony sternal segments in childhood and adolescence can cause deformities (Fig. 10.1) [9]. Abnormalities of rib or cartilage morphogenesis and growth are also likely causes [20]. It is possible that costal bending in childhood may be a precursor of deformity (Fig. 10.2).

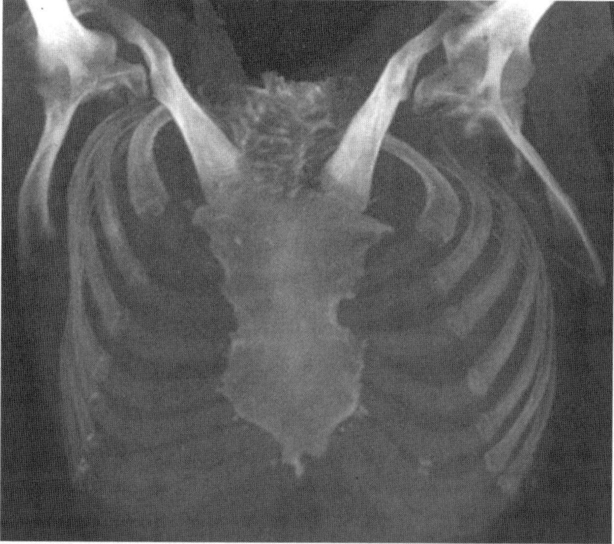

**Fig. 10.1** Pectus carinatum, anterior VIP CT reconstruction of the SCC region in a 47-year-old man. The sternum is short and broad with ankylosis corresponding to the MSJ. There are accompanying alterations of the first costal cartilages, being less voluminous, and the first sternocostal joints are placed more distally than normal. The left second sternocostal joint is broad with subchondral osseous condensation as signs of osteoarthritis

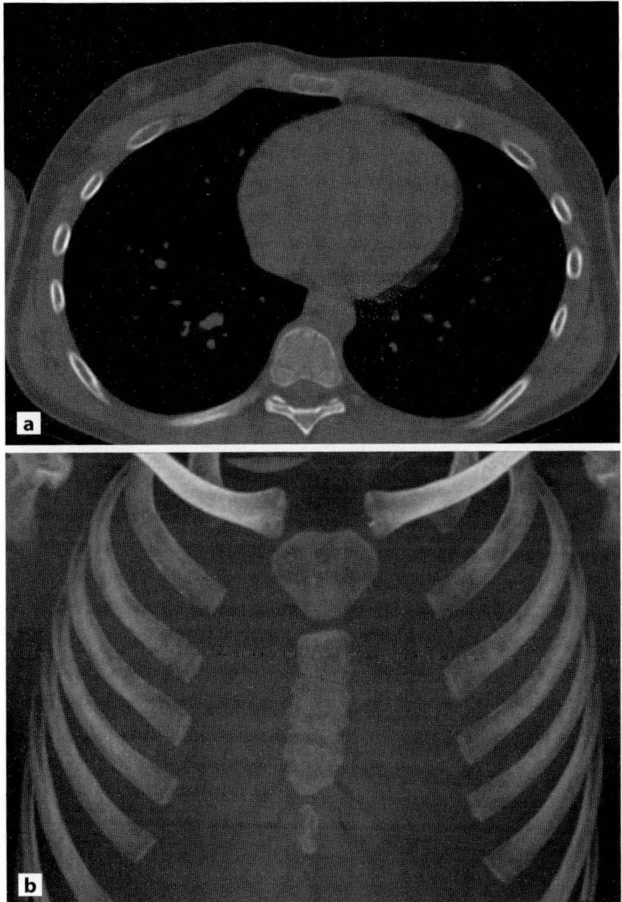

**Fig. 10.2** Costal bending misinterpreted as a tumour in an 11-year-old boy. **a** Axial CT slice showing prominent cartilage on the right side. **b** CT, VIP reconstruction shows asymmetric ossification of the sternal body segments causing slight rotation and cartilage prominence

## 10.2.2
## Imaging

The severity of the deformity can be accurately quantified using CT or MRI, to decide whether or not surgical correction is needed [18]. CT with three-dimensional (3D) reconstruction (Fig. 10.1) can be valuable to define the orientation of the ribs and costal cartilages and their relationship to the sternum. In addition it can provide exact preoperative measurement of the bony rib cage to be used for guiding individualised operative correction. This is especially valuable in children who have been operated on previously [17]. Breath-hold MRI can give valuable information regarding skeletal abnormalities, chest wall motion and accompanying diaphragmatic or cardiac changes [18].

## 10.3
## Sternal Fusion Anomalies

Fusion anomalies of the sternum vary greatly from total cleft formation to slight clefts at the ends or a persistent segmentation.

### 10.3.1
### Pathoanatomy

Failure in the normal midline fusion of cartilage in the early embryo (Chapter 1) can result in *vertical/sagittal cleft sternum*. This is a rare congenital anterior chest wall defect. Depending on the degree of separation, there are complete and incomplete forms either superior or inferior (Fig. 10.3) [12, 16]. The clinical significance is that a cleft may leave the heart and great vessels unprotected [11, 22], which particularly is serious in the very rare occurrence of a complete cleft [16]. Sternal cleft is often associated with other malformations such as craniofacial haemangiomas, omphalocele and cardiovascular malformations [3, 6, 12], and may be part of a PHACES syndrome. PHACES is the acronym for a rare neurocutaneous disorder including the following features: *p*osterior fossa brain malformations, facial *h*aemangiomas, *a*rterial, *c*ardiac, *e*ye, and *s*ternal cleft anomalies and/or *s*upraumbilical abdominal raphe [1, 25]. However, cleft sternum can occur without other abnormalities [11, 16, 23, 24].

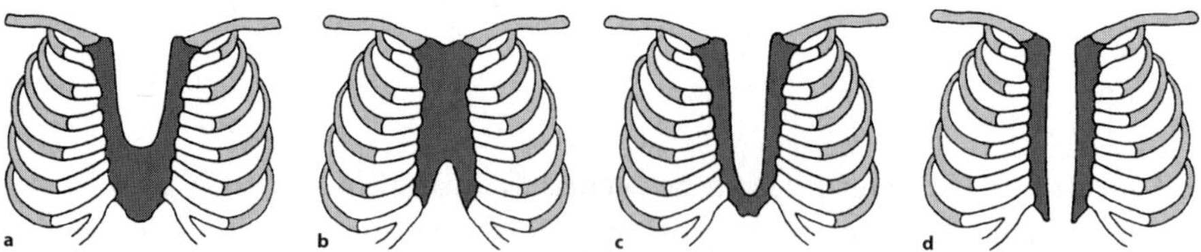

Fig. **10.3** Drawings of the most common forms of sternal cleft. **a** Superior. **b** Inferior. **c** Subtotal. **d** Total

## 10.3.2
## Imaging

Sternal fusion anomalies may be diagnosed by radiography (Fig. 10.4) [16], ultrasonography, CT or MRI [12, 14, 23]. Ultrasonography can be used to diagnose complete cleft sternum [24], but also minor abnormalities such as superior sternal cleft [1, 14]. Prenatal diagnosis of cleft sternum is also possible [6, 24] and can be important for planning of therapy. Surgical correction should be performed during the neonatal period when the direct suturing of the sternal halves often is possible and the thorax can accommodate the thoracic viscera. At an older age, surgical repair is feasible, but it may require additional chondrotomies of the adjacent costal cartilages and notching of the sternal bars, to facilitate the approximation.

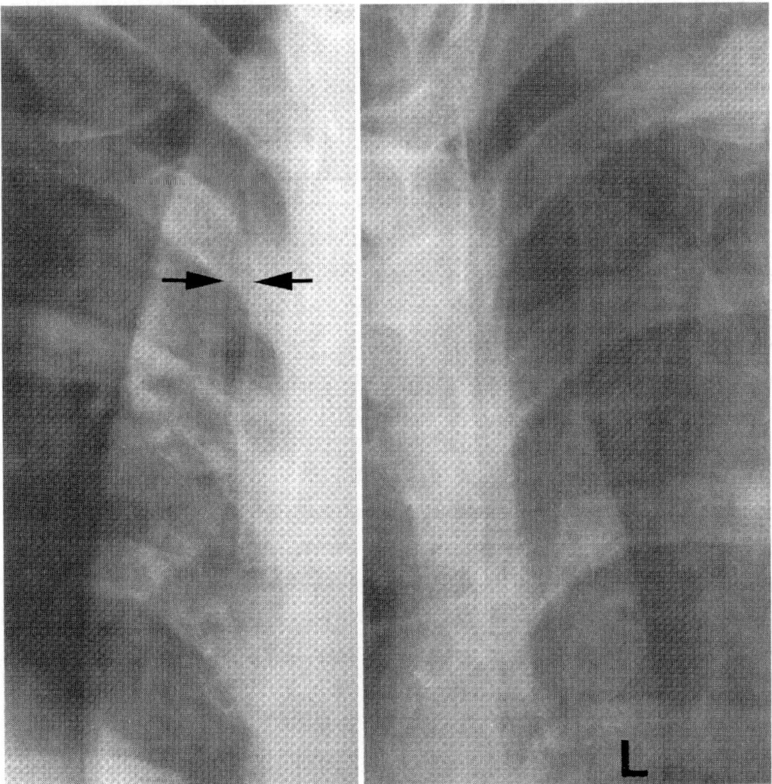


**Fig. 10.4** Complete sternal cleft in a 27-year-old woman without SCC complaints, detected by chest radiography. Oblique views show complete cleft (*arrows*) with the left side of the sternum being less than the right side [16]

Computed tomography and MRI can be important imaging modalities in the case of associated vascular dysplasia or PHACES syndrome including other ventral developmental defects [22].

## 10.4
## Other Sternal Abnormalities

*Partial* or *complete lack of the sternum* is a very rare abnormality which is usually accompanied by partial lack of other SCC structures [3, 22] or occurs together with other malformations such as cardiac abnormalities, but it can be the only abnormality [2, 10].

Sternal abnormalities can occur as part of *skeletal dysplasia* [19]. Developmental anomalies of the manubrium are constantly present in diastrophic dysplasia, a rare skeletal dysplasia with autosomal recessive inheritance. This dysplasia is often diagnosed in infancy or childhood based on typical clinical and radiological findings of short-limbed stature, multiple contractures and early degeneration of joints, hitch-hiker's thumb and spinal and foot deformities. If there is diagnostic uncertainty the finding of an accessory ossification centre (a double-layered manubrium) or an anterior bulging of the manubrium on a lateral radiograph may help to establish the diagnosis [19]. The frequent double-layered manubrium sterni in children with diastrophic dysplasia is probably due to a divergent development in the embryo and have by some been regarded a fusion anomaly [4].

Osseous deformity due to *osteogenesis imperfecta* may also occur. Osteogenesis imperfecta is a heterogeneous group of disorders characterised by defective production of collagen. The major features of osteogenesis imperfecta are osteoporosis and abnormal bone fragility leading to fracture. Bowing of long bones is well known and may in rare cases cause pseudomass formation due to hyperplastic callus formation. A similar pseudomass formation may occur in the sternum [26] and in the pelvic bones [5].

Variations in the appearance of the xiphoid process are numerous, but *xiphoid anomalies* are rare and consist mainly of agenesis as part of an inferior sternal cleft anomaly.

## 10.5
## Clavicular Abnormalities

Clavicular abnormalities are rare, but complete absence of the clavicle or large clavicular defects have been described most frequently as part of *cleidocranial dysos-*

*tosis* [21]. Also developmental changes in hereditary disorders such as *dwarfism* can involve the clavicle (Fig. 10.5). Isolated hypoplasia of the clavicle with formation of *congenital pseudoarthrosis* may occur. It is located in the middle part of the clavicle and is usually right-sided and unilateral [7, 15]. Endochondral ossification has been observed on both sides of the pseudoarthrosis. This supports that it may be due to fusion failure of the primary ossification centres [7] although the location, which is situated between the lateral and middle thirds of the clavicle, does not correspond to the junction of the two centres of ossification in the embryo [15].

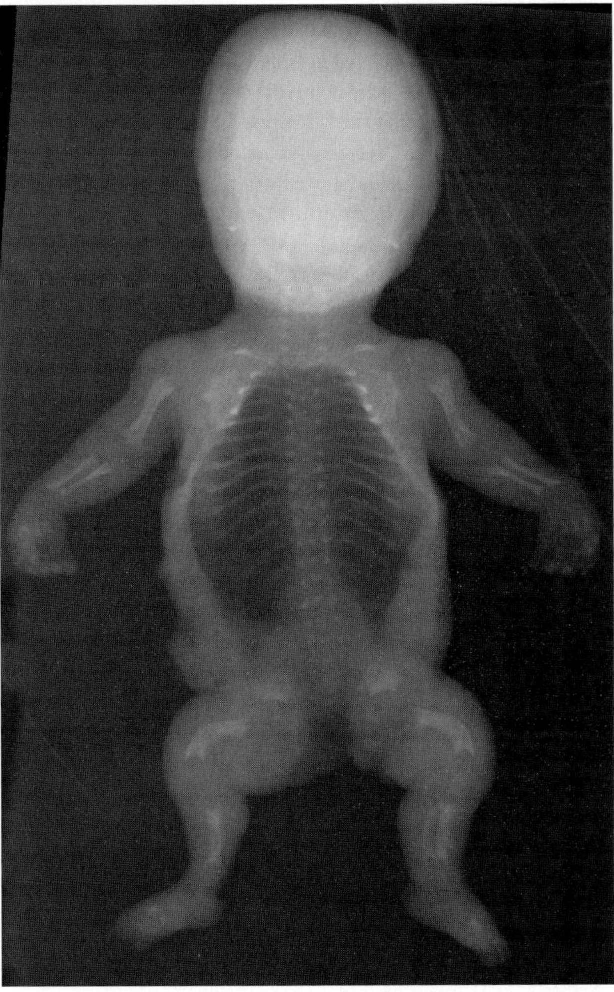

**Fig. 10.5** Seventeen-week-old fetus with deformities compatible with thanatophoric dwarfism. The ossified clavicles are short and bowed with irregular contours, especially laterally corresponding to the abnormalities present in tubular bones

## 10.6
## Conclusions

Congenital and developmental abnormalities influencing life are rare. They mainly consist of pectus deformities, sternal fusion abnormalities and clavicular pseudo-arthrosis. The most life-threatening abnormality is cleft sternum which may leave the heart and great vessels unprotected.

## References


1. Carles D, Pelluard F, Alberti EM, Maugey-Laulom B, Lin TY, Saura R, Roux D, Lacombe D (2005) Fetal presentation of PHACES syndrome. Am J Med Genet A 132:110
2. Chaukar AP, Mandke NV, Mehta SS, Pandey SR, Parulkar GB, Sen PK (1980) Surgical correction of absent sternum with homologous rib graft. J Postgrad Med 26:180B–185B
3. Cottrill CM, Tamaren J, Hall B (1998) Sternal defects associated with congenital pericardial and cardiac defects. Cardiol Young 8:100–104
4. Currarino G (2000) Double-layered manubrium sterni in young children with diastrophic dysplasia. Pediatr Radiol 30:404–409
5. Dobrocky I, Seidl G, Grill F (1999) MRI and CT features of hyperplastic callus in osteogenesis imperfecta tarda. Eur Radiol 9:665–668
6. Fokin AA (2000) Cleft sternum and sternal foramen. Chest Surg Clin N Am 10:261–276
7. Gomez-Brouchet A, Sales DG, Accadbled F, Abid A, Delisle MB, Cahuzac JP (2004) Congenital pseudarthrosis of the clavicle: a histopathological study in five patients. J Pediatr Orthop B 13:399–401
8. Haje SA, Bowen JR (1992) Preliminary results of orthotic treatment of pectus deformities in children and adolescents. J Pediatr Orthop 12:795–800
9. Haje SA, Harcke HT, Bowen JR (1999) Growth disturbance of the sternum and pectus deformities: imaging studies and clinical correlation. Pediatr Radiol 29:334–341
10. Haque KN (1984) Isolated asternia: an independent entity. Clin Genet 25:362–365
11. Herman TE, Siegel MJ (2001) Superior congenital sternal cleft. J Perinatol 21:334–335
12. Heron D, Lyonnet S, Iserin L, Munnich A, Padovani JP (1995) Sternal cleft: case report and review of a series of nine patients. Am J Med Genet 59:154–156
13. Keats T (1996) Atlas of normal roentgen variants that may simulate disease. Mosby, St. Louis
14. Mazzie JP, Lepore J, Price AP, Driscoll W, Bohrer S, Perlmutter S, Katz DS (2003) Superior sternal cleft associated with PHACES syndrome: postnatal sonographic findings. J Ultrasound Med 22:315–319
15. Ogata S, Uhthoff HK (1990) The early development and ossification of the human clavicle: an embryologic study. Acta Orthop Scand 61:330–334
16. Petersen KK, Rasmussen OS, Jurik AG (1989) Complete sternal cleft. Rontgenblatter 42:525–526

17. Pretorius ES, Haller JA, Fishman EK (1998) Spiral CT with 3D reconstruction in children requiring reoperation for failure of chest wall growth after pectus excavatum surgery. Preliminary observations. Clin Imaging 22:108–116
18. Raichura N, Entwisle J, Leverment J, Beardsmore CS (2001) Breath-hold MRI in evaluating patients with pectus excavatum. Br J Radiol 74:701–708
19. Remes VM, Helenius IJ, Marttinen EJ (2001) Manubrium sterni in patients with diastrophic dysplasia: radiological analysis of 50 patients. Pediatr Radiol 31:555–558
20. Sadler TW (2000) Embryology of the sternum. Chest Surg Clin N Am 10:237–244
21. Schmidt H, Freyschmidt J (1993) Kohler/Zimmer. Borderlands of normal and early pathologic findings in skeletal radiography. Thieme Medical, New York
22. Shalak L, Kaddoura I, Obeid M, Hashem H, Haidar R, Bitar FF (2002) Complete cleft sternum and congenital heart disease: review of the literature. Pediatr Int 44:314–316
23. Tastekin A, Kantarci M, Onbas O, Ermis B, Ors R (2003) Superior sternal cleft and minor hemangiomas in a newborn. Genet Couns 14:349–352
24. Twomey EL, Moore AM, Ein S, McAuliffe F, Seaward G, Yoo SJ (2005) Prenatal ultrasonography and neonatal imaging of complete cleft sternum: a case report. Ultrasound Obstet Gynecol 25:599–601
25. Vermeer S, van Oostrom CG, Boetes C, Verrips A, Knoers NV (2005) A unique case of PHACES syndrome confirming the assumption that PHACES syndrome and the sternal malformation-vascular dysplasia association are part of the same spectrum of malformations. Clin Dysmorphol 14:203–206
26. Yekeler E, Kumbasar B, Dursun M, Cantez S, Emiroglu HH, Tunaci M (2003) Pseudomass of the sternal manubrium in osteogenesis imperfecta. Skeletal Radiol 32:371–373

# 11 Traumatic and Post-traumatic Disorders

GIUSEPPE GUGLIELMI, MICHELE TONERINI
AND MARIANO SCAGLIONE

## Contents



## 11.1 Introduction

The sternocostoclavicular region is frequently injured during chest trauma and the injuries are characterised by a blunt trauma more often than a penetrating one. The most common causes are car accidents and falls causing a direct blow to the chest, or a crushing or deceleration injury [63, 82]. Sternocostoclavicular injuries are sometimes associated with mediastinal lesions, whose prompt identification can lead to life-saving therapies.

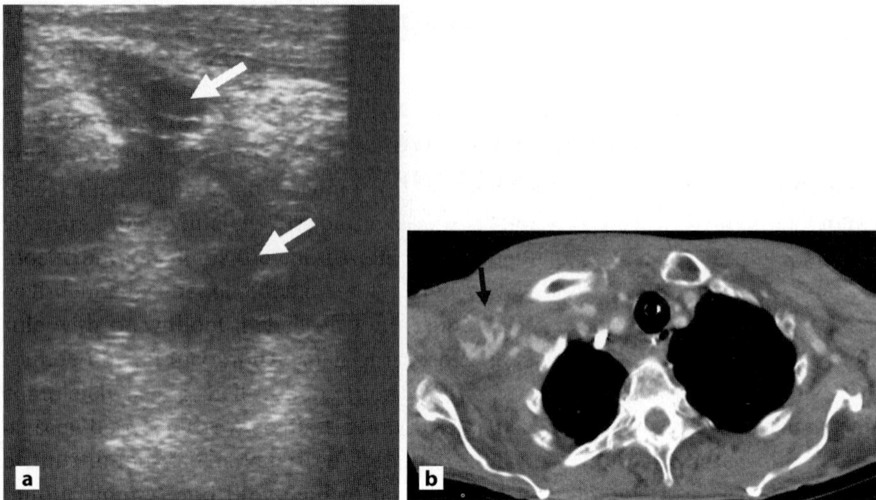

**Fig. 11.1** Complication of the insertion of a CVC in the right subclavian vein. **a** A 7.5-MHz axial sonographic scan shows a large haematoma in the soft tissue of the right subclavian region (*white arrows*). **b** A multirow CT scan clearly demonstrates the active bleeding originating from a penetrating injury tearing of the right subclavian artery (*black arrow*)

## 11.2
## Soft Tissue Injuries

Rarely soft tissue injuries to the anterior chest wall result in significant morbidity. Their entity is essentially dependent on the mechanism of trauma and the degree of protection of the thoracic wall [15]. Blunt trauma to the sternocostoclavicular region usually results in skin abrasions, burns, ecchymoses, lacerations, muscle tears and haematomas while a penetrating injury causes soft tissue tears, venous haemorrhages and pseudoaneurysms [84]. Blunt lesions are often the result of the restraining action of the seat belt which causes ecchymoses and friction burns on different sides in drivers and passengers, respectively. The compressive and shearing action of the seat belt may cause a rupture of the female breast tissue and a lactiferous duct avulsion in lactating women [52, 59]. Penetrating injuries may be the result of gunshots, stabbings or other sharp instruments such as central venous catheters (CVC). The insertion of CVCs in the subclavian or internal jugular veins for intravenous therapies may sometimes produce vascular tearing with hemorrhagic complications (Fig. 11.1) [40]. Soft tissues injuries are usually diagnosed clinically. Rarely large haematomas need to be imaged and drained by ultrasonography and/or computed tomography (CT) which is particularly useful in demonstrating great vessels injuries.

## 11.3
## Anterior Costal Fractures

Anterior costal fractures are very common in chest trauma and they are often multiple. The incidence is higher in elderly patients with less compliant chests compared with children; hence a major intrathoracic injury may occur in children without associated rib fractures [9, 69, 73]. They actually reflect the severity of a chest trauma and the likelihood of damage to certain thoracic or abdominal organs [25, 48, 50, 51]. In particular the involvement of the first three ribs is caused by a significant energy transfer because they are shorter, broader and more protected by the shoulder girdles and musculature. They are associated with clavicular fractures and brachial plexus, tracheal or vascular injuries in 3–15% of cases [23]. However the finding of fractures of the first three ribs in the absence of clinical and radiological evidence of vascular damage is not an indication for angiography [27]. In contrast the anterior portions of the fifth to seventh ribs are barely protected by thoracic muscles and they are thus commonly involved in blunt trauma. The fractured ribs rarely represent a life-threatening condition except for *flail chest* [14, 43, 60, 80], occurring in less than 10% of cases and especially in older patients with osteoporosis. The flail chest is a focal area of chest wall instability caused by one of the following conditions: (a) single fractures of five or more adjacent ribs in a row; (b) fractures of three or more adjacent ribs in two or more places; (c) contiguous combined rib and sternal or costochondral fractures [55]. Flail chest may be unilateral or, exceptionally, bilateral when anterior costochondral and/or sternal fractures cause a complete disruption of the anterior chest wall. The paradoxical motions of the "flail" segment impair respiratory mechanisms, produce atelectasis and induce respiratory failure [55, 60, 84]. The degree of respiratory impairment depends more on the underlying pulmonary injury than on the extent of the flail and the mortality rate can reach 40% [4, 15, 86]. Flail chest may tear the intercostal vessels and cause an *extrapleural haematoma* which develops between the parietal pleural surface and the thoracic cage [62]. Due to their extrapleural nature, such haematomas indent the parietal pleura focally and maintain a convex margin towards the lung. On chest plain films they appear as peripheral, lobulated areas of opacity which do not change with patient position, as will free pleural space fluid collections (Fig. 11.2) [50, 51]. On CT the localisation of a haematoma to the pleural or extrapleural space is usually based on the shape of the collection, but may sometimes be difficult. Its incorrect identification may determine an inappropriate chest tube placement. An extrapleural haematoma produces medial displacement of the fat layer that is just external to the parietal pleura and deep to the endothoracic fascia and inner intercostal muscles. The medial fat layer displacement aids in the localisation of a haematoma to the extrapleural region [2]. The fractured ribs can rarely tear the intercostal muscles producing a *traumatic lung hernia*, which

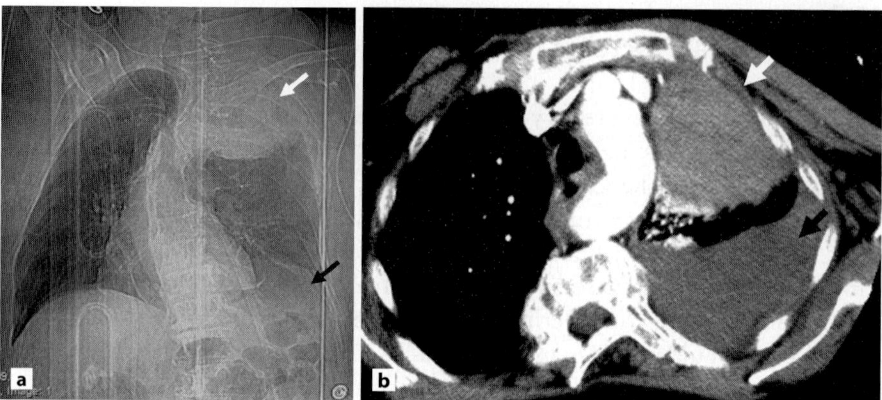

**Fig. 11.2** A 68-year-old male patient who had fallen from an olive tree. **a** Admission supine chest X-ray displays left-sided rib fractures and an apical extrapleural haematoma (*white arrow*) associated with free pleural effusion (*black arrow*). **b** Axial CT scan clearly shows both the extrapleural haematoma, which maintains a convex margin towards the lung (*white arrow*), and the free pleural effusion (*black arrow*)

may occur either anteriorly, near the sternum, or posteriorly, where there is only one single intercostal muscle layer. The diagnosis of traumatic lung hernia is suspected on chest plain films but it is more easily made with CT that clearly demonstrates lung tissue extending through fractured ribs into the chest wall [84]. The initial chest plain film overlooks anterior rib fractures, costochondral and chondrosternal dislocations in about 60% of cases, regardless of their location. Digital radiology is superior to conventional radiology in diagnosing these injuries owing to its capacity of modifying window settings after a single exposure [30, 70, 71]. Ultrasonography can correctly display the rib fractures and the dislocations [26, 85] but it cannot be proposed as a screening test for chest wall injuries in emergency departments. CT identifies the fractured ribs, the costochondral and chondrosternal dislocations and differentiates a haemothorax from an extrapleural haematoma [41, 46, 77].

## 11.4
## Costal Cartilage Injuries

Traumatic injuries of the costal cartilages are represented by fractures and by costochondral and sternochondral dislocations [65]. *Costal cartilage fractures* are rare lesions, which may be located at the chondrocostal or chondrosternal junction (Fig. 11.3). They are mostly observed in young male patients and probably occur

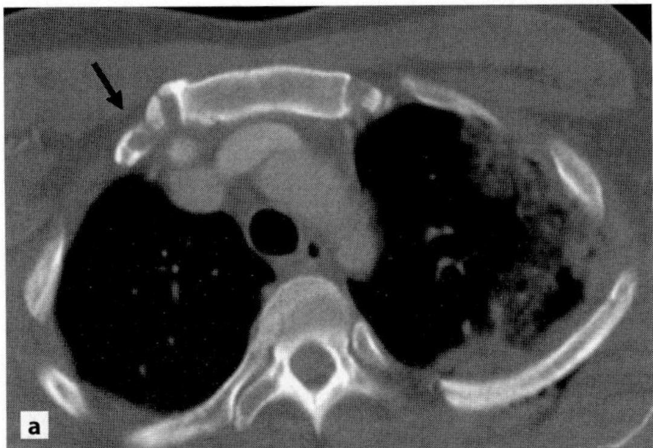

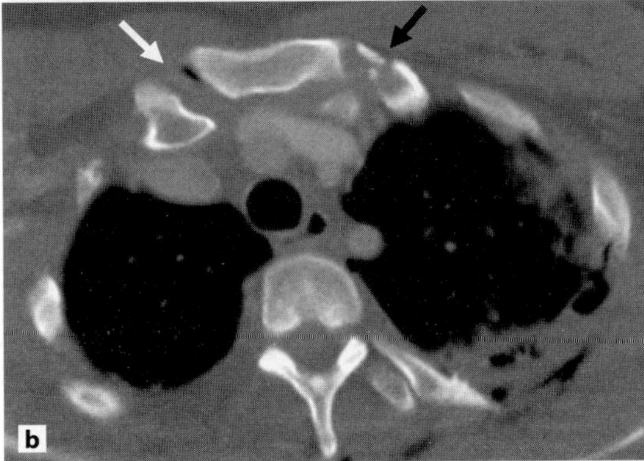

**Fig. 11.3** Seat-belted 35-year-old male car driver involved in a high-speed accident with a significant airbag collision. **a** Axial CT scan demonstrates the fracture of the first right calcified sternochondral junction (*black arrow*). **b** An upper CT scan shows the fracture of the first left calcified sternochondral junction (*black arrow*) and the post-traumatic diastasis of the right sternoclavicular joint with a vacuum phenomenon (*white arrow*)

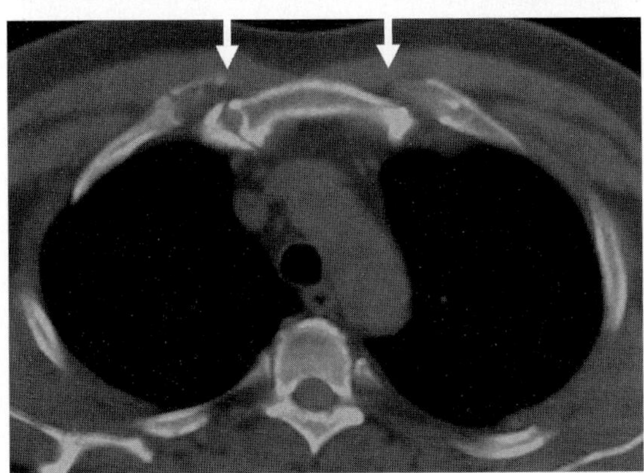

**Fig. 11.4** Unrestrained 53-year-old male driver with a significant airbag collision during a car accident with acute anterior thoracic pain. Axial CT scan clearly shows the anterior dislocation of the bilateral sternochondral articulation (*white arrows*)

more frequently than is recognised because of their difficult diagnosis. *Costochondral* and *sternochondral dislocations* may be encountered especially in children and, when multiple, they produce an anterior flail chest (Fig. 11.4) [64, 74]. These injuries are usually overlooked on radiographs unless they involve a strongly calcified cartilage [56]. However, costal cartilages are easily detected by ultrasonography or CT, which are indicated in cases of severe acute post-traumatic parasternal pain, or painful parasternal mass without an obvious recent trauma. On ultrasound examination the cartilages appear less echogenic than the adjacent muscle and are delineated by a thin echogenic anterior margin (Fig. 11.5). The cartilages are oriented along a horizontal or oblique axis and they present a round, ovoid, or ribbon-like pattern depending on the perpendicular or parallel orientation of the image scan [44]. Ultrasonography has the advantage of an easy multiplanar scanning capability, which is also obtained with multiplanar reformatted images from thin CT slices. There are few reports in the literature describing costal cartilage fractures diagnosed with ultrasonography [6, 13, 26] or CT [39]. Their diagnosis is based on the visualisation of a focal interruption in the relatively high costal cartilage density on CT images, or in the linear echogenic anterior margin of the hypoechogenic cartilages on ultrasonography. A significant displacement of the adjacent segments and a soft tissue swelling on CT images are associated in about 30% of patients. Two additional abnormalities may sometimes be observed: calcifications surrounding the fracture line several weeks after the trauma and accumulation of gas in the fracture cleft, probably the result of a vacuum phenomenon. Chronic symptoms may be caused by the inability of chondrocytes to respond effectively to cartilage fracture, contrary to bone cells that generate a neoformative process generally leading to consolidation of bony rib fractures within several weeks. Differential diagnosis includes other painful lesions of the costal cartilage, such as costochondritis and other seronegative chest wall syndromes (Chapters 12, 13 and 14) [34–36, 38]. In fact arthritis of the anterior chest wall may be found as part of ankylosing spondylitis, reactive arthritis and arthritis associated with psoriasis and/or pustulosis palmoplantaris. The chondral fractures with soft tissue

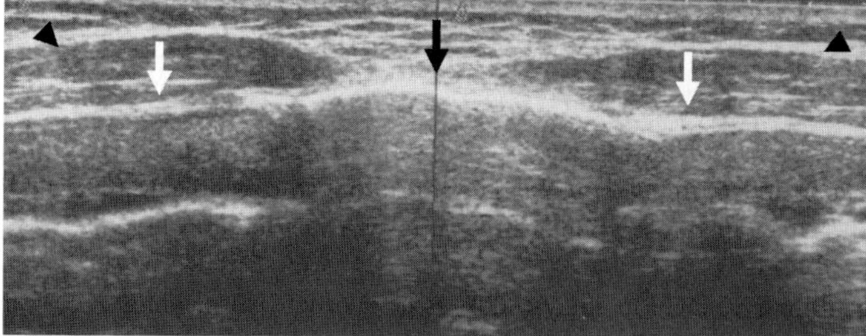

**Fig. 11.5** A normal 7.5-MHz sonographic axial scan of the sternal body (*black arrow*) and of the costal cartilages (*white arrows*) in a young male patient. The costal cartilages appear less echogenic than the adjacent muscle (*black arrowheads*) and are delineated by a thin echogenic anterior margin

swelling can be differentiated from these entities by visualisation of the fracture line (the curved multiplanar reformatted CT images are especially helpful in this evaluation), a step-off deformity and contained gas within the cartilage cleft, present in some cases. When the dominant symptom is a focal mass, tumoral or infectious lesions of the chest wall must be considered [56] and MRI can be relevant in this differential diagnosis (Chapters 16, 17 and 18) [18, 19].

## 11.5
## Sternal Fractures

Sternal fractures are rare injuries in blunt chest trauma (1.5–4% of cases). They often occur in car accidents and are caused by the action of the steering wheel, the airbag and/or the seat belts [3, 11, 17, 51, 55]. The association with seat belts is documented by the increased incidence (of about 100% in drivers and 150% in front seat passengers) since the introduction of seat belt legislation in the UK [66]. Crestanello et al. [17] noted that the fractures of the manubrium, rather than the sternal body, require high force. In rare cases the sternal fractures may result from cardiac resuscitation [8] and may arise indirectly from flexion associated with thoracic spine wedge compression fractures [17, 78, 79]. Sternal fractures are always the hallmark of a severe trauma with associated mediastinal injuries in more than 50% of cases and a mortality of 22% due to cardiac and great vessel lesions [57, 70]. Spontaneous sternal fractures may occur in osteoporotic, elderly people with a thoracic kyphosis [47]. The fracture lines are mostly transverse and their most common location (70% of cases) is in the sternal body, 2 cm from the manubriosternal joint. In 18% they occur at the manubriosternal joint [84] (Fig. 11.6). Fractures may be displaced or undisplaced and in the former the lower fragment in usually shifted posteriorly. The manubrial fractures may be associated with aortic and brachiocephalic vessels injuries, while the depressed sternal body fractures may determine myocardial injuries in 1.5–6% of patients [17, 31]. Thus echocardiography, CT and other cardiac tests are recommended to rule out pericardial effusion or other signs of myocardial injury in case of depressed, displaced sternal fractures [5, 24, 28, 68, 83]. In 40% of cases there are also compression fractures of the upper thoracic spine and more rarely of the cervical and lumbar spine. Clinically there is violent chest pain, tenderness, bruising and a stair-step sometimes palpable at the fracture line. In osteoporotic patients the pain following a spontaneous sternal fracture may mimic a myocardial ischaemia. A retrosternal haematoma, caused by a tearing of the internal mammary vessels or their branches, is frequently seen after a sternal fracture (Fig. 11.7) [60, 67]. It is confined by the parietal pleura and rarely produces a mediastinal widening. Thus an enlargement of the mediastinal silhouette on chest roentgenograms requires a CT scan to be

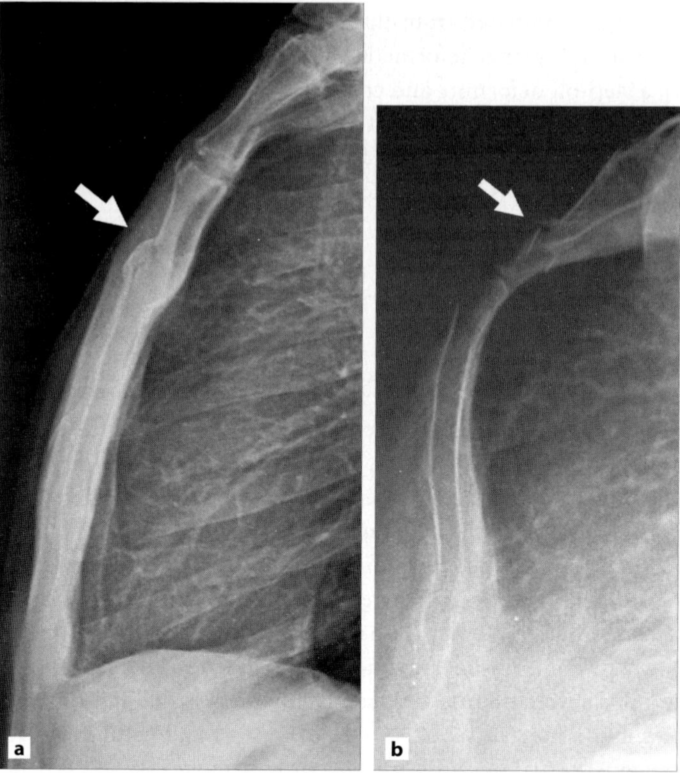

**Fig. 11.6** Lateral chest films displaying fractures (*white arrows*) of sternal body (**a**) and of sternal manubrium (**b**) after car collision

performed to exclude injuries to heart, thoracic aorta or other mediastinal great vessels [65, 75, 81]. When a retrosternal haematoma is seen on CT, the presence of a fat plane between the haematoma and the aorta implies that the haematoma is not aortic in origin (Fig. 11.8) [60]. Sternal fractures are not detected by frontal chest plain films unless associated with significant transverse displacement. Correct diagnosis requires lateral views or other special radiographic projections of the sternum [32, 87]. Early ultrasonography is more accurate than clinical and radiological evaluation in detecting sternal fractures (Fig. 11.9) [21, 61]. However, in multitrauma patients chest plain films and sonography are substituted by a chest CT scan, which identifies almost all sternal fractures, sternal displacements, internal thoracic injuries and retrosternal haematomas [50, 51]. Coronal and sagittal CT reformatted images are useful to visualise horizontal fracture lines, which may be missed on the axial scans (Fig. 11.10) [1, 37, 53].

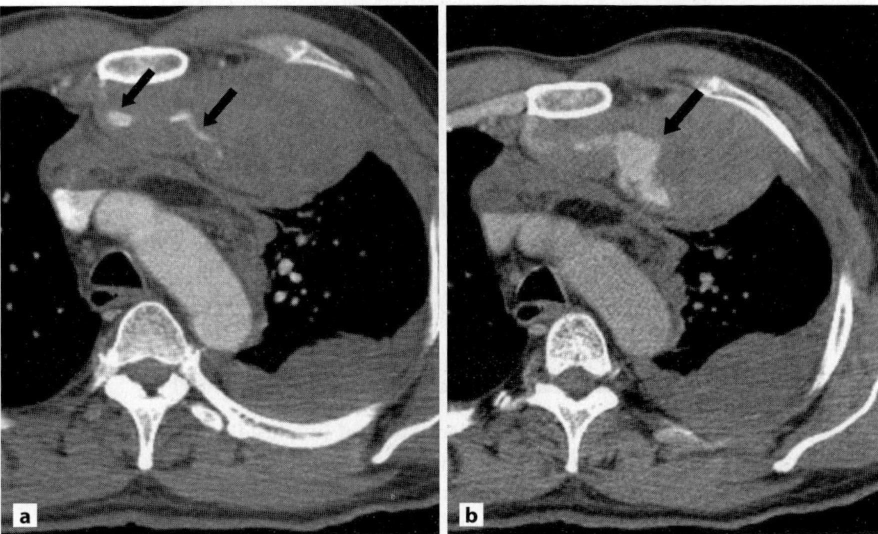

**Fig. 11.7** Seat-belted 63-year-old male patient involved in a frontal car crash. **a** Contrast-enhanced 16-row MSCT performed after 70 s of scan delay shows a "jet" of active extravasation within the haematoma (*arrows*). **b** At the same level, contrast-enhanced 16-row MSCT performed after 180 s shows a "pooling" of active extravasation within the retrosternal haematoma (*arrow*)

## 11.6
## Sternoclavicular Dislocations

Sternoclavicular dislocations are rare injuries consisting of a separation of the medial head of the clavicle from the sternal manubrium with a disruption of the ligaments of the sternoclavicular joint [7, 16, 22, 29]. They mostly occur in young adults, adolescents and children, and are often Salter type 1 or 2 medial clavicular epiphysiolysis, usually missed at the initial clinical examination [20]. A fall on the shoulder, occurring during a bicycle accident or in contact sports, is the typical cause [42]. Anterior dislocations are more frequent and result from an anterior blow to the shoulder that forces the lateral clavicle posteriorly. Posterior dislocations are determined by an anterior or a posterior impact that pushes the medial clavicle posteriorly and they may be associated with aortic, brachiocephalic, tracheal, oesophageal and brachial plexus injuries [10, 76]. Clinically there is pain, tenderness and a palpable or visible abnormality of the injured joint. The diagnosis is difficult on chest frontal plain films which may show the affected medial clavicle

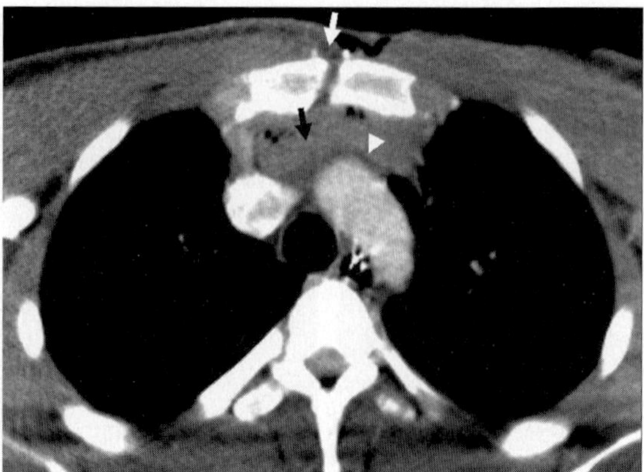

**Fig. 11.8** Seat-belted 45-year-old male patient involved in a head-on car crash. Axial CT shows a sternal body fracture (*white arrow*) with a retrosternal haematoma (*black arrow*). The presence of a fat plane between the haematoma and the thoracic aorta (*white arrowhead*) implies that the haematoma is not aortic in origin

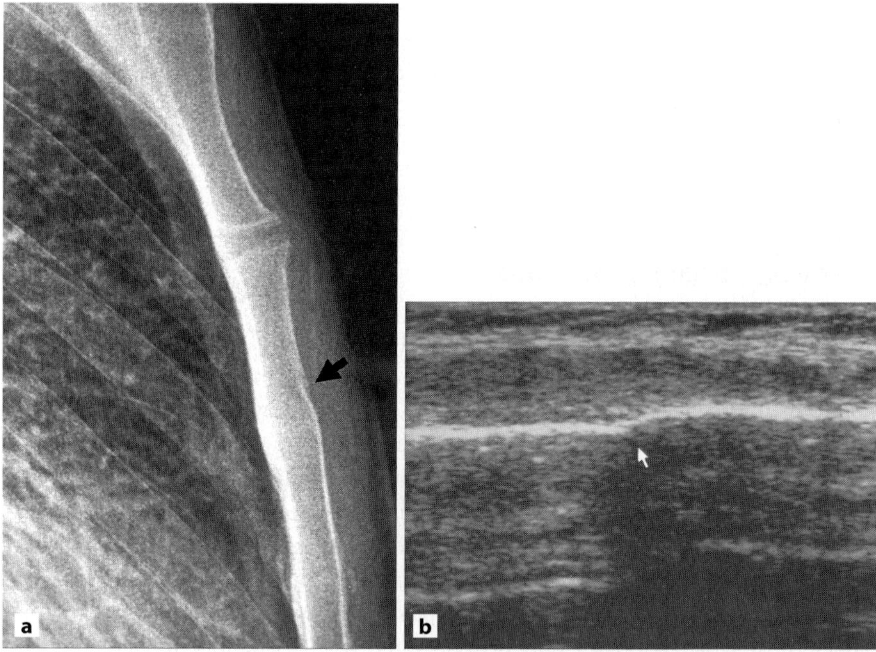

**Fig. 11.9** A 25-year-old male patient involved in a motorcycle accident. **a** Lateral sternal plain film shows an incomplete fracture of the anterior margin of the proximal portion of the sternal body (*black arrow*). **b** A 7.5-MHz, sagittal, sonographic scan clearly displays the traumatic break of the hyperechogenic line of the anterior sternal cortex (*white arrow*)

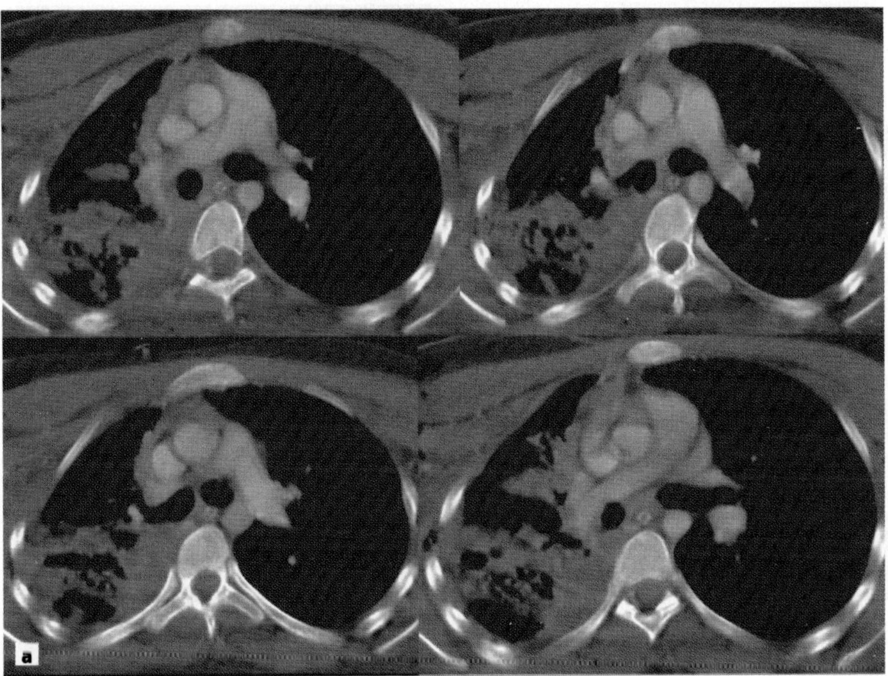

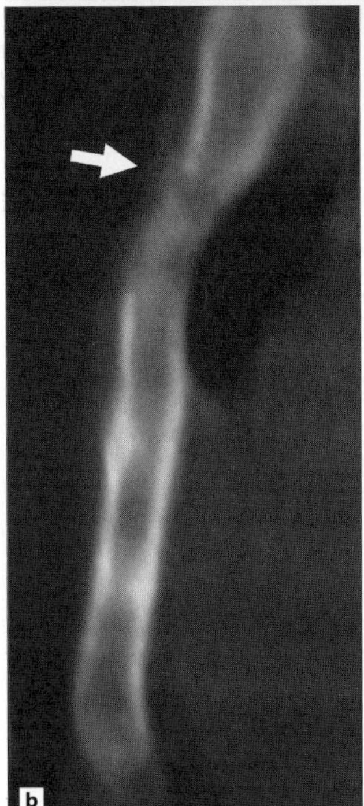

Fig. 11.10 Unrestrained 30-year-old car driver after a high-speed accident producing a steering-wheel impact. a The axial CT scans show a right lung contusion and no signs of sternal fracture: b The sagittal CT reformatted image well demonstrates the undisplaced horizontal fracture of sternal manubrium, missed on the axial scan

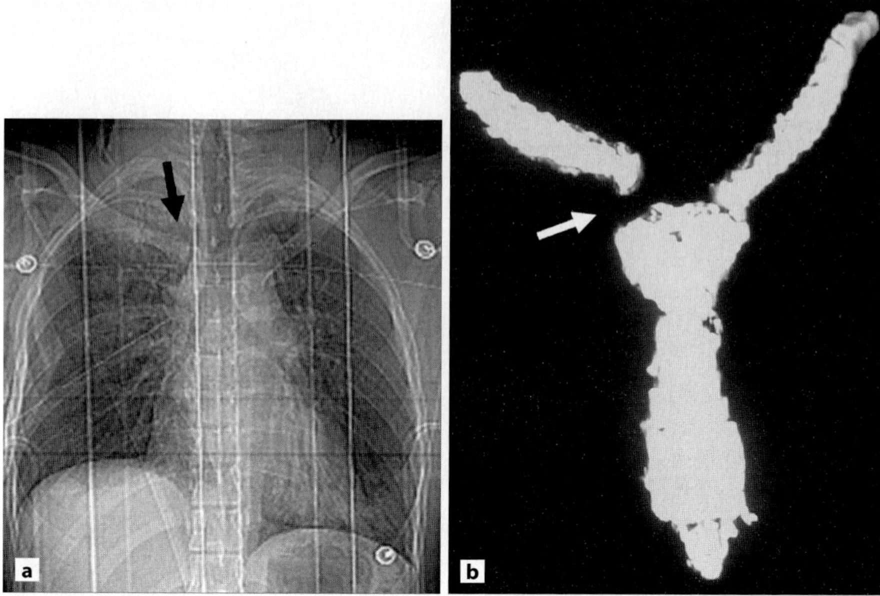

**Fig. 11.11** A 30-year-old male multitrauma patient after a high-speed motorcycle fall. Physical examination revealed an extensive haematoma in the right axilla, caused by a tearing of the right axillary artery. **a** Admission chest X-ray shows an anterior and superior dislocation of the right sternoclavicular joint (*black arrow*) associated with ipsilateral costal fractures. **b** A three-dimensional reconstruction clearly represents the dislocation of the right sternoclavicular joint (*white arrow*)

lying at a different level than the opposite site. Posterior dislocations may cause a retrosternal haematoma with mediastinal widening. Sternoclavicular dislocations are best identified by CT that can also evaluate great vessel, trachea and oesophagus injuries (Fig. 11.11) [20]. After a blunt chest trauma gas may be detected in the sternoclavicular joint ("vacuum" phenomenon) (Fig. 11.3). Patten et al. [58] noticed this finding more frequently in patients undergoing chest CT for blunt chest trauma than in those undergoing chest CT based on other indications. According to their report it does not represent a marker for significant mediastinal or thoracic injury.

## 11.7
## Manubriosternal Dislocations

Manubriosternal dislocations are rare lesions usually resulting from a high-energy trauma [12]. Sometimes they are determined by a minor trauma in patients with a pre-existing manubriosternal disease, as rheumatoid arthritis or seronegative chest wall syndromes [34–36, 54]. Anatomically the manubriosternal joint may have a synovial, synchondral or synosteal structure. The dislocations usually occur with the synovial type of joint, while synchondral and synosteal joints typically fracture through the manubrium rather than dislocate at the joint [72]. There are two types of manubriosternal dislocation: type 1, in which the sternum is dislocated posteriorly with respect to the manubrium, and type 2, more common, in which the manubrium is dislocated posteriorly with respect to the sternum. Type 1 dislocations are determined by a direct blow to the body of the sternum, while type 2 dislocations generally are caused by hyperflexion of the upper thoracic spine that discharges the traumatic energy on the first ribs and on the manubrium [33]. The diagnosis of manubriosternal dislocations is based first of all on the physical examination, as their detection on frontal chest plain film is usually difficult. An abnormal horizontal interface, projecting over the superior mediastinum, has been described as a clue to diagnosis, but there is no specific sign [54]. Lateral chest radiographic projections are necessary to identify the manubriosternal dislocation. CT examination can confirm the diagnosis and reveal any associated mediastinal injury [77], which can include potentially life-threatening injuries to the aorta, great vessels, trachea and oesophagus. It is important to underline that the identification of an internal mammary artery injury without a known manubriosternal dislocation or sternal fracture warrants further evaluation of these structures. Investigations, such as catheter angiography, oesophageal contrast studies or bronchoscopy should be performed if there is any suspicion of injury to the corresponding mediastinal structure [12].

## References


1.  Alkadhi H, Wildermuth S, Marincek B, et al (2004) Accuracy and time efficiency for the detection of thoracic cages fractures: volume rendering compared with transverse computed tomography images. J Comput Assist Tomogr 28:378–385
2.  Aquino SL, Chiles C, Oaks T (1997) Displaced extrapleural fat as revealed by CT scanning: evidence of extrapleural hematoma. AJR 169:687–689
3.  Athanassiadi K, Gerazounis M, Moustardas M, et al (2002) Sternal fractures: retrospective analysis of 100 cases. World J Surg 26:1243–1246

4. Balci AE, Ozalp K, Duran M, et al (2004) Flail chest due to blunt trauma: clinical features and factors affecting prognosis. Ulus Travma Derg 10:102–109

5. Bar I, Friedman T, Rudis E, et al (2003) Isolated sternal fractures: a benign condition? Isr Med Assoc J 5:105–106

6. Battistelli JM, Anselem B (1993) Apport de l'échographie dans les traumatismes des cartilages costaux. J Radiol 74:409–412

7. Benitez CL, Mintz DN, Potter HG (2004) MR imaging of the sternoclavicular joint following trauma. Clin Imaging 28:59–63

8. Black CJ, Busuttil A, Robertson C (2004) Chest wall injuries following cardiopulmonary resuscitation. Resuscitation 63:339–343

9. Bliss D, Silen M (2002) Pediatric thoracic trauma. Crit Care Med 30(11 suppl):409–415

10. Brinker MR, Simon RG (1999) Pseudo-dislocation of the sternoclavicular joint. J Orthop Trauma 13:222–225

11. Byard RW (2002) Shoulder-lap seat belts and thoracic transaction. J Clin Forensic Med 9:92–95

12. Cheng SG, Glickerman DJ, Karmy-Jones R, et al (2003) Traumatic sternomanubrial dislocation with associated bilateral internal mammary artery occlusion. AJR 180:810

13. Choi YW, Im JG, Song CS, et al (1995) Sonography of the costal cartilage: normal anatomy and preliminary clinical application. J Clin Ultrasound 23:243–250

14. Ciraulo DL, Elliott D, Mitchell KA, et al (1994) Flail chest as a marker for significant injuries. J Am Coll Surg 178:466–470

15. Collins J (2000) Chest wall trauma. J Thorac Imaging 15:112–119

16. Cope R, Riddervold HO, Shore JL, et al (1991) Dislocations of the sternoclavicular joint: anatomic basis, etiologies and radiologic diagnosis. J Orthop Trauma 5:379–384

17. Crestanello JA, Samuels LE, Kaufman MS, et al (1999) Sternal fracture with mediastinal hematoma: delayed cardiopulmonary sequelae. J Trauma 47:161–164

18. Demondion X, Boutry N, Drizenko A, et al (2000) Thoracic outlet anatomic correlation with MR imaging. AJR 175:417–422

19. Demondion X, Bacqueville E, Paul C (2003) Thoracic outlet: assessment with MR imaging in asymptomatic and symptomatic populations. Radiology 227:461–468

20. Eich GF, Kellenberger CJ, Willi UV (2002) Radiology of the chest wall. In: Baert Al, Sartor K (eds) Pediatric Chest Imaging. Springer, Berlin Heidelberg New York, pp 265–284

21. Engin G, Yekeler E, Guloglu R, et al (2000) US versus conventional radiography in the diagnosis of sternal fractures. Acta Radiol 41:296–299

22. Ernberg LA, Potter HG (2003) Radiographic evaluation of the acromioclavicular and sternoclavicular joints. Clin Sports Med 22:255–275

23. Fermanis GC, Deane SA, Fitzgerald PM (1985) The significance of first and second rib fractures. Aust N Z J Surg 55:383–386

24. Gouldman JW, Miller RS (1997) Sternal fracture: a benign entity? Am Surg 63:17–19

25. Greene R (1987) Lung alterations in thoracic trauma. J Thorac Imaging 2:1–11

26. Griffith JF, Rainer TH, Ching ASC, et al (1999) Sonography compared with radiography in revealing acute rib fracture. AJR 173:1603–1609

27. Guttenttag AR, Salwen JK (1999) Keep the eyes on the ribs: the spectrum of normal variants and disease that involves the ribs. Radiographics 19:1125–1142

28. Harley DP, Mena I (1986) Cardiac and vascular sequelae of sternal fractures. J Trauma 26:553–555

29. Harris JH Jr (2000) Chest. In: Harris JH Jr, Harris WH (eds) The Radiology of Emergency Medicine, 4th edn. Lippincott Williams & Wilkins, Philadelphia, pp 437–581

30. Hehir MD, Hollands MJ, Deane SA (1990) The accuracy of the first chest X-ray in the trauma patient. Aust N Z J Surg 60:529–532

31. Ho AM, Griffith JF, Joynt GM, et al (2004) Cardiac tamponade and sternal fracture. J Trauma 56:212–213

32. Huggett JM, Roszler MH (1998) CT findings of sternal fracture. Injury 29:623–626

33. Jones HK, McBride GG, Mumby RC (1989) Sternal fractures associated with spinal injury. J Trauma 29:360–364

34. Jurik AG (1991) Seronegative arthritides of the anterior chest wall: a follow-up study. Skeletal Radiol 20:517–525

35. Jurik AG (1992) Anterior chest wall involvement in seronegative arthritides. A study of the frequency of changes at radiography. Rheumatol Int 12:7–11

36. Jurik AG (1992) Seronegative anterior chest wall syndromes. A study of the findings and course at radiography. Acta Radiol Suppl 381:1–42

37. Jurik AG, Albrechtsen J (1994) Spiral CT with three-dimensional and multiplanar reconstruction in the diagnosis of anterior chest wall joint and bone disorders. Acta Radiol 35:468–472

38. Jurik AG, Justesen T, Graudal H (1987) Radiographic findings in patients with clinical Tietze syndrome. Skeletal Radiol 16:517–523

39. Kemp SPT, Targett SGR (1999) Injury to the first rib synchondrosis in a rugby footballer. Br J Sports Med 33:131–132

40. Knutstad K, Hager B, Hauser M (2003) Radiologic diagnosis and management of complications related to central venous access. Acta Radiol 44:508–516

41. Kuhlman JE, Pozniak MA, Collins J, et al (1998) Radiographic and CT findings of blunt chest trauma: aortic injuries and looking beyond them. Radiographics 18:1085–1106; discussion: 1107–1108

42. Lewonosky K, Basset GS (1992) Complete posterior sternoclavicular epiphyseal separation. A case report and review of the literature. Clin Orthop 281:84–88

43. Liman ST, Kuzucu A, Tastepe AI (2003) Chest injury due to blunt trauma. Eur J Cardiothorac Surg 23:374–378

44. Malghem J, Bruno C, Vande Berg FE, et al (2001) Costal cartilage fractures as revealed on CT and sonography. AJR 176:429–432

45. Martino F, D'Amore M, Angelelli G, et al (1991) Echographic study of Tietze's syndrome. Clin Rheumatol 10:2–4

46. Marts B, Durham R, Shapiro M, et al (1994) Computed tomography in the diagnosis of blunt thoracic injury. Am J Surg 168:688–692

47. Mayba II (1986) Sternal injuries. Orthop Rev 15:364–372

48. Mayberry JC, Trunkey DD (1997) The fractured rib in chest wall trauma. Chest Surg Clin N Am 2:239–261

49. Milgram JW (1990) Fracture healing. In: Milgram JW (ed) Radiologic and Histologic Pathology of Nontumorous Diseases of Bones and Joints. Northbrook Publishing, Northbrook, IL, pp 215–254

50. Mirvis SE (2003) Diagnostic imaging of thoracic trauma. In: Mirvis SE, Shanmuganathan K (eds) Imaging in Trauma and Critical Care, 2nd edn. Saunders, Philadelphia, pp 297–368

51. Mirvis SE (2004) Diagnostic imaging of acute thoracic injury. Semin Ultrasound CT MR 25:156–179

52. Murday AJ (1982) Seat belt injury of the breast: a case report. Injury 14:276–277

53. Nakae H, Tajimi K, Kodama H (2003) Diagnosis of a fractured manubrium aided by three-dimensional computed tomographic scanning. J Trauma 55:139–140

54. Nicholson AA, Holt ME, Jessop JD (1988) Dislocation of the manubriosternal joint: detection on frontal chest radiographs. Br J Radiol 61:643–645

55. Novelline RA (2004) Thoracic injury. In: Rhea JT, Ptak T, Sandri-Tafazoli F, Small AB (eds) ER Trauma Top 100 Diagnoses. Saunders, Philadelphia, pp 107–148

56. Ontell FK, Moore EH, Shepard JO, et al (1997) The costal cartilages in health and disease. Radiographics 17:571–577

57. Pate JW (1989) Chest wall injuries. Surg Clin North Am 69:59–70

58. Patten RM, Dobbins J, Gunberg SR (1999) Gas in the sternoclavicular joints of patients with blunt chest trauma: significance and frequency of CT findings. AJR 172:1633–1635

59. Pennes DR, Philips WA (1987) Auto seat restraint soft-tissue injury (letter). AJR 148

60. Primack SL, Collins J (2002) Blunt nonaortic chest trauma: radiographic and CT findings. Emerg Radiol 9:5–12

61. Rainer TH, Griffith JF, Lam E, et al (2004) Comparison of thoracic ultrasound, clinical acumen and radiography in patients with minor chest injury. 56:1211–1213

62. Rashid MA, Wikstrom T, Ortenwall P (2000) Nomenclature, classification, and significance of traumatic extrapleural hematoma. J Trauma 49:286–290

63. Reuter M (1996) Trauma of the chest. Eur Radiol 6:707–716

64. Rice D, Bikkasani N, Espada R, et al (2002) Seat belt-related chondrosternal disruption with lung herniation. Ann Thorac Surg 73:1950–1951

65. Rogers LF (1982) The thoracic cage. In: Rogers LF (ed) Radiology of Skeletal Trauma. Churchill Livingstone, New York, pp 339–375

66. Rutherford WH, Greenfield T, Hayes HRM, et al (1985) The medical effects of seat belt legislation in the United Kingdom. DHSS (Office of the Chief Scientist). HMSO Research Report number 13

67. Saab M, Kurdy NM, Birkinshaw R (1997) Widening of the mediastinum following a sternal fracture. Int J Clin Pract 51:256–257

68. Sadaba JR, Oswal D, Munsch CH (2000) Management of isolated sternal fractures: determining the risk of blunt cardiac injury. Ann R Coll Surg Engl 82:161–166

69. Sartorelli KH, Vane DW (2004) The diagnosis and management of children with blunt trauma of the chest. Semin Pediatr Surg 13:98–105

70. Schnyder P, Lacombe P (1991) Imaging of the chest: an update. In: Trauma of the Chest Syllabus, European Congress of Radiology, Vienna, pp 141–154

71. Schnyder P, Gamsu G, Essinger A, et al (1992) Trauma of the chest, volume 1: thorax and neck. In: Moss AA, Gamsu G, Genant HK (eds) Computed Tomography of the Body with Magnetic Resonance. Saunders, Philadelphia, pp 311–323

72. Schwagten V, Beaucourt L, Van Schil PV (1994) Traumatic manubriosternal joint disruption: case report. J Trauma 36:747–748

73. Shorr RM, Crittenden M, Indeck M, et al (1987) Blunt thoracic trauma: analysis of 515 patients. Ann Surg 206:200–205

74. Smeets AJ, Robben SJ, Meradji M (1990) Sonographically detected costo-chondral dislocation in an abused child. A new sonographic sign to the radiological spectrum of child abuse. Pediatr Radiol 20:566–567

75. Sturm JT, Luxenberg MG, Moundry BM, et al (1989) Does sternal fractures increase the risk for aortic rupture? Ann Thorac Surg 48:697–698

76. Thomas DP, Davies A, Hoddinott HC (1999) Posterior sternoclavicular dislocations: a diagnosis easily missed. Ann R Coll Surg Engl 81:201–204

77. Van Hise ML, Primack SL, Israel RS, et al (1998) CT in blunt chest trauma: indications and limitations. Radiographics 18:1071–1084

78. Vioreanu MH, Quinlan JF, Robertson I, et al (2005) Vertebral fractures and concomitant fractures of the sternum. Int Orthop 5:1–4

79. Von Garrell T, Ince A, Junge A, et al (2004) The sternal fracture: radiographic analysis of 200 fractures with special reference to concomitant injuries. J Trauma 57:837–844

80. Wanek S, Mayberry JC (2004) Blunt thoracic trauma: flail chest, pulmonary contusion and blast injury. Crit Care Clin 20:71–81

81. Westaby S, Brayler N (1990) ABC of major trauma. Thoracic trauma I. BMJ 300:1639–1643

82. Wicky S, Wintermark M, Schnyder P, et al (2000) Imaging of blunt chest trauma. Eur Radiol 10:1524–1538

83. Wiener Y, Achildiev B, Karni T, et al (2001) Echocardiogram in sternal fractures. Am J Emerg Med 19:403–405

84. Wintermark M, Schnyder P (2000) Trauma of the chest wall. In: Baert AL, Sartor K, Youker JE (eds) Radiology of Blunt Trauma of the Chest. Springer, Berlin Heidelberg New York, pp 9–27

85. Wustner A, Gehmacher O, Hammerle S, et al (2005) Ultrasound diagnosis in blunt thoracic trauma. Ultraschall Med 26:285–290

86. Ziegler DW, Agarwal NN (1994) The morbidity and mortality of rib fractures. J Trauma 37:975–979

87. Zinck SE, Primack SL (2000) Radiographic and CT findings in blunt chest trauma. J Thorac Imaging 15:87–96

# 12 Seronegative Arthritis and Sternocostoclavicular Syndromes

ANNE GRETHE JURIK

## Contents



## 12.1 Introduction

Seronegative arthritides or spondylarthropathies (SpA) encompass the disorders ankylosing spondylitis, reactive and enteropathic arthritis and arthritis associated with psoriasis, including pustulosis palmoplantaris [17]. The sternocostoclavicular (SCC) region is often involved in SpA [22], but pain indicating involvement may be referred to areas distant from the SCC region, such as the shoulder and neck [31, 48] or may be overshadowed by spinal or sacroiliac joint symptoms. This potentially leads to delayed or missed diagnosis of SCC involvement in SpA.

The frequency and appearance of sternoclavicular joint (SCJ) involvement may vary depending on the type of SpA, in addition to its duration and severity. Pronounced changes with osseous hyperostosis can usually be detected by conventional radiography (Fig. 12.1) [49] and is therefore seldom missed, but cross-sectional imaging (CT or MRI) or conventional tomography is usually needed for

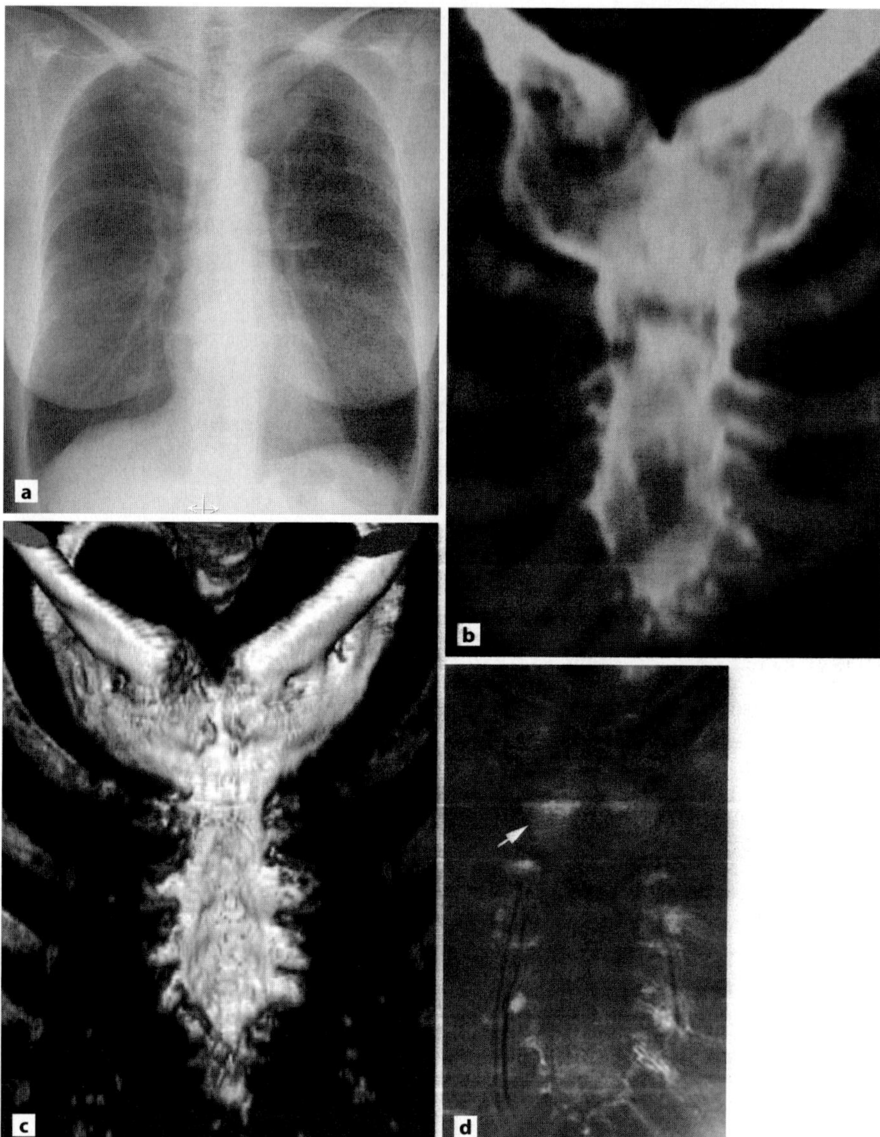

Fig. 12.1 Sternocostoclavicular hyperostosis. **a** PA chest radiograph of a 56-year-old woman with PPP shows osseous hyperostosis and sclerosis around the SCJs extending to the medial part of the clavicles, especially on the left side. **b** Coronal CT reconstruction displayed sclerosis and hyperostosis of the entire sternum and the medial part of the clavicles. **c** Three-dimensional (3D) surface reconstruction shows a hyperostotic ossified plate in the SCC region. **d** MRI, coronal postcontrast T1 FS shows only vascularised activity in the upper part of the manubrium sterni (*arrow*) and at the medial part of the right clavicle in addition to some enhancement in the costal cartilages

detecting subtle changes [10]. Involvement of the manubriosternal joint (MSJ) in SpA is generally frequent [22, 41], and the imaging features usually correspond to those of intervertebral SpA lesions. The sternocostal joints also seem frequently involved when looked for at cross-sectional imaging or conventional tomography [77]. Apart from hyperostotic involvement of the first sternocostal joint often occurring together with arthritis of the SCJ, the imaging features mostly correspond to those of other joints.

The clinical and radiological findings of SCC involvement in SpA may vary depending on the type of SpA, but this aspect has generally gained little attention, although differences related to different forms of SpA have be reported [40, 60]. Instead involvement of the SCC region has been extensively described as separate syndromes, such as SAPHO syndrome, sternocostoclavicular hyperostosis, etc. The SCC changes reported in different syndromes are often accompanied by other signs of SpA and could then have been termed in accordance with the basic disorder.

This chapter encompasses a summary of the findings in the different well-known SpA forms, in addition to an overview of the syndromes including SCC lesions.

## 12.2
## Ankylosing Spondylitis

Ankylosing spondylitis (AS) is a chronic inflammatory disease that primarily involves the sacroiliac and spinal joints and their adjacent ligamentous structures. As a rule changes of the sacroiliac joint progress to ankylosis, and the involvement of vertebrale, apophyseal joints, intervertebral ligaments or entheses may result in spinal ankylosis. The disease occurs predominantly in males and is frequently associated with the tissue type HLA-B27 [39–41].

## 12.2.1
## Features Related to Sternocostoclavicular Involvement

Involvement of SCC joints as part of AS occurs in all adult age groups and seems related to long disease duration [40, 79]. In accordance with this, SCC involvement usually occurs after the appearance of other skeletal lesions [39, 40, 44]. It may, however, be the first manifestation [37] or appear early in the disease [44] sometimes simultaneously with sacroiliitis [40, 79]. The symptoms of SCC involvement may be interpreted as, or overshadowed by pain due to spinal involvement or can present as referred pain to the shoulders [73]. Radiographic changes of the SCJs and especially of the MSJ can therefore occur without recognised SCC symptoms [16, 39, 40, 81].

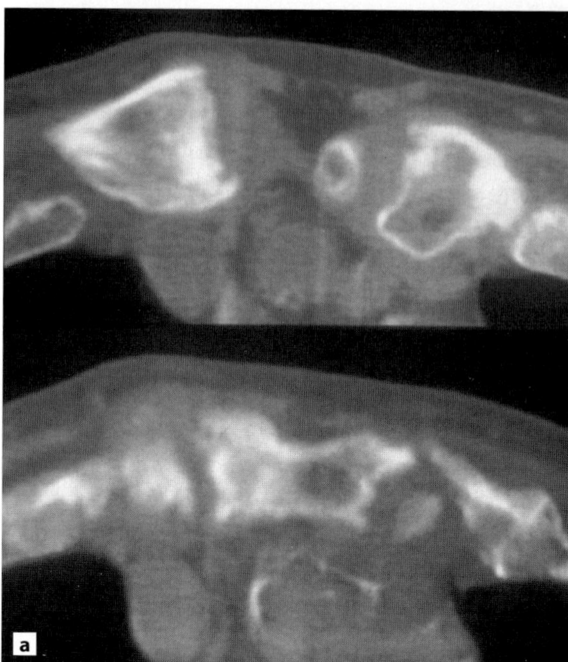

**Fig. 12.2a** Ankylosing spondylitis. CT slices of relatively early changes of the SCJs. There is erosion with subchondral sclerosis and joint space widening, especially on the right side

## 12.2.2
## Imaging Features

Changes in the SCJ at radiography or CT vary with the disease duration and severity. Early changes consist of erosion with slight or moderate subchondral sclerosis and often joint space widening or narrowing (Fig. 12.2a). Later, some degree of ankylosis with slight or moderate surrounding osseous hyperostosis occurs (Fig. 12.2b). There is usually concomitant involvement of the first SCJ and ossification of the adjacent costal cartilage (Fig. 12.2c) [39, 40, 73]. Lesions characterised by pronounced osseous hyperostosis and/or ligamentous ossification have, however, also been reported in AS. Such changes, often termed "sternocostoclavicular hyperostosis" (SCCH) or "intersternocostoclavicular ossification" (ISCCO), have been described in patients with AS of a rather long duration [12, 40, 49, 72, 77, 92]. It is, however, possible that some of the patients reported with AS and SCCH/ISCCO do not have typical AS, but AS-like axial lesions or sacroiliitis as part of other forms of SpA. In accordance with this HLA-B27 seems less frequent than in typical AS patients [41, 77, 92].

The radiographic features of MSJ involvement are usually like those of the sacroiliac joints. In the early stages they consist of osteoporosis followed by erosion

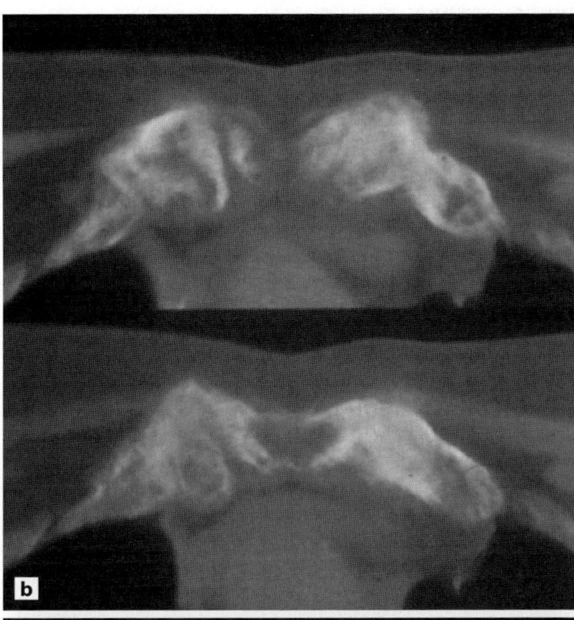

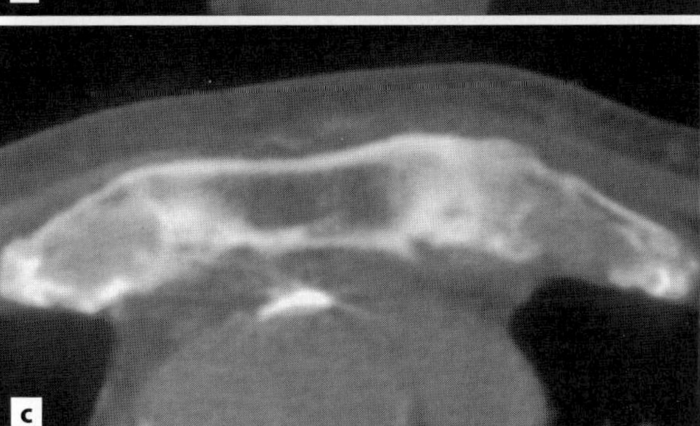

**Fig. 12.2b,c** Ankylosing spondylitis. CT slices of advanced changes with ankylosis of the left SCJ and partial ankylosis on the right side. There is concomitant ankylosis of both first sternocostal joints with pronounced ossification of the costal cartilages

of the joint facets with subchondral sclerosis and later on ankylosis with irregular osseous structure (Fig. 12.3) [39, 40, 79]. Accompanying erosion, irregularity and broadening of the second SCJs may occur, as may similar changes of the third SCJs [39].

Magnetic resonance imaging can be valuable in the detection of both disease activity and structural changes in the SCC region, but has not been systematically analysed in AS. Involvement of the MSJ is, however, often observed in AS patients evaluated at MRI for spinal involvement, if the SCC region is not obscured by MR saturation bands (personal experience) (Fig. 12.3).

Scintigraphy may sometimes be used to visualise the activity of AS especially corresponding to the spine and sacroiliac joints. Activity in the SCC region may

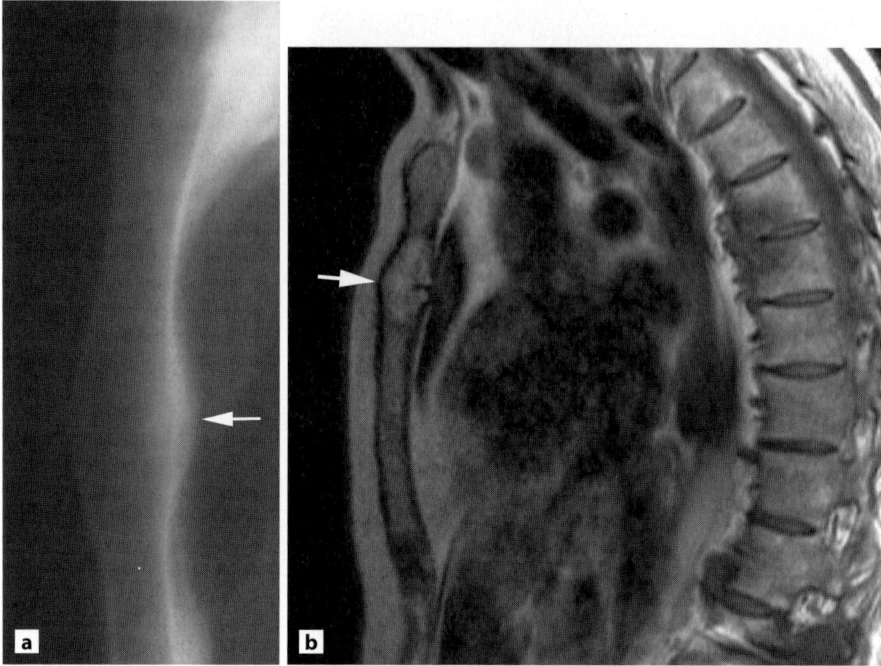

Fig. 12.3 Ankylosing spondylitis. **a** Lateral radiograph of the manubriosternal joint in a 45-year-old man with severe chronic AS. There is osseous ankylosis with a slightly irregular structure across the joint and some degree of hyperostosis (*arrow*) as signs of previous inflammation. **b** T1-weighted sagittal MR image obtained at spinal imaging shows ankylosis, but also surrounding fatty marrow changes (*arrow*) due to sequelae of inflammation

be difficult to detect due to overshadowing spinal activity. It seems, however, to be frequent, reported in 50% of patients [22]. In six AS patients with available views of the sternum, increased uptake was present in five at the MSJ and in five at the SCJs [13]. MRI is, however, preferable with regard to the SCC region as, in addition to signs of activity, it delineates structural abnormalities.

## 12.2.3
## Frequency of Sternocostoclavicular Involvement

Signs of SCC involvement have been found present in 5–25% of patients with AS [1, 29, 40, 75], but may be more common. When specially looked for the MSJ has thus been reported involved by history or physical examination in 5–60% [16, 29, 30, 37, 40, 75, 97] and the SCJs in 1–14% of AS patients [16, 29, 37, 40, 75, 97].

Radiographic changes of SCC joints occur in over half of patients with AS of varying severity and duration, and slightly more frequently in men than in women. The changes are located predominantly to the MSJ [40]. The frequency of radiographic changes at the SCJs has mainly been evaluated based on radiography [16, 40, 75, 89]. In three series abnormalities occurred in 16–28% of the patients [16, 40, 89], but in one group with AS of rather long duration only 2% of the patients had changes [75].

Radiographic changes of the MSJ have been found to occur in 39–85% of AS patients [16, 40, 57, 61, 66, 75, 79, 81, 84]. The wide range of frequencies seems mainly due to differences regarding disease duration and severity [40, 41, 79]. The radiographic method can, however, also play a part, but this has not been verified [41].

## 12.2.4
## Associated Skeletal Lesions and Other Findings

The presence of SCC involvement is related to long disease duration and signs of severe disease such as advanced sacroiliitis, spinal changes and involvement of root joints [40, 79]. The presence of inflammatory spondylodiscitis with erosion of nearly the whole vertebral plate seems to increase the likelihood for SCC involvement [40].

## 12.2.5
## Conclusion

Patients with AS often have radiographic changes of SCC joints. They are located predominantly to the MSJ, but involvement of the SCJs also occurs. Changes of the MSJ are usually like those of the sacroiliac joints. Early involvement of the SCJs is characterised by erosion, but later some degree of ankylosis usually occurs accompanied by involvement of the first SCJ and ossification of the adjacent costal cartilage. The presence of SCC involvement is related to long disease duration and radiographic signs of severe disease in the form of advanced sacroiliitis, spinal changes and involvement of root joints.

## 12.3
## Osteoarthropathy Associated with Pustulosis Palmoplantaris

Pustulosis palmoplantaris (PPP) is a rare chronic skin disease, mainly occurring in middle-aged women. It is characterised by recurrent eruptions of sterile pustules with erythema and exfoliation situated on the palms and/or soles. The relationship of PPP to psoriasis is controversial. It is not certain whether PPP can be regarded as a variant of pustular psoriasis or not. PPP, however, differs from psoriasis vulgaris by a frequent occurrence of accompanying skeletal lesions often located to the SCC region [63, 87]. In an analysis of 23 age- and gender-matched patients with skeletal disorder associated with PPP and psoriasis, 83% of the patients with PPP had signs of SCC involvement compared to 44% of the patients with psoriasis [63].

### 12.3.1
### Features Related to Sternocostoclavicular Involvement

Sternocostoclavicular involvement associated with PPP may occur in all age groups, but usually starts between the ages of 30 and 50 years [11, 41, 87]. It is seen predominantly in women and can appear before, simultaneously with, or after the skin disease and other skeletal abnormalities [41, 51, 87]. Symptoms of SCC involvement have been reported present in 83% of patients, located to the SCJ in 61%, to the MSJ in 22% and to the sternocostal joint in 30% of these patients [63]. The presence of radiographic SCC changes seems always to be accompanied by symptoms [41, 47].

The course of SCC involvement is prolonged over several years and fluctuates with recurrent pain and swelling usually accompanied by exacerbation of the skin disorder [11, 41, 45, 51, 87]. The exacerbations are often more acute in children/ adolescents than in adults, and the location of changes differs depending on age [41]. Children/adolescents usually appear with pain, tenderness and swelling located to the clavicle, often with accompanying slight inflammation of the overlaying dermal structures and sometimes slight malaise and fever. Children/adolescents are mostly healthy during remissions [45]. Adults have swelling of SCC joints and their adjacent bones, cartilages or ligamentous structures usually without dermal inflammation, malaise and fever [38–40, 43, 46, 56, 87]. Their disease often starts with swelling in the region of one joint and spreads to other joint regions during the course of several years [39, 43, 46]. Associated shoulder pain is frequent and there is usually persistence of some SCC discomfort between exacerbations [38–40, 43, 46, 87]. Otherwise the well-being of the patients is good, except for pain. Complicating subclavian vein obstruction or thrombosis can occur, but is rare [50, 58].

## 12.3.2
## Imaging Features

The most characteristic SCC lesions encountered at radiography or CT are those characterised primarily by osseous sclerosis. In adults they usually present as sclerosis and hyperostosis of the manubrium sterni. Sclerotic and hyperostotic clavicular lesions occur especially in children/adolescents, but have been observed in adults. Such osseous lesions may also occur in patients without PPP and are therefore described separately in Chapter 13.

Adults with PPP can also present with primary joint and/or ligamentous involvement. Based on analyses in our department, changes in the region of SCC joints seem more frequent than osseous lesions in adults, whereas the lesions of children/adolescents are nearly always osseous [41].

The primary joint changes of adults can be located to the SCJs, the MSJ and/or the upper sternocostal joints [38–40, 56, 63, 94]. In the early stages involvement of the SCJ is usually unilateral and radiographically characterised by erosion with pronounced subchondral sclerosis and ossification of the adjacent cartilage, sometimes also in the region of the costoclavicular ligament (Fig. 12.4a,b) [39, 40, 63, 67, 82]. Bilateral involvement mostly occurs with time [39]. The changes usually progress and can then present as joint erosion or ankylosis with subchondral sclerosis and surrounding new bone formation causing hyperostosis. Involvement of the medial part of the clavicle, the sternum and the anterior aspect of the upper ribs accompanied by soft tissue calcification, including the costoclavicular ligament, may result in a hyperostotic SCC plate [28, 39, 40, 58, 62]. Such changes can usually be detected by conventional radiography (Fig. 12.1), but tomography or cross-sectional imaging (CT or MRI) is needed for further characterisation. Such advanced changes seem to be rather characteristic for PPP-associated SCC arthritis in Caucasians [12, 39, 40, 77, 92, 94]. In Japanese patients pronounced ligamentous ossification without accompanying joint changes have been reported [10, 11, 85, 87].

Changes of the MSJ in the early stages are characterised by erosion, usually with pronounced subchondral sclerosis and associated irregularity of the second sternocostal joint [50]. Later ankylosis may supervene [38–40, 43].

Involvement of sternocostal joints mainly occur at the first sternocostal joints (Fig. 12.4c,d). In this region involvement can appear as the only abnormality or together with changes of the SCJ [10, 38–40, 44, 94]. Isolated abnormalities at the first sternocostal joint can appear as erosion or ankylosis with subchondral sclerosis and ossification of the adjacent costal cartilage or as predominantly osseous sclerosis adjacent to an irregular sternocostal joint facet [38, 44]. Changes of the

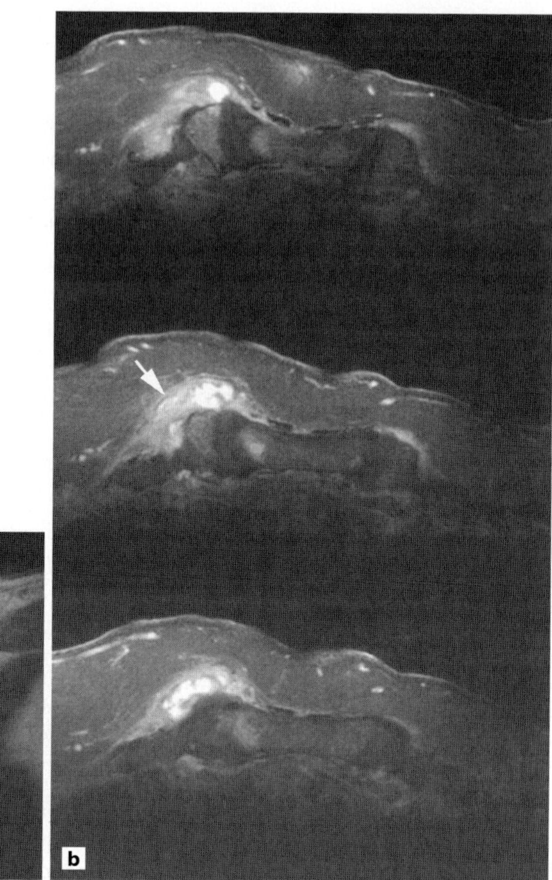

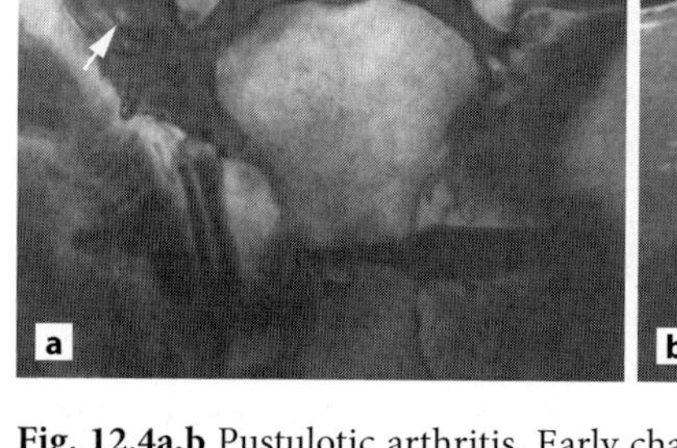

**Fig. 12.4a,b** Pustulotic arthritis. Early changes located to the SCJ in a 53-year-old woman with PPP during 4 years and swelling in the region of the right SCJ. MRI, coronal T1-weighted (**a**) and axial postcontrast T1 FS (**b**) show swelling of the right SCJ with slight subchondral enhancement. There is a mass corresponding to the costoclavicular ligament with pronounced enhancement (*arrows*)

second sternocostal joint also occur, but often accompanied by involvement of the MSJ. There may be changes of lower sternocostal joints, but less frequently [39]. This suggests a relationship between the presence of PPP lesions and changes in the region of the first sternocostal joint.

At MRI the appearance depends on the activity, duration and severity of the disease. In the active stage there are signs of oedema and enhancement corresponding to areas of activity. On T1-weighted images the lesions often have irregular

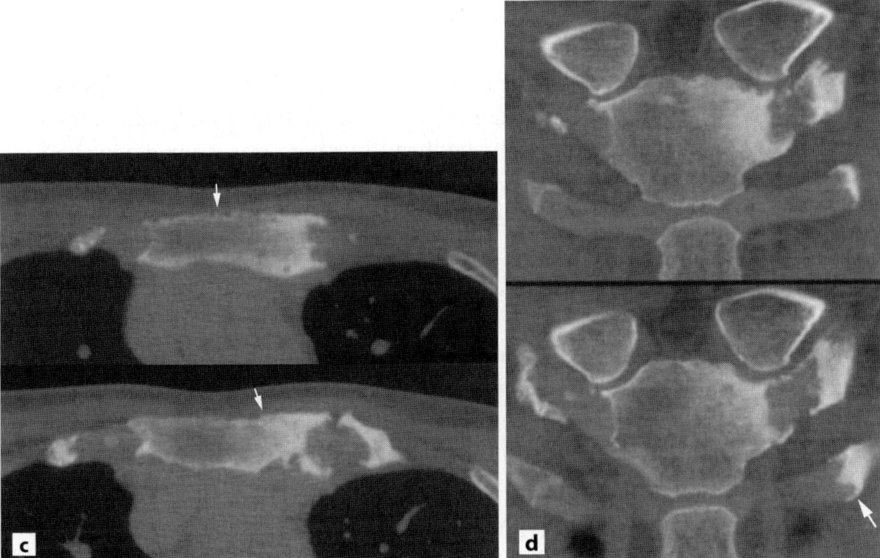

**Fig. 12.4c,d** Pustulotic arthritis. Early changes located to the first sternocostal joint in a 57-year-old woman with PPP and increasing swelling at the left first sternocostal joint. **c** Axial CT slices at the first sternocostal joint show erosion of the joint facet with pronounced subchondral sclerosis and calcification at the peripheral part of the costal cartilage. Osseous proliferation on the surface of the bone is clearly delineated (*arrow*). **d** Coronal CT reconstructions display the erosion and subchondral sclerosis and also an osseous lesion at the second costochondral junction (*arrow*)

borders and display low and slightly inhomogeneous signal intensity depending on the content of fatty marrow changes caused by previous inflammation. On T2-weighted images the signals may remain relatively low, but there is contrast enhancement corresponding to active areas [26, 56]. Erosions are not always demonstrated as well as by tomography or CT [26].

Scintigraphy has been widely used in the evaluation of patients with skeletal disorders associated with PPP, often termed pustulotic arthro-osteitis (PAO). During exacerbations there is usually increased activity in the SCC region and the presence of other lesions may be detected [23, 35, 53, 58, 63, 68, 76, 94]. Increased uptake in the SCC region has been reported to occur in 52% of patients with PPP being located to the SCJ in 48% and to the MSJ in 4% of the patients [63]. A characteristic "bullhead-like" tracer uptake in the SCC region has been described [23]. In this appearance the manubrium sterni represents the upper skull and the inflamed SCJs the horns of the bullhead (Fig. 9.2). The bullhead sign has been regarded not only as the typical and highly specific scintigraphic appearance of advanced PAO, but also of SCCH [23, 26]. Whole-body scintigraphy may in addition show a possible existence of other skeletal lesions. In an analysis of 49 patients with SCCH and/or PAO examined with scintigraphy and radiography, 43 of 49 patients showed a characteristic bullhead-like high tracer uptake in the SCC region. Additional skeletal manifestations (spondylitis, sacroiliitis, osteitis) were revealed in 33 of the patients, sometimes in unexpected locations. The finding of a bullhead sign at scintigraphy can be important in patients without skin disease at the time of presentation to avoid unnecessary biopsies. PPP may develop later and, therefore, it can be justified to classify the disorders as incomplete PAO with high risk to develop other skeletal manifestations later in the course of the disease [23]. The bullhead sign is, however, not specific for PAO as it occur in patients with SCCH. Besides, there can be other appearances, such as predominant uptake corresponding to the clavicle [68], and the bullhead sign may not be present in early or inactive stages of the disorders.

Bone scintigraphy has been reported used to monitor the course and to assess therapeutic efficiency (e.g. of biphosphonate) in patients with SCC lesions [14, 68]. The method can be an easy way to monitor the disease if the changes are part of a multifocal disease. When limited to the SCC region it is more appropriate to monitor by MRI, as a STIR sequence will give the same information about activity as scintigraphy and will provide further pathoanatomical details. In addition, MRI is without any inherent radiation risk.

The use of FDG PET to visualise metabolically active tissue has been reported in only two cases [53, 68] and its value has to be evaluated further.

### 12.3.3
### Frequency of Sternocostoclavicular Involvement

Radiographic SCC changes occur in about 20% of adult Danes with PPP of varying severity [38]. Half of the patients have predominantly osseous sclerotic lesions and half have joint changes located to the SCJs, the two upper sternocostal joints and/ or the MSJ [38]. The frequency of radiographic SCC changes is apparently lower in Japanese with PPP, reported to be present in about 10% [86]. Ethnic diversities and a different composition of patients regarding age and sex can possibly explain some of the differences. It is possible that SCC involvement is more frequent in Scandinavians than in other Caucasians with PPP. The finding of increased scintigraphic SCC activity in 7.4% of a German group of PPP patients compared with 22% of a Swedish group supports this [32]. Significant relationships between SCC involvement and other features of patients with PPP have not been detected [32, 38], except that severe skin disease increases the risk of SCC involvement [38].

Sternocostoclavicular involvement occurs frequently in patients appearing with arthropathy associated with PPP. It has been found present in 68–82% of Caucasians [9, 39, 40] and in 93–100% of Japanese patients [51, 87].

The radiographic SCC changes found during surveys on adults with PPP are generally minimal compared with those of patients appearing with manifest arthropathy associated with PPP [32, 38–40, 43, 46, 51, 87]. Based on the finding in epidemiological studies of PPP in 0.01–0.05% of Scandinavians, and the result of the Danish frequency study, such minor changes can be estimated to occur in 0.002–0.01% of the population [38]. Thus, advanced SCC changes associated with PPP must be rare.

## 12.3.4
## Associated Skeletal Lesions and Other Findings

Adults with SCC changes primarily in the region of joints often have accompanying pelvospondylitis [9, 19, 32, 39, 40, 43, 45–47, 51, 59, 67, 77, 82, 87].

Spinal changes are usually characterised by erosion of vertebral plates with subchondral sclerosis, sometimes involving the entire vertebral body [9, 38, 39, 51, 59, 82, 87]. The erosion may be located to one side of the intervertebral space only [39], but involvement of both vertebral plates accompanied by disc space narrowing or paravertebral ossification is also seen [38, 47, 51]. Occasionally there are syndesmophytes, either located to single intervertebral spaces or extending over several levels [9, 38, 39, 87], and bulky paravertebral ossifications [43, 67, 77, 87]. There can be associated unilateral or bilateral sacroiliitis, which usually is slight and thereby differs from the changes in AS [9, 19, 32, 38–40, 51, 87], but ankylosis has been reported [50]. Sclerosis of pelvic bones adjacent to irregular joint margins at the pubic symphysis or at the sacroiliac joints may also occur, but is rare [9, 39, 47, 51]. Peripheral joint complaints, arthritis or tenosynovitis may be present, but as a rule without erosion [9, 32, 38, 39, 43, 67, 82, 87]. Involvement of the shoulders and hips (root joints) is rare [41, 87].

Biochemical findings are non-specific [38, 39, 43–46, 87]. They mainly consist of elevated erythrocyte sedimentation rate (ESR) or C-reactive protein (CRP) [35, 38, 39, 43–46, 58] and protein electrophoretic signs of active inflammatory disease during exacerbations [39, 43, 45, 46]. Abnormal white blood cell and differential counts are rare [51]. Tests for rheumatoid factor and antinuclear antibodies are generally negative [36, 39, 43, 45, 46, 50]. In adults appearing with joint involvement the frequency of HLA-B27 may be slightly increased compared to the normal population [19, 39, 40], but it does not occur in patients with primarily osseous SCC lesions. SCC lesions associated with PPP can therefore generally be regarded not associated with HLA-B27.

Histopathological findings are also non-specific. In adults with primary joint involvement non-specific synovial and soft tissue inflammation or fibromatosis have been detected, in addition to changes in the subchondral bone similar to those of patients with primary osseous lesions [11, 19, 49, 58, 87]. Inflammatory changes of the costoclavicular ligament merging into the bone, consistent with inflammation of the enthesis, have also been observed [87]. Bacterial cultures are generally negative [11, 43, 45, 46, 59, 87]. *Propionibacterium acnes* [19] and a non-specified corynebacterium [59] have been detected in a few patients, but are probably due to contamination, as such species are normal skin/nose parasites.

The process leading to hyperostosis probably relates to periosteal, endosteal and/or heterotrophic reactive bone formation including enthesopathic ossification of the costoclavicular ligament. The costoclavicular ligament merges with the SCJ capsule [8], and it is likely that ossification is due to enthesopathy associated with arthritis of this joint. It does not occur in healthy individuals [91].

The nomenclature of PPP-associated skeletal lesions has varied considerably. In the first studies, which confirmed a connection between SCC involvement and PPP, the changes were named PAO [34, 35, 62, 86, 87, 94]. This term was sometimes used in subsequent reports on adult patients [67, 82], but several other names have been used including SCCH [36], "sternocostoclavicular arthro-osteitis" [19], "spondarthritis hyperostotica pustulo-psoriatica" [80], SAPHO syndrome (synovitis-acne-pustulosis-hyperostosis-osteitis) [9, 14, 15, 28, 53, 56, 64, 68, 76], "juxtasternal arthritis" [49] and "bone and joint lesions, or arthritis and osteitis associated with PPP" [32, 51, 59]. This may be confusing, and it is proposed that the skeletal abnormalities associated with PPP are termed PAO.

### 12.3.5
### Conclusion

Changes in the SCC region associated with PPP may have different radiographic features. The most characteristic lesions are primarily located to the bones. They appear as sclerosis and hyperostosis, which in adults are located to the sternum or clavicle and in children/adolescents predominantly to the clavicle. Such lesions can occur as part of a multifocal osseous disease. Erosive changes of SCC joints also occur in adults, but generally not in children/adolescents. Radiographically they are usually characterised by joint erosion or ankylosis with pronounced subchondral sclerosis and hyperostosis of the adjacent bones. Concomitant ossification of the first costal cartilage and the costoclavicular ligament usually occurs as part of SCJ involvement. Changes of SCC joints are often accompanied by spondylodiscitis with sclerosis of adjacent bone, sometimes involving the entire vertebra. Accompanying paravertebral ossifications, syndesmophytes, sacroiliitis, sclerosis of pelvic bones and peripheral non-erosive arthritis may also occur, but are less frequent.

## 12.4
## Psoriatic Arthritis

Common psoriatic arthritis is associated with the dermal disease psoriasis vulgaris. It is a chronic skin disease characterised by sharply demarcated brownish-red papules and plaques often covered with layers of fine silvery scales [63]. It is mostly located on the extensor prominences and the scalp. Accompanying peripheral arthritis may occur and sometimes also pelvospondylitis.

### 12.4.1
### Features Related to Sternocostoclavicular Involvement

Sternocostoclavicular involvement associated with psoriasis vulgaris is often clinically silent and may remain undiagnosed. It is seen in all age groups [40], and appears equally often in men and women, just as psoriasis and psoriatic arthritis [40]. SCC changes at imaging can occur without significant local symptoms [40, 54] (Fig. 12.5). Their presence is related to long disease duration and SCC abnormalities therefore usually follow other skeletal manifestations [40, 54], but they can appear simultaneously [54] or be the first lesion [43, 44].

### 12.4.2
### Imaging Features

Radiographic changes of the SCJ may vary from unilateral or bilateral erosion with joint space narrowing accompanied by slight subchondral sclerosis and/or osteophytes to pronounced hyperostotic changes [40, 49, 93]. Hyperostotic changes are, however, rare in patients with psoriasis vulgaris only. The patients reported with hyperostotic lesions and psoriasis often had accompanying PPP lesions [12, 21, 25, 39, 40, 42, 49, 88].

Changes of the MSJ associated with psoriasis vulgaris are characterised by joint erosion with slight subchondral sclerosis and joint space narrowing or widening [40, 54]. The erosive changes may progress to ankylosis [40]. Patients with both psoriasis and PPP usually have more pronounced subchondral sclerosis [3, 39], just as patients with PPP only [39, 43].

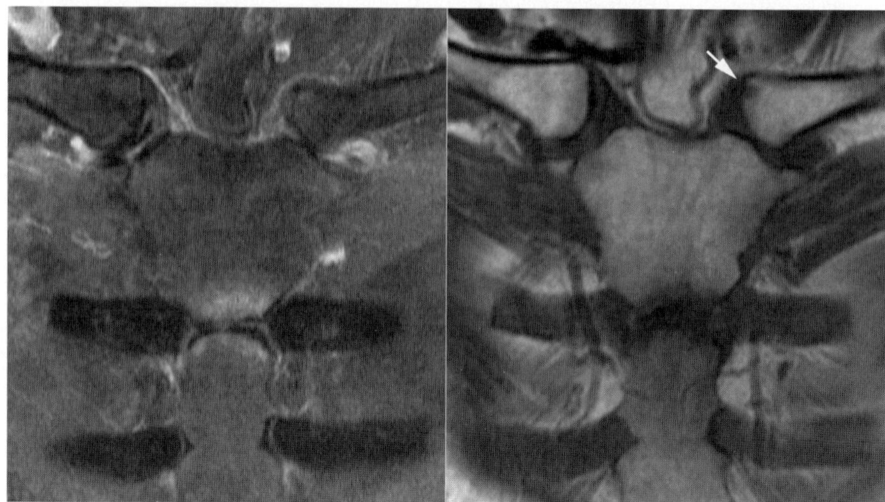

**Fig. 12.5** Psoriatic arthritis. MRI of a 48-year-old woman with psoriatic arthritis and pain in the lower neck, left shoulder and upper arm. Radiological examination of the neck and shoulder were normal and because of slight swelling at the left sternoclavicular region an MRI screening examination was performed. Coronal STIR (*left*) and T1-weighted image (*right*) show fluid in the left SCJ with erosion of the left clavicle (*arrow*) and also erosion with surrounding oedema at the MSJ as signs of arthritis

## 12.4.3
### Frequency of Sternocostoclavicular Involvement

The reported frequency has varied considerably, which may be due to inclusion of patients with PPP in some analyses. When specially looked for clinical involvement of SCC joints has been found to be present in 44% of 23 patients with psoriatic arthritis being located to the SCJ in 30% and to the MSJ and sternocostal joints in 9% and 17%, respectively [63]. In comparison the frequency of SCC involvement was 82% in patients with arthropathy associated with PPP [63]. In another study including separation of patients with regard to dermal disease, clinical involvement occurred in only 1% of patients with psoriasis vulgaris, but in 27% of the patients with both psoriasis and PPP, and in 50% of the patients with PPP only [40]. These results are not directly comparable with other clinical studies of patients with non-specified psoriasis and arthritis. In such groups the SCJs have been found involved by history or physical examination in 0–15% and the MSJ in 1–68% of the patients [54, 61].

Based on plain radiographs, abnormalities of SCC joints occur in about a quarter of patients with peripheral arthritis associated with psoriasis vulgaris [40] and are predominantly located to the MSJ [40]. Changes of the MSJ have been reported present in 24% of patients, and changes of the SCJs in 9% of the patients [40].

Involvement of the SCJs may, however, be more frequent. In an analysis of 10 patients with non-specified psoriatic arthritis, changes at CT occurred in 9 patients. They consisted of erosion, subchondral cysts, sclerosis and joint space narrowing sometimes associated with osteophytes. Ankylosis did not occur [93]. Joint space narrowing, sclerosis and osteophytes, however, also occurred in a few control persons.

The MSJ has received more attention with radiographic changes reported present in 0–100% of patients with psoriatic arthritis [54, 61, 66, 81]. The wide range is probably due to differences regarding the composition of patient groups. The type of dermal disease and the duration and severity of arthritis are important factors. The radiographic method may also play a part, but it has not been proved [41].

Increased SCC uptake at scintigraphy occurs in 30–50% of patients with psoriatic arthritis [22, 63, 71], being located to the SCJs in 17% and to the MSJ in 13% [63].

## 12.4.4
## Associated Skeletal Lesions and Other Findings

The presence of SCC involvement is related to signs of advanced generalised psoriatic arthritis, such as peripheral erosive polyarthritis and involvement of root joints [40, 54]. Radiographic changes of peripheral and root joints are similar in patients with, and those without, SCC involvement, except for the degree [40]. The same applies to abnormalities of the spine and the sacroiliac joints.

Biochemical and histopathological findings are non-specific [40, 43]. SCC involvement associated with psoriasis vulgaris is not related to HLA-B27, but it may be the case in patients with both psoriasis and PPP [40]. SCC changes have been analysed histologically in only a few patients with psoriasis. Some of them had hyperostotic SCC lesions and accompanying PPP [21, 25]. Their changes consisted of increased bone remodelling, periosteal, entheseal or heterotopic bone formation, and subacute osseous and soft tissue inflammation [21, 25]. Evaluation of non-hyperostotic sternoclavicular changes has apparently been performed in only one patient, in whom the joint was replaced by scar tissue [83].

### 12.4.5
### Conclusion

Radiographic changes of SCC joints occur in about a quarter of patients with arthritis associated with psoriasis vulgaris. They are located predominantly to the MSJ, but changes of the SCJs also occur. The MSJ involvement is characterised by erosion with slight subchondral sclerosis and joint space narrowing or widening, or by ankylosis. Changes in the region of the SCJs are usually slight. They consist of joint space narrowing and erosion with slight subchondral sclerosis and minimal or no hyperostosis. The presence of SCC abnormalities is related to peripheral erosive polyarthritis and involvement of root joints. Patients with both psoriasis and PPP often have SCC and associated skeletal lesions somewhat similar to those of patients with PPP only.

## 12.5
## Reactive Arthritis

Reactive arthritis (ReA) is a non-pyogenic arthritis that develops soon after or during infections elsewhere in the body, often non-gonococcal urethritis or cervicitis and intestinal infections [2, 55]. It is usually transient, but recurrences and development of chronic peripheral erosive arthritis or pelvospondylitis may occur [55, 69, 70].

### 12.5.1
### Features Related to Sternocostoclavicular Involvement

Sternocostoclavicular involvement as part of ReA occurs in all adult age groups, but appears predominantly in men, as does ReA [39, 40, 70]. Radiographic changes may occur without significant local symptoms [40, 55]. Their presence is related to long disease duration. Consistent with this the involvement usually occurs after other skeletal manifestations [39, 40], but can appear early in the disease or be one of the first manifestations [40].

### 12.5.2
### Imaging Features

Changes of the SCJs in the early stages are usually unilateral and consist of erosion with slight or moderate subchondral sclerosis and joint space narrowing, but

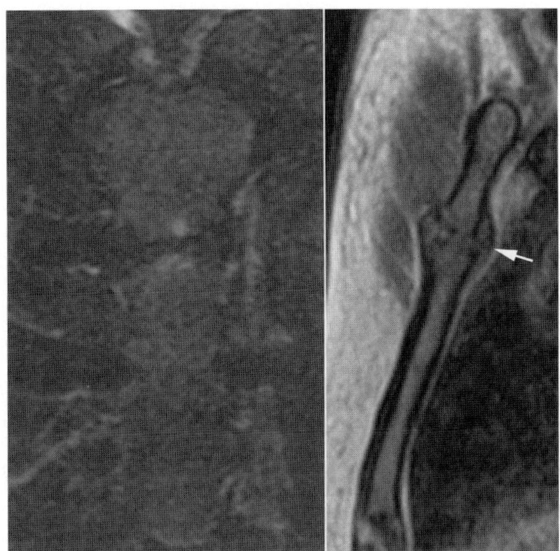

**Fig. 12.6** Reactive MSJ arthritis. MRI of a 28-year-old-man with pain and swelling at the MSJ during 3 months following an episode of urethritis; coronal STIR (*left*) and sagittal T1-weighted image (*right*). There is erosion of the joint facets with signs of inflammatory activity in the form of oedema on the STIR image and extension of the capsule (*arrow*)

usually minimal or no hyperostosis [39, 40]. Bilateral involvement may occur with time, and the involvement in chronic ReA may progress to joint ankylosis with moderate degrees of osseous sclerosis and hyperostosis. Such changes are accompanied by involvement of the first SCJ and ossification of the adjacent costal cartilage [39, 40]. Pronounced hyperostotic and sclerotic involvement of the SCJ has, to the author's knowledge, not been verified in ReA. It is, however, possible that some of the patients described with hyperostotic SCC lesions accompanied by AS-like pelvospondylitis had ReA initially and develop AS-like changes at a later date [39].

The imaging features of MSJ involvement in the early stages are characterised by erosion with subchondral sclerosis, sometimes progressing to ankylosis [39, 40, 66] (Fig. 12.6). Accompanying erosion, irregularity and broadening of the second SCJs may occur, as may similar changes of the third SCJs [39].

## 12.5.3
### Frequency of Sternocostoclavicular Involvement

Clinically manifest SCC involvement occurred in 2–14% of patients with ReA [39, 40], being detected at the SCJs by history or physical examination in 2–14% [69, 70, 96] and at the MSJ in 0–10% of the patients [39, 40, 69, 70, 96].

Abnormalities of SCC joints have been found in 36% of patients with ReA at tomography [55] and in 20% of patients based on radiography [40]. Changes of the SCJs were found in 4–6% of the patients at plain radiography [40, 96]. Most analyses of the SCC region have been centred on the MSJ, which has been reported involved in 0–56% of the patients [61, 66, 81]. This wide range is probably due to differences regarding disease duration and severity. The radiographic method may also play a part, but it has not been proved [41].

## 12.5.4
### Associated Skeletal Lesions and Other Findings

The presence of SCC involvement is infrequent in patients with uncomplicated ReA, and occurs especially in those with a chronic or recurrent disease [39, 40, 55]. SCC changes are related to signs of advanced generalised arthritis in the form of peripheral erosive polyarthritis, sacroiliitis and spinal changes [39, 40]. The associated spinal changes mainly consist of parasyndesmophytes [39, 40, 61].

Biochemical findings are non-specific except a frequent association with HLA-B27, in patients both with and without SCC involvement [2, 40, 55].

## 12.5.5
### Conclusion

Sternocostoclavicular changes as part of ReA occur especially in patients with a chronic or recurrent illness resulting in peripheral erosive polyarthritis or pelvo-spondylitis. The involvement is located predominantly to the MSJ, but changes of the SCJs also occur. Abnormalities of the MSJ are radiographically characterised by erosions with subchondral sclerosis, occasionally progressing to ankylosis. Early changes of the SCJ consist of erosion and joint space narrowing with slight or moderate subchondral sclerosis, but usually minimal hyperostosis. They may progress to ankylosis with moderate surrounding hyperostosis and sclerosis. There is then accompanying involvement of the first sternocostal joint and ossification of the adjacent costal cartilage.

## 12.6
### Enteropathic Arthropathy

Spondylarthropathy associated with inflammatory bowel diseases such as Crohn's disease and ulcerative colitis is usually named enteropathic arthropathy. This disorder can present as an axial and/or peripheral arthropathy (Fig. 12.7).

**Fig. 12.7** Enteropathic arthropathy. CT of a 26-year-old man with inflammatory SCC and spinal symptoms during 1 year accompanied by huge weight loss (40 kg) due to colitis. **a** Axial CT slices through the SCJs shows erosion of the joint facet in both joints (*arrows*). **b** Axial slice at the third sternocostal joints reveals broadening of the left joint with subchondral sclerosis. **c** Coronal reconstruction clearly delineates the involvement at both the sternoclavicular and the sternocostal joints. In particular the left third sternocostal joint involvement is better delineated on the reconstruction. **d** MRI, coronal T1 FS after intravenous contrast shows enhancement in the erosion (*arrows*) and the synovia of both SCJs in addition to enhancement at the third sternocostal joint (*arrow*)

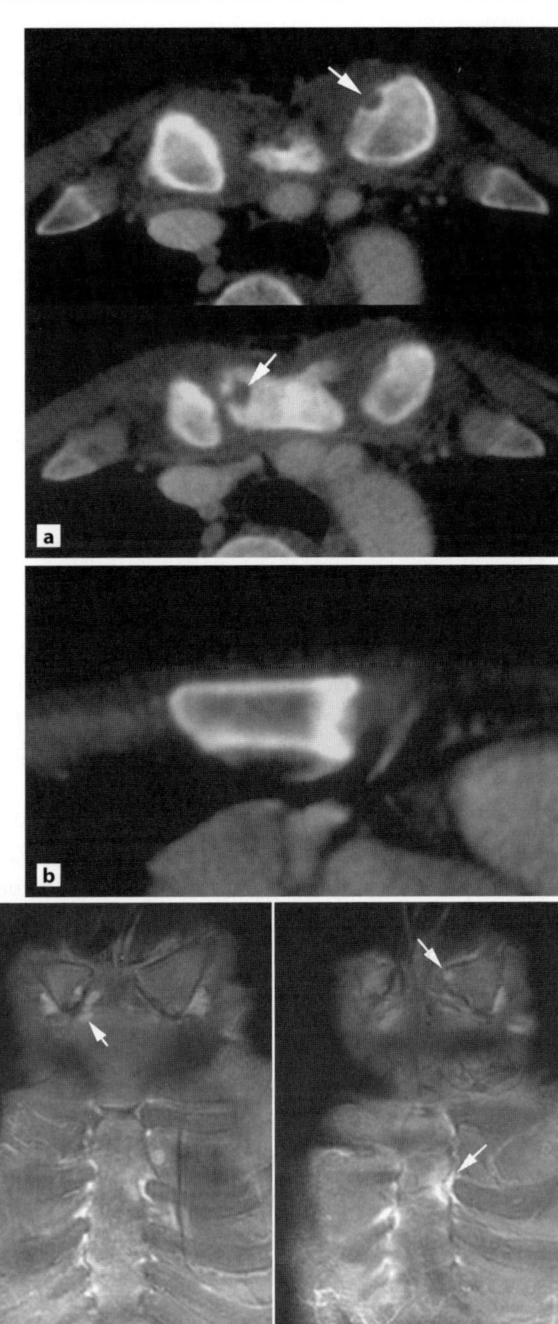

Sternocostoclavicular involvement as part of enteropathic arthropathy has not been systematically evaluated, but has been described in case reports. SAPHO syndrome including SCC involvement has been reported associated with Crohn's disease [27] and non-specified inflammatory bowel disease [98]. Also, SCCH changes corresponding to the clavicle and manubrium have been observed together with colitis [74]. The presence of such manifest changes implies that preliminary minor changes can occur. In accordance with this, clavicular periosteal new bone formation [95] and ligamentous ossification have been described associated with ulcerative colitis [92].

## 12.7
## SAPHO, Sternocostoclavicular Hyperostosis and Other "Syndromes"

Hyperostotic osteoarticular involvement of the SCC region can occur as a dominant disease manifestation. It is a rare abnormality that has received many names. The most frequently used names today are SAPHO syndrome (synovitis-acne-pustulosis-hyperostosis-osteitis), SCCH (sternocostoclavicular hyperostosis), ISCCO (intersternocostoclavicular ossification) and PAO (pustulotic arthro-osteitis) when associated with PPP. Many other names have been used, including "acquired hyperostosis syndrome", "hyperostotic pustular psoriatic spondathritis", juxtasternal arthro-osteitis [49], etc.

*SAPHO syndrome* is a term coined for diseases that manifest sterile inflammatory bone lesions together with skin eruptions [4, 7, 90]. It groups together several separately well described osteoarticular disorders such as chronic recurrent multifocal osteomyelitis (CRMO), PAO and arthro-osteitis associated with acne and different forms of psoriasis [6, 7, 9, 18, 33, 90]. The SAPHO syndrome is mostly considered to belong to the group of SpA disorders. Most hyperostotic SCC changes can in accordance with this be classified as belonging to one of the common forms of SpA [17]. These do not include acne arthropathy. The SCC lesions associated with acne are, like those associated with PPP, often characterised by more osseous sclerosis than generally seen in other forms of seronegative arthritis [5, 9, 20, 43, 45, 49]. It seems appropriate to name the arthropathy in accordance with the accompanying dermal disease as acne arthropathy. SAPHO syndrome must not be regarded a disease entity itself, but more a combination of signs, which may guide the way to a more specific diagnosis. The use of the term SAPHO may therefore confuse the classification of the different disorders included.

*Sternocostoclavicular hyperostosis* is a term often used to designate SCC changes radiographically characterised by hyperostosis in the region of the SCJs with joint erosion or ankylosis, and varying degrees of calcification of the upper costal cartilages. Such changes were first reported in Caucasians by Köhler in 1975 [52]. Since then many case reports and also series of patients with SCCH have been published [41]. The findings on radiographic examination have varied considerably. Some of the adults described with SCCH had pronounced changes of the SCJs with ankylosis, but others had less advanced erosive joint changes [36, 41, 52, 74]. Quite different, predominantly osseous sclerotic and hyperostotic lesions of the manubrium sterni or the clavicle [24, 25, 65] and predominantly ligamentous changes [10, 11, 85] have also been described under the term SCCH.

*Intersternocostoclavicular ossification* was initially described in Japanese patients [85]. The features of ISCCO differ somewhat from those of SCCH in Caucasians [12]. ISCCO changes consist of ossification in the region of the costoclavicular ligament graduated in three stages: stage 1: ossification localised to the area of the costoclavicular ligament; stage 2: pronounced ossification filling the space between the clavicle and the first rib accompanied by irregularity of the inferior margin of the clavicle and the superior margin of the first rib; and stage 3: additional hyperostosis of the medial part of the clavicle, and in severe cases also of the manubrium sterni [85]. It was claimed that the disease always progresses from stage 1 to 3, but the radiographic method used mainly consisted of plain radiographs, and most of the patients had stage 1–2 changes [85]. By the use of tomography, joint changes were sometimes detected in subsequent Japanese studies, but ossification of the costoclavicular ligament occurred in most of the patients and seemed to be a more dominant trait than in Caucasians [10, 11]. Ligament ossification also occurs in Caucasians, but apparently less frequently [12, 78].

The changes in SCCH/ISCCO have often been reported accompanied by other skeletal abnormalities [49, 77, 85, 92]. Four radiographic types of associated spinal lesions have been described: spondylodiscitis with erosion of vertebral plates usually with some degree of subchondral sclerosis, and sometimes also syndesmophytes or paravertebral ossifications; AS-like lesions; parasyndesmophytes or pronounced paravertebral ossifications resembling those of diffuse idiopathic skeletal hyperostosis (DISH); and diffuse metastasis-like vertebral sclerosis [41]. Changes of the sacroiliac joint have been reported to vary from unilateral or bilateral mild sacroiliitis to advanced symmetrical involvement in patients with AS or AS-like lesions. Peripheral lesions have also been described, consisting of hyperostosis of tubular bones, erosive arthritis sometimes accompanied by para-articular new bone formation, non-erosive arthritis and ossification in the region of ligament attachments [41]. In addition, associated involvement of the mandible and pelvic bones has been reported [9].

A connection between ISCCO/SCCH and the dermal disease PPP was already noticed in the early Japanese study [85] and later mentioned in Caucasians. Co-existence of PPP and psoriasis or severe acne have been reported in Caucasians [41].

## 12.8
## Conclusions

Hyperostotic SCC lesions can occur in nearly all forms of SpA. They have been described under several names such as SAPHO syndrome, SCCH and ISCCO. Conditions included under such syndrome terms may therefore represent different disorders. The described changes either encompass a spectrum of erosive, sclerotic and hyperostotic changes in the region of the sternoclavicular and upper sternocostal joints or consist of predominantly osseous sclerotic or ligamentous lesions. The SCC involvement either occurred as an isolated skeletal lesion occasionally associated with PPP, or appeared together with other abnormalities suggesting generalised arthritis or DISH. A close analysis of patients with such "SCC syndromes" will often reveal other lesions seen as part of SpA. A hyperostotic SCC lesion may thus be a manifestation of different arthritic, enthesopathic and/or osteitic conditions. Their presence therefore demands a search for one of the classified SpA disorders. If this is diagnosed, the SCC lesion should be named accordingly.

The SCC joints are often forgotten in patients with known SpA. The frequency and features of involvement are therefore not fully established. The SCC region thus deserves more attention in patients with inflammatory disorders, including modern imaging to establish the features of SCC involvement in the different forms of SpA.

## References


1.  Adler E, Carmon A (1961) Ankylosing spondylitis: a review of 115 cases. Acta Rheum Scand 7:219–232
2.  Aho K, Leirisalo-Repo M, Repo H (1985) Reactive arthritis. Clin Rheum Dis 11:25–40
3.  Becker NJ, Smet AA, Chathcart-Rake W, Stechschulte DJ (1986) Psoriatic arthritis affecting the manubriosternal joint. Arthritis Rheum 29:1029–1031
4.  Beretta-Piccoli BC, Sauvain MJ, Gal I, Schibler A, Saurenmann T, Kressebuch H, Bianchetti MG (2000) Synovitis, acne, pustulosis, hyperostosis, osteitis (SAPHO) syndrome in childhood: a report of ten cases and review of the literature. Eur J Pediatr 159:594–601
5.  Bookbinder SA, Fenske NA, Clement GB, Espinoza LR, Germain BF, Vasey FB (1982) Clavicular hyperostosis and acne arthritis. Ann Intern Med 97:615–616
6.  Boutin RD, Resnick D (1998) The SAPHO syndrome: an evolving concept for unifying several idiopathic disorders of bone and skin. Am J Roentgenol 170:585–591
7.  Caravatti M, Wiesli P, Uebelhart D, Germann D, Welzl-Hinterkorner E, Schulthess G (2002) Coincidence of Behcet's disease and SAPHO syndrome. Clin Rheumatol 21:324–327

8.  Cave AJ (1961) The nature and morphology of the costoclavicular ligament. J Anat 95:170–179

9.  Chamot AM, Benhamou CL, Kahn MF, Beraneck L, Kaplan G, Prost A (1987) [Acne-pustulosis-hyperostosis-osteitis syndrome. Results of a national survey. 85 cases.] Rev Rhum Mal Osteoartic 54:187–196

10. Chigira M, Shimizu T (1989) Computed tomographic appearances of sternocostoclavicular hyperostosis. Skeletal Radiol 18:347–352

11. Chigira M, Maehara S, Nagase M, Ogimi T, Udagawa E (1986) Sternocostoclavicular hyperostosis. A report of nineteen cases, with special reference to etiology and treatment. J Bone Joint Surg Am 68:103–112

12.  Colhoun EN, Hayward C, Evans KT (1987) Inter-sterno-costo-clavicular ossification. Clin Radiol 38:33–38

13. Collie DA, Smith GW, Merrick MV (1993) 99mTc-MDP scintigraphy in ankylosing spondylitis. Clin Radiol 48:392–397

14. Courtney PA, Hosking DJ, Fairbairn KJ, Deighton CM (2002) Treatment of SAPHO with pamidronate. Rheumatology (Oxford) 41:1196–1198

15. Davies AM, Marino AJ, Evans N, Grimer RJ, Deshmukh N, Mangham DC (1999) SAPHO syndrome: 20-year follow-up. Skeletal Radiol 28:159–162

16. Dilsen N, McEwen C, Poppel M, Gersh WJ, DiTata D, Carmel P (1962) A comparative roentgenologic study of rheumatoid arthritis and rheumatoid (ankylosing) spondylitis. Arthritis Rheum 5:341 368

17. Dougados M, van der Linden S, Juhlin R, Huitfeldt B, Amor B, Calin A, Cats A, Dijkmans B, Olivieri I, Pasero G (1991) The European Spondylarthropathy Study Group preliminary criteria for the classification of spondylarthropathy. Arthritis Rheum 34:1218–1227

18. Earwaker JW, Cotten A (2003) SAPHO: syndrome or concept? Imaging findings. Skeletal Radiol 32:311–327

19. Edlund E, Johnsson U, Lidgren L, Pettersson H, Sturfelt G, Svensson B, Theander J, Willén H (1988) Palmoplantar pustulosis and sternocostoclavicular arthro-osteitis. Ann Rheum Dis 47:809–815

20. Ellis BI, Shier CK, Leisen JJ, Kastan DJ, McGoey JW (1987) Acne-associated spondylarthropathy: radiographic features. Radiology 162:541–545

21. Fallet GH, Arroyo J, Vischer TL (1983) Sternocostoclavicular hyperostosis: case report with a 31-year follow-up. Arthritis Rheum 26:784–790

22. Fournie B, Boutes A, Dromer C, Sixou L, Le Guennec P, Granel J, Railhac JJ (1997) Prospective study of anterior chest wall involvement in ankylosing spondylitis and psoriatic arthritis. Rev Rhum Engl Ed 64:22–25

23. Freyschmidt J, Sternberg A (1998) The bullhead sign: scintigraphic pattern of sternocostoclavicular hyperostosis and pustulotic arthroosteitis. Eur Radiol 8:807–812

24. Geake T (1988) Sterno-costoclavicular hyperostosis. A report of two new cases and review. Australas Radiol 32:440–443

25. Gerster JC, Lagier R, Nicod L (1985) Case report 311 (sterno-costoclavicular hyperostosis). Skeletal Radiol 14:53–60

26. Ginalski JM, Landry M, Rappoport G, Chamot AM, Gerster JC (1992) MR imaging of sternocostoclavicular arthro-osteitis with palmoplantar pustulosis. Eur J Radiol 14:221–222

27. Girelli CM, Scarpellini M (2001) Gastric Crohn's disease and SAPHO syndrome. Clin Exp Rheumatol 19:356

28. Gmyrek R, Grossman ME, Rudin D, Scher R (1999) SAPHO syndrome: report of three cases and review of the literature. Cutis 64:253–258

29. Good AE (1963) The chest pain of ankylosing spondylitis. Its place in the differential diagnosis of heart pain. Ann Intern Med 58:926–937

30. Hart FD, Bogdanovitch A, Nichol WD (1950) The thorax in ankylosing spondylitis. Ann Rheum Dis 9:116–131

31. Hassett G, Barnsley L (2001) Pain referral from the sternoclavicular joint: a study in normal volunteers. Rheumatology (Oxford) 40:859–862

32. Hradil E, Gents C-F, Matilainen T, Möller H, Sanzén L, Udén A (1988) Skeletal involvement in pustulosis palmoplantaris with special reference to the sterno-costo-clavicular joints. Acta Derm Venereol (Stockh) 68:65–73

33. Hyodoh K, Sugimoto H (2001) Pustulotic arthro-osteitis: defining the radiologic spectrum of the disease. Semin Musculoskelet Radiol 5:89–93

34. Ikegawa S, Urano F, Suzuki S, Fujisawa N, Nishii Y (1999) Three cases of pustulotic arthro-osteitis associated with episcleritis. J Am Acad Dermatol 41:845–846

35. Jang KA, Sung KJ, Moon KC, Koh JK, Choi JH (1998) Four cases of pustulotic arthro-osteitis. J Dermatol 25:201–204

36. Johnston KA, Elston DM (1998) Palmoplantar pustulosis associated with sternocostoclavicular hyperostosis. Cutis 62:75–76

37. Julkunen H (1962) Rheumatoid spondylitis. Clinical and laboratory study of 149 cases compared with 182 cases of rheumatoid arthritis. Acta Rheumatol Scand Suppl 4:1–110

38. Jurik AG (1990) Anterior chest wall involvement in patients with pustulosis palmoplantaris. Skeletal Radiol 19:271–277

39. Jurik AG (1991) Seronegative arthritides of the anterior chest wall: a follow-up study. Skeletal Radiol 20:517–525

40. Jurik AG (1992) Anterior chest wall involvement in seronegative arthritides. A study of the frequency of changes at radiography. Rheumatol Int 12:7–11

41. Jurik AG (1992) Seronegative anterior chest wall syndromes. A study of the findings and course at radiography. Acta Radiol Suppl 301:1–42

42. Jurik AG, de Carvalho A (1985) Sterno-clavicular hyperostosis in a case with psoriasis and HLA-B27 associated arthropathy. Rofo 142:345–347

43. Jurik AG, Graudal H (1987) Monarthritis of the manubriosternal joint. A follow-up study. Rheumatol Int 7:235–241

44. Jurik AG, Graudal H (1988) Sternocostal joint swelling: clinical Tietze's syndrome. Report of sixteen cases and review of the literature. Scand J Rheumatol 17:33–42

45. Jurik AG, Moller BN (1987) Chronic sclerosing osteomyelitis of the clavicle. A manifestation of chronic recurrent multifocal osteomyelitis. Arch Orthop Trauma Surg 106:144–151

46. Jurik AG, Moller BN, Jensen MK, Jensen JT, Graudal H (1986) Sclerosis and hyperostosis of the manubrium sterni. Rheumatol Int 6:171–178

47. Jurik AG, Helmig O, Graudal H (1988) Skeletal disease, arthro-osteitis, in adult patients with pustulosis palmoplantaris. Scand J Rheumatol Suppl 70:3–15

48. Kalke S, Perera SD, Patel ND, Gordon TE, Dasgupta B (2001) The sternoclavicular syndrome: experience from a district general hospital and results of a national postal survey. Rheumatology (Oxford) 40:170–177

49. Katz ME, Shier CK, Ellis BI, Leisen JC, Hardy DC, Jundt JW (1989) A unified approach to symptomatic juxtasternal arthritis and enthesitis. Am J Roentgenol 153:327–333

50. Kawabata T, Morita Y, Nakatsuka A, Kagawa H, Kawashima M, Sei T, Yamamura M, Makino H (2005) Multiple venous thrombosis in SAPHO syndrome. Ann Rheum Dis 64:505–506

51. Kawai K, Doita M, Tateshi H, Hirobata K (1988) Bone and joint lesions associated with pustulosis palmaris et plantaris. J Bone Joint Surg Br 70:117–122

52. Köhler H, Uehlinger E, Kutzner J, Weihrauch TR, Wilbert L, Schuster R (1975) Sterno-kosto-klavikuläre Hyperostose, ein bisher nicht beschriebenes Krankheitsbild. Dtsch Med Wochenschr 100:1535–1536

53. Kohlfuerst S, Igerc I, Lind P (2003) FDG PET helpful for diagnosing SAPHO syndrome. Clin Nucl Med 28:838–839

54. Kormano M, Karvonen J, Lassus A (1975) Psoriatic lesion of the sternal synchondrosis. Acta Radiol Diagn (Stockh) 16:463–468

55. Kousa M (1978) Clinical observations on Reiter's disease with special reference to the venereal and non-venereal aetiology. Acta Derm Venereol Suppl (Stockh) 81:1–36

56. Laiho K, Soini I, Martio J (2001) Magnetic resonance imaging findings of manubri-osternal joint involvement in SAPHO syndrome. Clin Rheumatol 20:232–233

57. Laitinen H, Saksanen S, Suoranta H (1970) Involvement of the manubrio-sternal articulation in rheumatoid arthritis. Acta Rheum Scand 16:40–46

58. Lazzarin P, Punzi L, Cesaro G, Sfriso P, De Sandre P, Padovani G, Todesco S (1999) Thrombosis of the subclavian vein in SAPHO syndrome. A case report. Rev Rhum Engl Ed 66:173–176

59. Le Goff P, Brousse A, Fauquert P, Guillet G, Leroy JP (1985) Arthropathies érosives thoraciques antérieures et intervertébrales associées à la pustulose palmoplantaire. Rev Rhum 52:391–396

60. Louvel JP, Duvey A, Da Silva F, Primard E, Mejjad O, Henry J, le Loet X (1997) Computed tomography of sternoclavicular joint lesions in spondylarthropathies. Skeletal Radiol 26:419–423

61. McEwen C, DiTata D, Lingg C, Porini A, Good A, Rankin T (1971) Ankylosing spondylitis and spondylitis accompanying ulcerative colitis, regional enteritis, psoriasis, and Reiter's disease. A comparative study. Arthritis Rheum 14:291–318

62. McGee TC, Field RS, Loebl DH, Bailey JP Jr, Sizemore KR (1993) Pustulotic arthro-osteitis: a cause of atypical chest pain and a new arthritic syndrome. South Med J 86:469–472

63. Mejjad O, Daragon A, Louvel JP, Da Silva LF, Thomine E, Lauret P, le Loet X (1996) Osteoarticular manifestations of pustulosis palmaris et plantaris and of psoriasis: two distinct entities. Ann Rheum Dis 55:177–180

64. Orion E, Brenner S (1999) Stress-induced SAPHO syndrome. J Eur Acad Dermatol Venereol 12:43–46

65. Otsuka N, Fukunaga M, Sone T, Nagai K, Tomomitsu T, Yanagimoto S, Muranaka A, Ono S, Morita R (1986) Usefulness of bone imaging in diagnosis of sterno costo-clavicular hyperostosis. Clin Nucl Med 11:651–652

66. Parker VS, Malhotra CM, Ho G, Kaplan SR (1984) Radiographic appearance of the sternomanubrial joint in arthritis and related conditions. Radiology 153:343–347

67. Patterson AC, Bentley-Corbett K (1985) Pustulotic arthro-osteitis. J Rheumatol 12:611–614

68. Pichler R, Weiglein K, Schmekal B, Sfetsos K, Maschek W (2003) Bone scintigraphy using Tc-99m DPD and F18-FDG in a patient with SAPHO syndrome. Scand J Rheumatol 32:58–60

69. Popert AJ, Gill AJ, Laird SM (1964) A prospective study of Reiter's syndrome. An interim report on the first 82 cases. Br J Vener Dis 40:160–165

70. Prohaska E, Ellegast H, Petershofer H, Hawel R, Obererlacher J (1984) Besondere discovertebrale Verlaufsformen bei der Spondylitis ankylosans. Z Rheumatol 43:303–310

71. Punzi L, Pianon M, Rossini P, Schiavon F, Gambari PF (1999) Clinical and laboratory manifestations of elderly onset psoriatic arthritis: a comparison with younger onset disease. Ann Rheum Dis 58:226–229

72. Resnick D, Vint V, Poteshman NL (1981) Sternocostoclavicular hyperostosis. A report of three new cases. J Bone Joint Surg Am 63:1329–1332

73. Reuler JB, Girard DE, Nardone DA (1978) Sternoclavicular joint involvement in ankylosing spondylitis. South Med J 71:1480–1481

74. Ringe JD, Faber H, Farahmand P (2006) Rapid pain relief and remission of sternocostoclavicular hyperostosis after intravenous ibandronate therapy. J Bone Miner Metab 24:87–93

75. Rosen PS, Graham DC (1962) Ankylosing (Strümpell-Marie) spondylitis (a clinical review of 128 cases. Arch Intern Am Rheumatol 5:158–233

76. Rutten HP, van Langelaan EJ (2002) The SAPHO syndrome: a report of 2 patients. Acta Orthop Scand 73:590–593

77. Sartoris DJ, Schreiman JS, Kerr R, Resnik CS, Resnick D (1986) Sternocostoclavicular hyperostosis: a review and report of 11 cases. Radiology 158:125–128

78. Satoris DJ, Schreiman JS, Kerr R, Resnik CS, Resnick D (1986) Sternocostoclavicular hyperostosis: a review and report of 11 cases. Radiology 158:125–128

79. Savill DL (1951) The manubrio-sternal joint in ankylosing spondylitis. J Bone Joint Surg Br 33:56–64

80. Schilling F, Kessler S (1998) [Spondarthritis hyperostotica pustulo-psoriatica: nosologic study with clinical and radiologic presentation in relation to the SAPHO syndrome.] Fortschr Geb Rontgenstr Neuen Bildgeb Verfahr 169:576–584

81. Sebes JI, Salazar JE (1983) The manubriosternal joint in rheumatoid disease. Am J Roentgenol 140:117–121

82. Seppälä J, Forssman L, Hypen M (1987) Pustulotic arthro-osteitis. A report of two cases. Scand J Rheumatol 16:135–138

83. Sokoloff F, Gleason IO (1954) The sternocostoclavicular articulation in rheumatic disease. Am J Clin Pathol 24:406–416

84. Solovay J, Gardner C (1951) Involvement of the manubriosternal joint in Marie-Strümpell disease. Am J Roentgenol 65:749–759

85. Sonozaki H, Azuma A, Okai K, Nakamura K, Fukuoka S, Tateishi A, Kurosawa H, Mannoji T, Kabata K, Mitsui H, Seki H, Abe I, Furusawa S, Matsuura M, Kudo A, Hoshino T (1979) Clinical features of 22 cases with "inter-sterno-costo-clavicular ossification". A new rheumatic syndrome. Arch Orthop Trauma Surg 95:13–22

86. Sonozaki H, Kawashima M, Hongo O, Yaoita H, Ikeno M, Matsuura M, Okai K, Azuma A (1981) Incidence of arthro-osteitis in patients with pustulosis palmaris et plantaris. Ann Rheum Dis 40:554–557

87. Sonozaki H, Mitsui H, Miyanaga Y, Okitsu K, Igarashi M, Hayashi Y, Matsuura M, Azuma A, Okai K, Kawashima M (1981) Clinical features of 53 cases with pustulotic arthro-osteitis. Ann Rheum Dis 40:547–553

88. Spar I (1978) Psoriatic arthritis of the sternoclavicular joint. Conn Med 42:225–226

89. Spencer DG, Park WM, Dick HM, Papazoglou SN, Buchanan WW (1979) Radiological manifestations in 200 patients with ankylosing spondylitis: correlation with clinical features and HLA B27. J Rheumatol 6:305–315

90. Sugimoto H, Tamura K, Fujii T (1998) The SAPHO syndrome: defining the radiologic spectrum of diseases comprising the syndrome. Eur Radiol 8:800–806

91. Sutro CJ (1974) The sternoclavicular joint and attached structures (costoclavicular ligament). Bull Hosp Jt Dis 35:168–201

92. Sutro CJ, Sutro WH (1984) Hyperostosis of the clavicle and ossification of the costoclavicular ligament in association with ankylosing spondylitis. Bull Hosp Jt Dis 44:65–71

93. Taccari E, Spadaro A, Riccieri V, Guerrisi R, Guerrisi V, Zoppini A (1992) Sternoclavicular joint disease in psoriatic arthritis. Ann Rheum Dis 51:372–374

94. Tamai K, Saotome K (1999) Panclavicular ankylosis in pustulotic arthroosteitis. A case report. Clin Orthop Relat Res 146–150

95. Verbruggen LA, Buyck R, Handelberg F (1985) Clavicular periosteal new bone formation in ulcerative colitis. Clin Exp Rheumatol 3:163–166

96. Weldon WV, Scalettar R (1961) Roentgen changes in Reiter's syndrome. Am J Roentgenol 86:344–350

97. Wilkinson M, Bywaters EGL (1958) Clinical features and course of ankylosing spondylitis as seen in a follow-up of 222 hospital referred cases. Ann Rheum Dis 17:209–228

98. Yamasaki O, Iwatsuki K, Kaneko F (2003) A case of SAPHO syndrome with pyoderma gangrenosum and inflammatory bowel disease masquerading as Behcet's disease. Adv Exp Med Biol 528:339–341

# 13 Predominant Osseous Inflammatory Lesions

ANNE GRETHE JURIK

**Contents**



## 13.1
## Introduction

Predominant osseous lesions in the sternocostoclavicular (SCC) region occur in the form of non-pyogenic osseous inflammation involving the clavicle, the sternum or costae. Inflammatory sclerotic involvement of the clavicle mainly occurs in children, adolescents and young adults and may be part of "chronic recurrent multifocal osteomyelitis" (CRMO). In adults osseous lesions of the sternum and/or the clavicle are often associated with dermal diseases, especially pustulosis palmoplantaris (PPP). A fluctuating clinical course occurs both in children and adolescents and in adults accompanied by a gradual development of the sclerotic and hyperostotic osseous lesions that display signs of inflammatory activity clinically and at MRI or scintigraphy during exacerbations.

Although it is possible that the disorders of children and adolescents and adults are similar, just with age-related differences, the description in this chapter includes a separation. The disorders in children and adolescents are described under the heading CRMO, and those of adults as osteoarthropathy followed by a section about terminology.

## 13.2
## Chronic Recurrent Multifocal Osteomyelitis

Chronic recurrent multifocal osteomyelitis is a well-established, relatively rare, skeletal disorder of unknown aetiology mainly occurring in children and adolescents. It affects girls more often than boys [28, 40, 55] and occurs predominantly in children and adolescents, but has occasionally been described in adults [40]. CRMO is a diagnosis of exclusion based on the characteristic features listed in Table 13.1. The lesions of CRMO are predominantly located to tubular bones followed by the clavicle, the spine and pelvic bones, but involvement of ribs, the sternum, the mandible and small tubular bones may also occur [32]. The lesions are often multiple and sometimes symmetrical, but the disease can manifest in only one location [23, 32]. There may be accompanying skin disease, most frequently PPP, but an association with acne, psoriasis vulgaris and pyoderma gangrenosum has also been reported [3, 10, 15, 16, 23, 26, 27, 32, 33, 40, 48, 51, 52, 55]. The presence of skin disease supports the diagnosis, which usually is based on a characteristic clinical course and conventional radiography supplemented by bone scintigraphy and/or MRI. Histopathological and microbiological examinations may be necessary to exclude tumour and infectious diseases.

**Table 13.1** Characteristic features of CRMO

| | |
|---|---|
| **Clinical signs** | Local pain with gradual onset<br>Improvement by anti-inflammatory drugs<br>Sometimes accompanying dermal disease |
| **Clinical course** | Prolonged and fluctuating with recurrent pain episodes during several years corresponding to the bones involved |
| **Location of lesions** | Atypical compared to infectious osteomyelitis with a frequent involvement of the clavicle and often multifocal lesions |
| **Radiographic appearance** | Suggests subacute or chronic osteomyelitis |
| **Scintigraphic appearance** | Clinically silent lesions may be revealed |
| **Laboratory findings** | Compatible with non-specific subacute or chronic inflammation, e.g. elevated CRP and/or ESR |
| **Bacterial culture** | Negative |
| **Histopathological findings** | Non-specific subacute or chronic inflammation |

## 13.2.1
## Clavicular Lesions

Non-pyogenic inflammatory sclerotic clavicular lesions are generally rare findings. They mainly occur in children and adolescents with CRMO, but can also appear in young adults. Irrespective of age there is a female predominance [37].

### 13.2.1.1
### Clinical features

Clavicular lesions are characterised by recurrent episodes of pain, swelling and slight redness of the skin in the region of the clavicle without suppuration or fistula formation [6, 37, 41, 50, 52, 54]. Accompanying malaise and low-grade fever occur occasionally [10, 37, 40, 49, 50, 55], but eliciting infections are usually absent. The course is prolonged over several years, but the patients are usually without symptoms of the lesion during remissions except the presence of a clavicular prominence [37]. Complicating subclavian vein obstruction or fracture may occur, but is rare [49, 53]. The disorder is sometimes accompanied by PPP or acne [6, 37].

### 13.2.1.2
### Imaging Features

The radiographic features of clavicular lesions in the early active stages are characterised by lytic medullary destruction in the medial part of the clavicle and periosteal new bone formation, occasionally like onion skin simulating malignancies (Fig. 13.1) [10, 16, 32, 36, 41, 54, 56]. During periods of remission the clavicular destruction tends to heal with the formation of sclerosis, and the periosteal new bone to organise, sclerose and fuse with the clavicular bone (Fig. 13.1) [22, 33, 36, 37, 40, 50, 54, 55]. If the periosteal new bone formation is mineralised peripherally a "bone within bone" appearance can occasionally be seen, especially at CT or MRI [56, 60] (Fig. 13.1g,h). The course usually implies several exacerbations during which new lytic osseous destruction and sometimes periostal new bone formation occur, similarly healing with sclerosis. This may results in progressive clavicular sclerosis and hyperostosis [33, 36]. It can be difficult by conventional radiography to detect activity in such hyperostotic and sclerotic bone lesions unless there is periosteal new bone formation or areas with lytic destruction.

The hyperostotic and sclerotic clavicular changes usually persist for several years and gradually extend laterally [10, 15, 16, 36]. Although some spontaneous regression occurs during remissions, complete healing is rare. The features of the

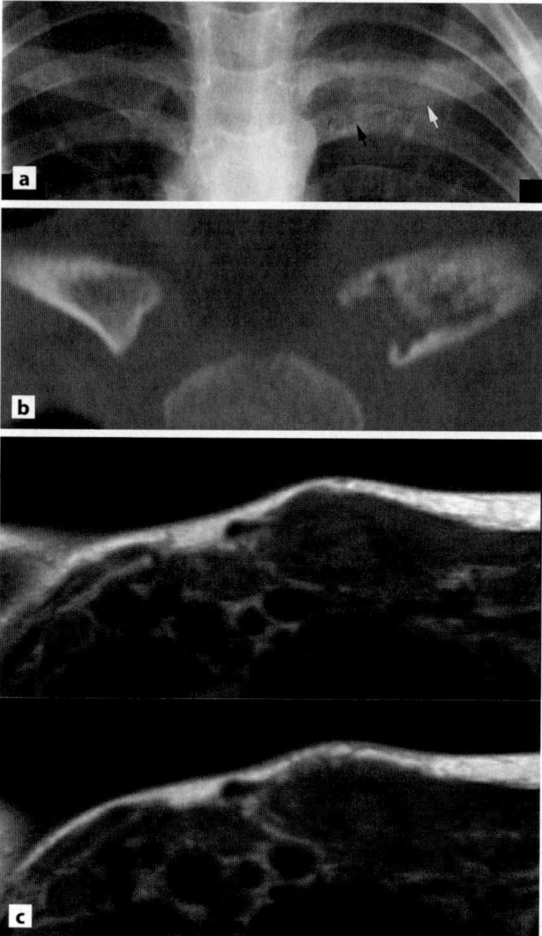

**Fig. 13.1** Clavicular lesions in CRMO: non-specific appearance. **a** AP radiograph of the medial part of the clavicles in a 6-year-old girl with left-sided clavicular pain and swelling during 3 months. There are lytic destruction (*black arrow*) and periosteal new bone formation (*white arrow*) at the medial part of the clavicle. **b** Coronal CT reconstruction showed lytic destruction of the medial part of the bone including the joint facet with irregular medullary and periosteal new bone formation. **c,d** MRI, axial T1 (**c**) and semiaxial STIR (**d**) show a mass with low signal intensity at T1 and high signal intensity at STIR both corresponding to the bone and in the surrounding soft tissue. **e** Scintigraphy revealed increased uptake at the clavicle and at the upper growth plate of the left tibia (*arrow*). Biopsy revealed non-specific inflammatory changes. **f** AP radiograph 6 months later showed smoothing of the osseous contours and more pronounced sclerosis. **g,h** Bone within bone appearance in a 15-year-old girl with pain and swelling during 4 months. Coronal T1 (**g**) and postcontrast T1 FS sequence (**h**) showing a characteristic bone (*arrow*) within the periosteal new bone formation

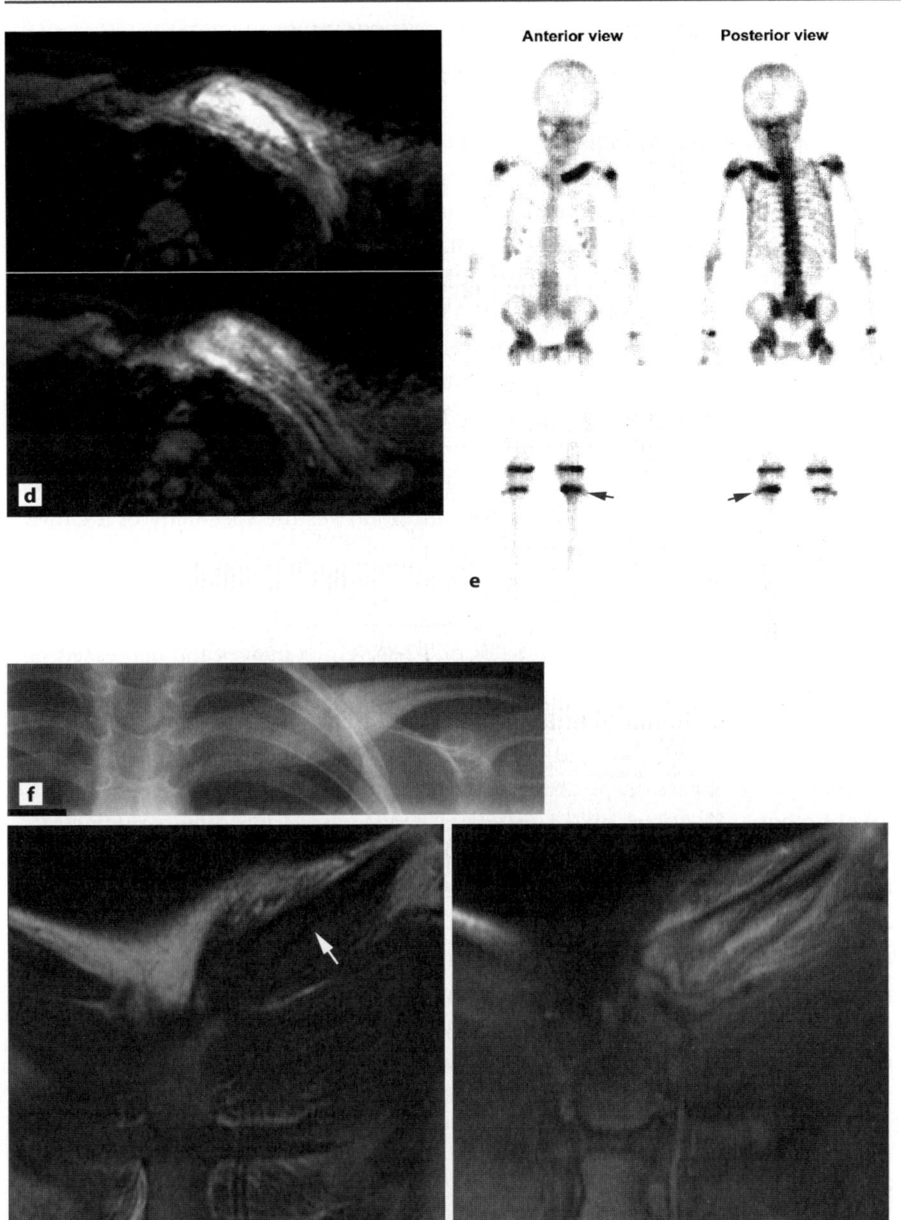
Anterior view
Posterior view
d
e
f
g
h

disorder can therefore be seen also in adults. In contrast to the adult disease, the sternoclavicular joint, sternum and rib are rarely involved in childhood and adolescence [16].

The appearance at MRI in the early stage is often non-specific. On T1-weighted images the lesion appears as a rather homogeneous mass of low signal intensity containing the bone marrow, cortical bone and the periosteal new bone formation. On STIR or T2-weighted images the mass displays high signal intensity corresponding to the bone and periosteal new bone with concomitant high signal intensity in the surrounding soft tissue (Fig. 13.1). After the administration of gadolinium (Gd), a marked, somewhat inhomogeneous, signal enhancement is seen both in the bone lesions and the adjacent soft tissue [22], but there is no delineated soft tissue mass or abnormalities suggesting abscess formation or tumour (Fig. 13.1) [16, 33]. Sometimes the bone within bone appearance is seen at MRI (Fig. 13.1g,h). The addition of this MRI appearance to the clinical and radiographic features aids the attainment of a definitive diagnosis and improves the specificity of a CRMO diagnosis [3]. In addition MRI can be used to indicate the most appropriate biopsy site for the highest potential diagnostic yield. MRI can also be helpful in disease monitoring, especially with regard to disease activity [33]. Active lesions present with increased signal intensity on STIR or T2-weighted images and decreased signal intensity on T1 images.

In later, more chronic stages, the MRI appearance includes sequels of previous inflammation. On both T1-weighted and STIR or T2 FS images an inactive sclerotic clavicular lesion presents with low signal intensity corresponding to the sclerotic bone. However, on T1-weighted images the lesion often contains scattered high signal intensity areas (fatty marrow degeneration) as sign of sequels of inflammation (fatty marrow degeneration). Despite these chronic changes MRI can be valuable in detecting activity. During exacerbations high signal intensity areas will occur corresponding to inflammatory areas on STIR or T2 FS images. For the delineation of such areas it is important to use fat suppressed sequences such as STIR, and when contrast is needed a T1 FS sequence to secure suppression of signals from fatty areas in the chronic lesions [16, 33].

## 13.2.2
### Sternocostal Lesions

Sternal and costal lesions are far less common than clavicular involvement, but involvement of ribs [48, 51, 52, 54], the sternum [27] or the manubriosternal joint (MSJ) [26, 51, 52] has been reported (Fig. 13.2). Such lesions mainly occur in adolescents and young adults.

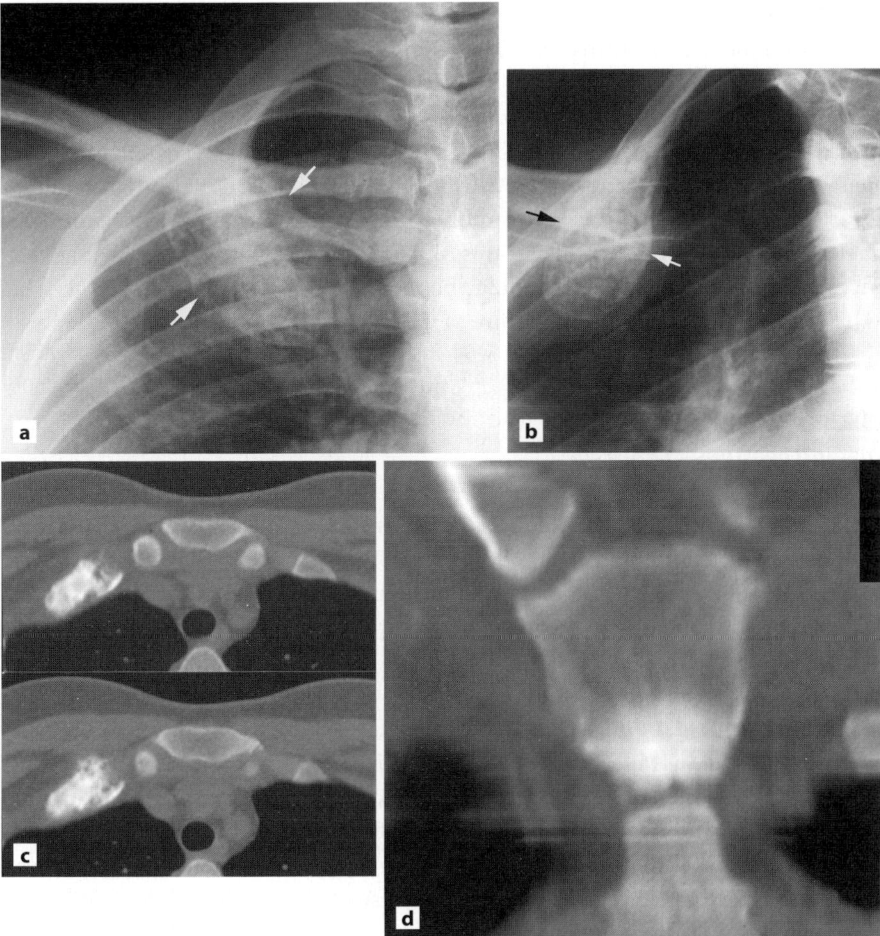

**Fig. 13.2** Rib and sternal lesion in a 27-year-old woman with pain and swelling at the first right rib. **a,b** AP and oblique radiograph show a hyperostotic irregular osseous mass simulating the clavicular lesions, presenting irregular hyperostosis. **c,d** CT, axial slices (**c**) and coronal CT reconstruction (**d**) showed an irregular hyperostotic lesion of the rib, but also a predominant osseous sclerotic lesion at the lower part of the manubrium sterni

At imaging, the sternal changes often consist of sclerotic osseous inflammation adjacent to the MSJ with concomitant irregular joint facets (Fig. 13.2). Rib lesions usually occur at the costochondral junction. They can be predominantly sclerotic as in the sternal lesions, but can also appear inhomogeneous as in the clavicular lesions (Fig. 13.2).

### 13.2.3
### Associated Skeletal Lesions and Other Findings

In children and adolescents there may be accompanying lesions of other bones in accordance with the description of CRMO [6, 32, 52]. Although clavicular involvement is a characteristic feature of CRMO, the lesions are, based on all patients reported, predominantly located to tubular bones followed by the spine and the clavicle [23, 32, 37]. Pelvic bone lesions [49, 52] and sacroiliitis [6, 52] also occur, but are infrequent as are short tubular bone and mandibular lesions [32, 49, 52, 54]. Peripheral arthritis is not a feature of CRMO.

### 13.2.3.1
### Imaging Features

Bone scintigraphy can be helpful in assessing the extent of lesions as some of them can be asymptomatic [11, 22, 24, 28, 41, 45, 55, 57]. Active lesions display a high tracer uptake (Fig. 13.1). The diagnosis of tubular bone lesions can, however, be difficult in childhood due to the normal high uptake in growth plates. It can therefore be difficult to make a certain diagnosis of such lesions, especially when they are symmetrical.

Changes of tubular bones usually have a characteristic although not pathognomonic appearance at radiography [33, 40]. Initially the lesion consists of eccentrically located lytic metaphyseal destruction adjacent to the growth plate with a sclerotic rim demarcating it from normal bone, but no periosteal new bone formation or sequesters (Fig. 13.3) [6, 37, 49, 50]. Concomitant involvement of the epiphyseal bone seems rare [11, 33, 46]. The destruction usually heals with sclerosis followed by normalisation of the osseous structure [37, 49]. Progressive sclerosis and hyperostosis of adjacent metaphyseal and diaphyseal bone occasionally occur linking the changes to those previously described under the term Garré osteomyelitis [32, 37, 49].

Magnetic resonance imaging is useful in assessing the extent and activity of tubular bone lesions. In the early stages it usually reveals more pronounced involvement of the metaphyseal bone marrow than deemed by conventional radiography. Delineated abscess formation often seen in infectious lesions does not occur, but there may be slight surrounding soft tissue inflammation [32].

Spinal lesions may appear as a lytic osseous destruction occasionally with collapse of the vertebral body or as a spondylodiscitis-like lesion with erosion of vertebral plates sometimes accompanied by reduced intervertebral space and/or subchondral sclerosis [6, 32, 37, 52]. Such changes can heal with minimal sequels or

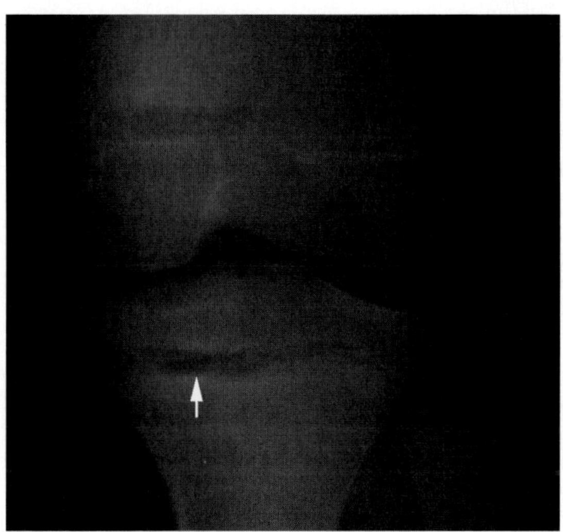

**Fig. 13.3** Tubular bone lesions. AP radiographs of the left knee show characteristic lytic metaphyseal destruction adjacent to the growth plates with surrounding osseous sclerosis (*arrow*)

with the formation of vertebral fusion [37]. MRI can be of help in differentiating the lesion from tumour or infection [32].

Pelvic lesions either present as destruction at joint facets or synchondroses with surrounding sclerosis or as predominant osseous sclerotic lesions, which may heal with minimal sequels [32, 52].

### 13.2.3.2
### Biochemical and Histopathological Features

Biochemical findings in most patients with CRMO include an elevated erythrocyte sedimentation rate (ESR) or C-reactive protein (CRP) during exacerbations, but they have normal white blood cell (WBC) and differential counts [6, 9, 10, 20, 23, 28, 37, 40, 49, 50, 55, 60]. Rheumatoid factor, antinuclear antibodies and HLA-B27 are usually negative [6, 23, 37, 49, 50].

Histopathological findings usually consist of non-specific subacute or chronic inflammation with intertrabecular spaces filled with fibrovascular material containing inflammatory cells, mainly lymphocytes, but also plasma cells, macrophages, histiocytes, multinucleated giant cells and some polymorphonuclear leukocytes [9, 10, 15, 23, 28, 37, 49, 54, 55]. More acute changes may occur especially corresponding to clavicular lesions [9, 55]. Organisms, eosinophils, granulomatous foci, abscess formation or sequesters are generally absent and bacterial cultures are negative [23, 28, 37, 49]. Later spongiosclerosis, signs of remodelling and predominantly chronic inflammation may occur, corresponding to the changes of adults [37]. The sclerosis is probably elicited by osteitis, which can cause increased endosteal, medullary or periosteal new bone formation. The detection of inflammatory changes, however, depends upon the disease duration and the activity at the time of biopsy [37].

## 13.2.4
## Long-term Outcome

The characteristic course of CRMO is prolonged with periods of exacerbation, often involving the same osseous lesion (or lesions) affected previously, or alternatively occurring in an entirely new site [4, 11, 19, 40]. The patients may be symptom-free between attacks except for persistence of a hard non-tender swelling corresponding to hyperostotic lesions.

The long-term clinical course is generally unpredictable [23]. Most cases are self-limited and their lesions eventually resolve without major sequels or functional impairment [1, 5, 20, 23, 28, 32, 40, 52, 55]. Sequels due to premature closure of the epiphysis, bone deformity and kyphosis may occur, but are rare [11, 40, 55]. The duration of symptoms may be in the range of 7–25 years [14, 27, 40], but there may be long periods without symptoms and the symptoms related to the initial lesion may have been replaced by other symptomatic lesions [40]. However, in two analyses with follow-up after skeletal maturity noticeable deformity and leg-length inequality were found to be relatively frequent [14, 27]. Continued symptoms as a result of CRMO occur in about a quarter of the patients, sometimes due to associated medical problems such as arthritis, sacroiliitis, psoriasis, recurrent pustular rashes and inflammatory bowel diseases [27]. These associated disease manifestations also occur in seronegative spondylarthropathy (SpA), indicating that CRMO can progress to a form of SpA. This is supported by the finding of CRMO evolving to SpA in another study [62].

## 13.2.5
## Cause and Pathophysiology

The pathophysiology of CRMO is poorly understood. Haematogenous spread of an infection seems unlikely because pathogens are generally not cultured from the blood, bones or joints. Occasionally an organism has been isolated, usually *Staphylococcus epidermidis* and *Propionibacterium acnes*. It has generally been considered a result of contamination rather than true infection [32, 55]. In accordance with this, the course of the disease is not altered by antibiotic therapy, but it remains possible that a slow-growing unknown organism with fastidious growth requirements, not detected on common media, causes CRMO.

Chronic recurrent multifocal osteomyelitis is more likely an autoimmune disorder as it has been reported associated with several autoimmune diseases, including chronic inflammatory bowel diseases, Wegener's granulomatosis, psoriasis and Takayasu's vasculitis [3, 7, 9, 27, 28, 32, 55]. It is possible that CRMO represents a juvenile form of SpA. This is supported by the occasional occurrence of the following findings: (1) association with disease manifestations seen in adults with SpA such as PPP, inflammatory bowel disorders and psoriasis, (2) observed familiar relation to SpA, PPP and psoriasis vulgaris and (3) observed proceeding of CRMO to SpA [3, 26–28, 40, 52, 55, 62]. CRMO has clinical and radiographic similarities with pustulotic arthro-osteitis (PAO) of adults and dissimilarities may be explained by different phases of bone development with the absence of tubular bone synchondrosis in adults. It is therefore possible that some CRMO patients have a juvenile form of PAO. The occurrence of CRMO-like lesions in adults with PAO and a rather frequent occurrence of PPP in patients with CRMO are consistent with this [32].

## 13.2.6
## Differential Diagnoses

The differential diagnosis mainly includes infectious osteomyelitis, juvenile idiopathic arthritis and tumour or tumour-like lesions [28, 55]. Biopsy may be needed to exclude by histological examination the rare case of a tumour presenting with a similar picture, for example Ewing sarcoma and leukaemia or histiocytosis X/eosinophilic granuloma, and to provide material for microbiological studies. In the differential diagnosis the CRMO features listed in Table 13.1 should be taken into account. The presence of skin disease strongly supports the diagnosis, so biopsy and culture may be unnecessary.

## 13.3
## Adult Osteoarthropathy

Inflammatory predominant osseous lesions of the sternum or the clavicle also occur in adults, sometimes as part of a multifocal disease. The clavicular lesions seem similar to those of children and adolescents apart from the occasional concomitant ossification of the first costal cartilage, whereas sternal lesions occur mainly in adults.

### 13.3.1
### Sclerotic and Hyperostotic Sternocostoclavicular Lesions

#### 13.3.1.1
#### Sclerosis and Hyperostosis of the Sternum

Diffuse inflammatory osseous sclerosis of the manubrium sterni is a rare finding [2, 13, 21, 29, 30, 34, 38, 39, 42, 47]. Less pronounced, localised changes are more common [17, 25, 29, 35, 59] and they probably represent early changes in patients who later develop diffuse sclerosis [30, 34, 38, 39]. The lesions may occur in all adult age groups, but are predominantly seen in women.

Clinically the involvement is characterised by recurrent attacks of pain and swelling in the region of the manubrium sterni and the surrounding joints, often with accompanying shoulder pain, but rarely malaise and fever [39]. The symptoms usually start in the region of one SCC joint and gradually spread in the bone to the region of other joints. The course is fluctuating and prolonged over several years, often with persistence of slight SCC discomfort during remissions [39]. Accompanying PPP occurs in about half of the patients [29, 34, 39, 42, 47].

The findings at conventional or computed tomography in the early stages are characterised by osseous sclerosis of the manubrium sterni adjacent to uneven joint facets, often those of the sternoclavicular and first sternocostal joints, but the sclerosis may also start at the MSJ (Figs. 13.4 and 13.5) [30, 34, 39, 43]. Gradually the sclerosis spreads to involve nearly the entire manubrium. Periosteal new bone formation and lytic areas within the sclerosis are occasionally seen during exacerbations, best delineated at CT (Fig. 13.5) [38, 39]. The disease sometimes crosses the MSJ and the first sternocostal joints, which may ankylose. Changes adjacent to the sternoclavicular joints seem to be different. The joint facets may be uneven, but erosion of the opposite clavicular facets conforming to ordinary arthritis or development of ankylosis is rare. It seems as though the intra-articular disc can resist spread of the disease [30, 34], but accompanying clavicular sclerosis analogous to that of the sternum can occur [30, 34, 38, 39]. Degenerative changes of the sternoclavicular joints in the form of joint space narrowing and/or osteophytes are, however, a frequent finding in late stages [30, 38, 39], and there is usually accompanying ossification of the first costal cartilages, and sometimes also slight ossification of the costoclavicular ligaments [30, 38, 39]. The osseous sclerosis persists for many years and although regression has been observed the bone will never return to normal [38, 39]. Nearly diffuse sclerosis of the manubrium sterni may also occur together with advanced arthritis of the sternoclavicular joints, but it is usually uncertain whether their sclerosis evolved primarily or was secondary to arthritis.

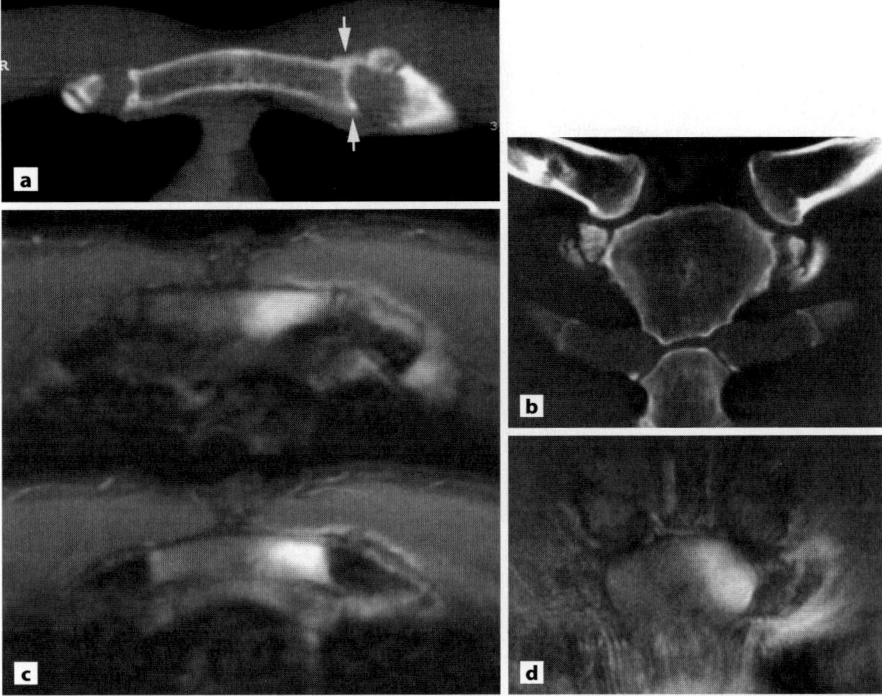

**Fig. 13.4** Early adult osteoarthropathy in a 38-year-old man with pain and swelling corresponding to the left first sternocostal joint during 9 months. **a,b** Axial CT slice (**a**) and coronal reconstruction (**b**) show slight broadening of the sternocostal joint (*arrow*) with irregular joint facet and concomitant calcification of the costal cartilage. **c,d** MRI, axial (**c**) and coronal postcontrast T1 FS (**d**) images showed mainly enhancement of the upper part of the manubrium sterni, but also some enhancement around the adjacent costal cartilage

The findings at MRI depend on the degree and activity of the disease. Active inflammatory areas present as high signal intensity on STIR images and/or enhancement on postcontrast images (Fig. 13.4). There is not always correspondingly low signal intensity on T1-weighted images because sequels of inflammation may have caused fatty marrow changes presenting as high signal intensity. MRI can be used to locate active areas for biopsy, for example guided by CT [43].

Activity in sternal lesions can be detected by scintigraphy, which in addition may reveal concomitant lesions [12, 18].

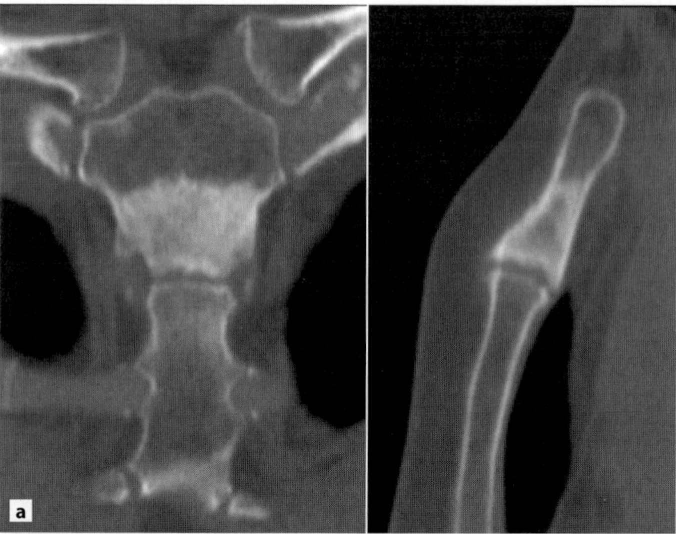

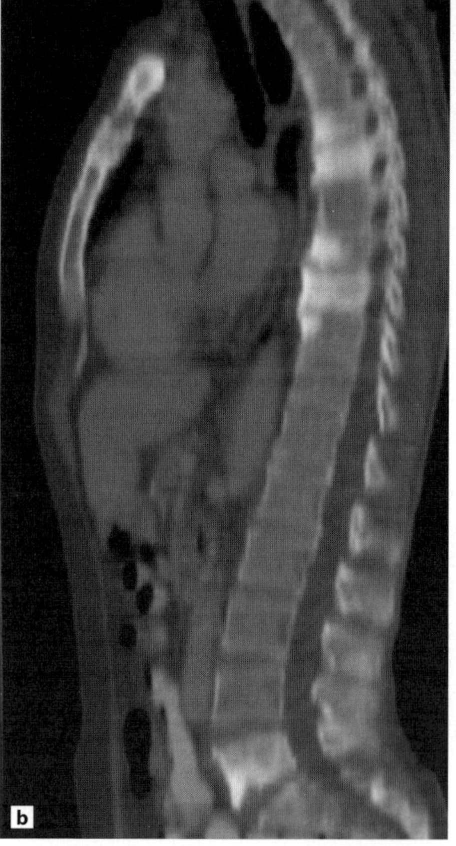

**Fig. 13.5** Advanced adult osteoarthropathy. **a** Coronal and sagittal CT reconstruction in a 47-year-old woman with SCC complaints during 3 years. Sclerosis and hyperostosis of the lower part of the manubrium sterni adjacent to the MSJ, but without changes on the other side of the joints. **b** Ten years later sagittal CT reconstruction of a whole body CT shows diffuse osseous sclerosis of the manubrium sterni extending to the sternal body and accompanied by ankylosis of the MSJ. There are concomitant osseous sclerotic lesions of vertebral bodies with some erosion of the vertebral plates

## 13.3.1.2
## Sclerosis and Hyperostosis of the Clavicle

Adults can have sclerotic and hyperostotic clavicular lesions somewhat similar to those of children and adolescents [37, 42], but often accompanied by ossification of the first costal cartilage [30]. An association of such changes with PPP [42], acne [8] and inflammatory bowel diseases [61] has been described. CRMO-like lesions in adults have been regarded by some as a manifestation of SAPHO [3].

## 13.3.2
## Associated Skeletal Lesions and Other Findings

Sclerotic sternal lesions often occur as an isolated skeletal abnormality, but can be accompanied by vertebral or pelvic bone lesions [29, 38, 39]. Sclerotic lesions of tubular bones may also occur [12].

## 13.3.2.1
## Imaging Features

The vertebral lesions appear as diffuse metastasis-like sclerosis [38, 39] or as a spondylodiscitis with pronounced subchondral sclerosis [29] (Fig. 13.5). The pelvic lesions are usually characterised by pronounced sclerosis adjacent to an uneven joint facet at the pubic symphysis or the sacroiliac joint, but sacroiliitis has also been observed [38, 39]. Hyperostotic and sclerotic clavicular lesions may be accompanied by similar lesions.

## 13.3.2.2
## Biochemical and Histopathological Features

Biochemical findings are non-specific. They mainly consist of elevated ESR or CRP [15, 34, 39, 47] and protein electrophoretic signs of active inflammatory disease during exacerbations. Abnormal WBC and differential counts, and positive serological reaction for bacterial agents are rare [39] (Fig. 13.5). The disorders are not associated with HLA-B27 [39], and tests for rheumatoid factor and antinuclear antibodies are negative [37] as are bacterial cultures for pathogens [37]. *Propionibacterium acnes* has been reported [43, 44], but is probably due to contamination.

The histopathological findings are also non-specific. They consist of spongiosclerosis with broad trabeculae of bone surrounding relatively small marrow spaces filled with a fibrovascular material that occasionally contains lymphocytes and plasma cells [2, 15, 34, 39]. The detection of inflammatory changes, however, depends upon the disease activity at the time of examination [37].


### 13.3.3
### Differential Diagnoses

The main differential diagnoses of inflammatory osseous lesions in adults are chronic infectious osteitis, benign and malignant osteoblastic bone tumours, metastatic and lymphoproliferative lesions, Paget's disease and metabolic disorders.


### 13.4
### Terminology

Hyperostotic and sclerotic SCC lesions in adults are generally rare findings. This may be the reason for the varying nomenclature. During recent years the two most frequent used terms are "pustulotic arthro-osteitis" (PAO) and SAPHO syndrome (synovitis acne-pustulosis-hyperostosis-osteitis) [12, 43]. The sternal lesions have, however, been described under the terms SCCH [21], "sternocostoclavicular arthro-osteitis" [17] and "acquired hyperostosis syndrome" [13]. They have also be named "skeletal lesions associated with PPP" [25, 42], "sternal hyperostosis" [2] and "sclerotic changes or sclerosis and hyperostosis of the manubrium sterni" [38, 39]. Sclerotic clavicular lesions occurring in adults have been named PAO, SCCH, SAPHO syndrome [54], "clavicular hyperostosis", "multiple hyperostosis with unilateral sacroiliitis" and "bone lesions associated with PPP" [42].

The lesions of children and adolescents have been described under several headings such as SAPHO [10, 16, 56, 60], "recurrent hyperostosis of the clavicle", "clavicular hyperostosis", "idiopathic cortical hyperostosis", "condensing osteitis of the clavicle", "sclerosing osteitis", "inflammatory metachronous hyperostosis of the clavicle", "chronic sclerosing osteomyelitis or inflammatory hyperostosis and sclerosis of the clavicle" [37], "tumour of the medial end of the clavicle" and "bone lesions associated with PPP or acne" [42]. When part of a multifocal disease, the changes have often been termed CRMO [6, 37, 52], but also "chronic multifocal cleido-metaphyseal osteomyelitis" [50] and "subacute and chronic symmetrical osteomyelitis".

The disorder of children and adolescents conforming to CRMO has by some been regarded a paediatric variant of the SAPHO syndrome, a term coined for diseases that manifest sterile inflammatory bone lesions together with skin eruptions [3, 58]. This only points to a connection with SpA in adulthood, but can be confusing.

The finding of PPP in some of the patients indicates that the lesions represent a manifestation of a seronegative osteoarthropathy, and the nomenclature should be in accordance with this.

The clinical, radiographic, laboratory and histopathological findings are similar in patients with and without PPP [6, 37–39, 52]. Irrespective of the presence of PPP, the abnormalities probably represent identical diseases. It may be hypothesised that some of the patients with osseous sclerotic SCC lesions, but no PPP, have a PPP-related involvement without manifest skin disease. The time lag often occurring between the skin and SCC lesions in patients with both findings implies that some patients for a period have only one of the findings [31]. Patients without accompanying PPP may later develop it.


# 13.5
# Conclusions

Chronic recurrent multifocal osteomyelitis is a clinical entity different from bacterial osteomyelitis. It mainly occurs in children and adolescents and is characterised by a prolonged, fluctuating course with recurrent episodes of pain occurring over several years. It is often multifocal and can involve the clavicle. The radiographic picture suggests subacute or chronic osteomyelitis. Histopathological and laboratory findings are non-specific and bacterial culture negative. CRMO lesions are often diagnosed by exclusion of the two main differential diagnoses, infectious diseases and tumours, by its characteristic course and the findings by conventional radiography, if necessary supplemented by scintigraphy and/or MRI. The MRI features of clavicular lesions may however be non-specific unless it displays a bone within bone appearance. Inflammatory predominant osseous SCC lesions also occur in adults located to the sternum or the clavicle. They may simulate tumour, Paget's disease, chronic infection and metabolic disorders. The presence of concomitant dermal disease supports the diagnosis. In case of doubt, complementary biopsy with histopathology and culture must be performed.

It is important to be aware of these rare disorders and make the diagnosis in order to avoid unnecessary diagnostic procedures, initiate an appropriate therapy with non-steroidal anti-inflammatory drugs and inform the patient about the relatively benign, but usually prolonged and recurrent course.

The occurrence of osseous sclerotic SCC lesions in both adults and children and adolescents sometimes accompanied by lesions of other bones and PPP indicates that they may be similar diseases just with a different location depending on age.

A female predominance in both groups supports this. Based on a frequent association with PPP, the lesions of adults can be regarded as a sign of a seronegative PPP-related osteoarthropathy, and the disorder of children and adolescents has to be classified accordingly.

## References


1. Andersson R (1995) Effective treatment with interferon-alpha in chronic recurrent multifocal osteomyelitis. J Interferon Cytokine Res 15:837–838
2. Bechtold RE, Karstaedt N, Wolfman NT (1990) MR appearance of sternal hyperostosis. J Comput Assist Tomogr 14:136–139
3. Beretta-Piccoli BC, Sauvain MJ, Gal I, Schibler A, Saurenmann T, Kressebuch H, Bianchetti MG (2000) Synovitis, acne, pustulosis, hyperostosis, osteitis (SAPHO) syndrome in childhood: a report of ten cases and review of the literature. Eur J Pediatr 159:594–601
4. Bjorksten B, Boquist L (1980) Histopathological aspects of chronic recurrent multifocal osteomyelitis. J Bone Joint Surg Br 62:376–380
5. Bjorksten B, Gustavson KH, Eriksson B, Lindholm A, Nordstrom S (1978) Chronic recurrent multifocal osteomyelitis and pustulosis palmoplantaris. J Pediatr 93:227–231
6. Björkstén B, Gustavson K-H, Eriksson B, Lindholm, Nordström S (1978) Chronic recurrent multifocal osteomyelitis and pustulosis palmoplantaris. J Pediatr 93:227–231
7. Bognar M, Blake W, Agudelo C (1998) Chronic recurrent multifocal osteomyelitis associated with Crohn's disease. Am J Med Sci 315:133–135
8. Bookbinder SA, Fenske NA, Clement GB, Espinoza LR, Germain BF, Vasey FB (1982) Clavicular hyperostosis and acne arthritis. Ann Intern Med 97:615–616
9. Bousvaros A, Marcon M, Treem W, Waters P, Issenman R, Couper R, Burnell R, Rosenberg A, Rabinovich E, Kirschner BS (1999) Chronic recurrent multifocal osteomyelitis associated with chronic inflammatory bowel disease in children. Dig Dis Sci 44:2500–2507
10. Caravatti M, Wiesli P, Uebelhart D, Germann D, Welzl-Hinterkorner E, Schulthess G (2002) Coincidence of Behçet's disease and SAPHO syndrome. Clin Rheumatol 21:324–327
11. Carr AJ, Cole WG, Roberton DM, Chow CW (1993) Chronic multifocal osteomyelitis. J Bone Joint Surg Br 75:582–591
12. Davies AM, Marino AJ, Evans N, Grimer RJ, Deshmukh N, Mangham DC (1999) SAPHO syndrome: 20-year follow-up. Skeletal Radiol 28:159–162
13. Dihlmann W, Hering L, Bargon GW (1988) Das akquirierte Hyperostose-Syndrom (AHS). Synthese aus 13 eigenen Beobachtungen von sternokostoklavikulärer Hyperostose und über 300 Fällen aus der Literatur, Teil 1. Fortschr Röntgenstr 149:386–391
14. Duffy CM, Lam PY, Ditchfield M, Allen R, Graham HK (2002) Chronic recurrent multifocal osteomyelitis: review of orthopaedic complications at maturity. J Pediatr Orthop 22:501–505

15. Dumolard A, Gaudin P, Juvin R, Bost M, Peoc'h M, Phelip X (1999) SAPHO syndrome or psoriatic arthritis? A familial case study. Rheumatology (Oxford) 38:463–467

16. Earwaker JW, Cotten A (2003) SAPHO: syndrome or concept? Imaging findings. Skeletal Radiol 32:311–327

17. Edlund E, Johnsson U, Lidgren L, Pettersson H, Sturfelt G, Svensson B, Theander J, Willén H (1988) Palmoplantar pustulosis and sternocostoclavicular arthro-osteitis. Ann Rheum Dis 47:809–815

18. Freyschmidt J, Sternberg A (1998) The bullhead sign: scintigraphic pattern of sternocostoclavicular hyperostosis and pustulotic arthroosteitis. Eur Radiol 8:807–812

19. Gallagher KT, Roberts RL, MacFarlane JA, Stiehm ER (1997) Treatment of chronic recurrent multifocal osteomyelitis with interferon gamma. J Pediatr 131:470–472

20. Gamble JG, Rinsky LA (1986) Chronic recurrent multifocal osteomyelitis: a distinct clinical entity. J Pediatr Orthop 6:579–584

21. Geake T (1988) Sterno-costoclavicular hyperostosis. A report of two new cases and review. Australas Radiol 32:440–443

22. Girschick HJ, Krauspe R, Tschammler A, Huppertz HI (1998) Chronic recurrent osteomyelitis with clavicular involvement in children: diagnostic value of different imaging techniques and therapy with non-steroidal anti-inflammatory drugs. Eur J Pediatr 157:28–33

23. Girschick HJ, Raab P, Surbaum S, Trusen A, Kirschner S, Schneider P, Papadopoulos T, Muller-Hermelink HK, Lipsky PE (2005) Chronic non-bacterial osteomyelitis in children. Ann Rheum Dis 64:279–285

24. Handrick W, Hormann D, Voppmann A, Schille R, Reichardt P, Trobs RB, Moritz RP, Borte M (1998) Chronic recurrent multifocal osteomyelitis: report of eight patients. Pediatr Surg Int 14:195–198

25. Hradil E, Gents C-F, Matilainen T, Möller H, Sanzén L, Udén A (1988) Skeletal involvement in pustulosis palmoplantaris with special reference to the sterno-costo-clavicular joints. Acta Derm Venereol (Stockh) 68:65–73

26. Huaux JP, Esselinckx W, Rombouts JJ, Maldague B, Malghem J, Devogelaer JP, Nagant dD (1988) Pustulotic arthroosteitis and chronic recurrent multifocal osteomyelitis in children. Report of three cases. J Rheumatol 15:95–100

27. Huber AM, Lam PY, Duffy CM, Yeung RS, Ditchfield M, Laxer D, Cole WG, Kerr GH, Allen RC, Laxer RM (2002) Chronic recurrent multifocal osteomyelitis: clinical outcomes after more than five years of follow-up. J Pediatr 141:198–203

28. Job-Deslandre C, Krebs S, Kahan A (2001) Chronic recurrent multifocal osteomyelitis: five-year outcomes in 14 pediatric cases. Joint Bone Spine 68:245–251

29. Jurik AG (1990) Anterior chest wall involvement in patients with pustulosis palmoplantaris. Skeletal Radiol 19:271–277

30. Jurik AG (1991) Seronegative arthritides of the anterior chest wall: a follow-up study. Skeletal Radiol 20:517–525

31. Jurik AG (1992) Seronegative anterior chest wall syndromes. A study of the findings and course at radiography. Acta Radiol Suppl 301:1–42

32. Jurik AG (2004) Chronic recurrent multifocal osteomyelitis. Semin Musculoskelet Radiol 8:243–253

33. Jurik AG, Egund N (1997) MRI in chronic recurrent multifocal osteomyelitis. Skeletal Radiol 26:230–238

34. Jurik AG, Graudal H (1987) Monarthritis of the manubriosternal joint. A follow-up study. Rheumatol Int 7:235–241

35. Jurik AG, Graudal H (1988) Sternocostal joint swelling: clinical Tietze's syndrome. Report of sixteen cases and review of the literature. Scand J Rheumatol 17:33–42

36. Jurik AG, Moller BN (1986) Inflammatory hyperostosis and sclerosis of the clavicle. Skeletal Radiol 15:284–290

37. Jurik AG, Moller BN (1987) Chronic sclerosing osteomyelitis of the clavicle. A manifestation of chronic recurrent multifocal osteomyelitis. Arch Orthop Trauma Surg 106:144–151

38. Jurik AG, Graudal H, de Carvalho A (1985) Sclerotic changes of the manubrium sterni. Skeletal Radiol 13:195–201

39. Jurik AG, Moller BN, Jensen MK, Jensen JT, Graudal H (1986) Sclerosis and hyperostosis of the manubrium sterni. Rheumatol Int 6:171–178

40. Jurik AG, Helmig O, Ternowitz T, Moller BN (1988) Chronic recurrent multifocal osteomyelitis: a follow-up study. J Pediatr Orthop 8:49–58

41. Jurriaans E, Singh NP, Finlay K, Friedman L (2001) Imaging of chronic recurrent multifocal osteomyelitis. Radiol Clin North Am 39:305–327

42. Kawai K, Doita M, Tateshi H, Hirobata K (1988) Bone and joint lesions associated with pustulosis palmaris et plantaris. J Bone Joint Surg Br 70:117–122

43. Kirchhoff T, Merkesdal S, Rosenthal H, Prokop M, Chavan A, Wagner A, Mai U, Hammer M, Zeidler H, Galanski M (2003) Diagnostic management of patients with SAPHO syndrome: use of MR imaging to guide bone biopsy at CT for microbiological and histological work-up. Eur Radiol 13:2304–2308

44. Kotilainen P, Merilahti-Palo R, Lehtonen OP, Manner I, Helander I, Mottonen T, Rintala E (1996) *Propionibacterium acnes* isolated from sternal osteitis in a patient with SAPHO syndrome. J Rheumatol 23:1302–1304

45. Mandell GA, Contreras SJ, Conard K, Harcke HT, Maas KW (1998) Bone scintigraphy in the detection of chronic recurrent multifocal osteomyelitis. J Nucl Med 39:1778–1783

46. Mortensson W, Edeburn G, Fries M, Nilsson R (1988) Chronic recurrent multifocal osteomyelitis in children. A roentgenologic and scintigraphic investigation. Acta Radiol 29:565–570

47. Otsuka N, Fukunaga M, Sone T, Nagai K, Tomomitsu T, Yanagimoto S, Muranaka A, Ono S, Morita R (1986) Usefulness of bone imaging in diagnosis of sterno-costo-clavicular hyperostosis. Clin Nucl Med 11:651–652

48. Paller AS, Pachman L, Rich K, Esterly NB, Gonzalez-Crussi F (1985) Pustulosis palmaris et plantaris: its association with chronic recurrent multifocal osteomyelitis. J Am Acad Dermatol 12:927–930

49. Pelkonen P, Ryoppy S, Jaaskelainen J, Rapola J, Repo H, Kaitila I (1988) Chronic osteomyelitis-like disease with negative bacterial cultures. Am J Dis Child 142:1167–1173

50. Probst FP (1976) Chronic multifocal cleido-metaphyseal osteomyelitis of childhood. Report of a case. Acta Radiol Diagn (Stockh) 17:531–537

51. Probst FP (1984) Chronic recurrent multifocal osteomyelitis. Case report and overview as a contribution to the knowledge about the disease. Radiologe 24:24–30

52. Probst FP, Bjorksten B, Gustavson KH (1978) Radiological aspect of chronic recurrent multifocal osteomyelitis. Ann Radiol (Paris) 21:115–125

53. Raja S, Goel A, Paul A (2003) Sternoclavicular hyperostosis with pathological fracture of the clavicle: a case report. Injury 34:464–466

54. Reith JD, Bauer TW, Schils JP (1996) Osseous manifestations of SAPHO (synovitis, acne, pustulosis, hyperostosis, osteitis) syndrome. Am J Surg Pathol 20:1368–1377

55. Schultz C, Holterhus PM, Seidel A, Jonas S, Barthel M, Kruse K, Bucsky P (1999) Chronic recurrent multifocal osteomyelitis in children. Pediatr Infect Dis J 18:1008–1013

56. Sidhu G, Andrews G, Forster B, Keogh C (2003) Residents' corner. Answer to case of the month #89. Chronic recurrent multifocal osteomyelitis as a presentation of SAPHO syndrome. Can Assoc Radiol J 54:189–191

57. Stanton RP, Lopez-Sosa FH, Doidge R (1993) Chronic recurrent multifocal osteomyelitis. Orthop Rev 22:229–233

58. Sugimoto H, Tamura K, Fujii T (1998) The SAPHO syndrome: defining the radiologic spectrum of diseases comprising the syndrome. Eur Radiol 8:800–806

59. Van Doornum S, Barraclough D, McColl G, Wicks I (2000) SAPHO: rare or just not recognized? Semin Arthritis Rheum 30:70–77

60. Vanin E, Drigo P, Martini G, Gigante C, Chiozza ML, Marcazzo L, Zulian F (2002) SAPHO syndrome and transient hemiparesis in a child: coincidence or new association? J Rheumatol 29:384–387

61. Verbruggen LA, Buyck R, Handelberg F (1985) Clavicular periosteal new bone formation in ulcerative colitis. Clin Exp Rheumatol 3:163–166

62. Vittecoq O, Said LA, Michot C, Mejjad O, Thomine JM, Mitrofanoff P, Lechevallier J, Ledosseur P, Gayet A, Lauret P, le Loet X (2000) Evolution of chronic recurrent multifocal osteitis toward spondylarthropathy over the long term. Arthritis Rheum 43:109–119

# 14 Other Rheumatic Inflammatory Disorders

ANNE GRETHE JURIK

**Contents**



## 14.1 Introduction

All rheumatic inflammatory disorders can involve the sternocostoclavicular (SCC) region. The most frequently encountered disorder is osteoarthritis (Chapter 15), but other manifestations of arthritides such as rheumatoid arthritis also occur. Moreover, involvement of SCC joints can occur as the only disease manifestation.

## 14.2 Rheumatoid Arthritis

Rheumatoid arthritis (RA) can involve any of the SCC joints, but especially the sternoclavicular joint [42]. The frequency of SCC involvement in RA is, however, low compared to that of seronegative spondylarthropathies (SpA). Clinical evidence of SCC joint involvement in RA occurs in only 10% of patients with RA, although symptoms of pain and swelling related to the sternoclavicular, MSJ and sternocostal articulations when looked for may be present in more than 70% of patients with erosive RA [28].

The pathoanatomical RA changes in the sternoclavicular joints are similar to those in other joints, including pannus formation and bony erosion [45]. The involvement of the MSJ in RA may be related to the occasional occurrence of synovia in the MSJ [29, 43, 44] or spread of inflammation from the adjacent synovial second sternocostal joints. At autopsy over half of RA patients have been found to have erosion of the MSJ [29].

The symptoms of joint involvement may be overlooked or misinterpreted as caused by shoulder or neck involvement [15]. RA involvement of the SCC joints is therefore seldom obtained at imaging.

## 14.2.1
## Sternoclavicular Joints

Clinical signs of sternoclavicular joint involvement consist of pain, tenderness and swelling. It has been reported present in 1–19% of patients with RA [9, 17, 30], but may be more frequent when specially looked for.

Radiographic features are like those of other synovial joints involved by RA characterised by subchondral and marginal erosions, and joint space narrowing (Fig. 14.1) [24]. However, involvement of the sternoclavicular joints in RA can manifest as large synovial cysts or a more solid tumour-like mass representing a rheumatoid nodule [1, 11]. Such lesions demands ultrasonography or MRI for obtaining the diagnosis.

## 14.2.2
## Manubriosternal Joint

Clinical signs of MSJ involvement consist of pain, swelling and tenderness. In comparison with the sternoclavicular joint, clinical involvement of the MSJ is relatively infrequent in RA, occurring in 2–9% of patients [9, 17]. Based on radiographic analysis the joint has been found more frequently involved [29]. The lack of specific symptoms referred to MSJ involvement may be due to symptoms presenting as referred pain or resembling pleuritic pain [10]. Involvement occurs especially in patients with an aggressive and destructive course. There can be complicating MSJ subluxation, described associated with severe cervical spine disease [31] or thoracic kyphosis [28]. Complicating septic arthritis can also occur (Chapter 16; Fig. 16.1).

On lateral radiographs the changes consist of diminution in height of the fibrocartilage with erosion or slight irregularity of the bony ends [10, 41]. The osseous

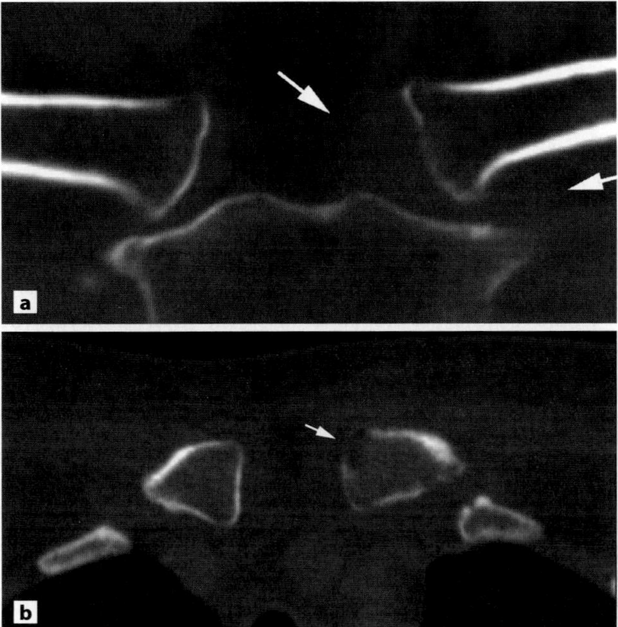

**Fig. 14.1** Rheumatoid arthritis in a 52-year-old woman with known seropositive erosive peripheral RA for 10 years and pain, swelling and tenderness corresponding to the left sternoclavicular joint during 2 months. **a** Initial CT, coronal reconstruction shows distension of the left sternoclavicular joint (*arrows*) and superficial erosion of the lower two thirds of the clavicular joint surface. **b** Six months later, axial CT slice shows clavicular erosion (*arrow*)

proliferation seen in SpA does not occur, but some of the abnormalities detected have also been observed in healthy persons [41]. Radiographic changes have been reported in 15–71% of RA patients [9, 14, 31, 44]. However, unequivocal radiographic abnormalities are also frequent in patients in the same age range, having osteoarthritis, found to occur in 32% of patients compared with 44% of patients with RA [46].

## 14.3
## Gout

Acute gout may involve the SCC region although rarely. The sternoclavicular joint [12, 40], the costochondral articulations [12] and the MSJ [27] can be affected.

The appearance by radiography is not specific and may simulate degenerative changes [27]. The definite diagnosis is obtained by arthrocentesis followed by polarising microscopy showing needle-shaped crystals, or by histology in the rare occurrence of tophus formation [45].


## 14.4
## Pseudogout – Chondrocalcinosis

Calcium pyrophosphate deposition disease (CPPD) mainly occurs in the knees, wrists, hips, glenohumeral and acromioclavicular joints, but can involve the SCC region. Involvement of the sternoclavicular joint predominantly occurs in the polyarticular form of chondrocalcinosis.

The radiological changes consist of calcification in the articular disc and usually a gradual development of secondary degenerative changes with marginal osteophytes, particular on the clavicles [37, 49]. Involvement of the MSJ may also occur, probably corresponding to the occasional involvement of the pubic symphysis [37]. The rare occurrence of tophaceous CPPD in the soft tissue of the SCC region simulating chondrosarcoma have been described [38].


## 14.5
## Monarthritis

Monarthritis of the SCC region is rare, but can occur corresponding to the sternoclavicular, manubriosternal and sternocostal joints. Such involvement should always be considered as a differential diagnosis of chest and shoulder pain and/or swelling in the SCC region. Involvement of the SCC joints may manifest as pain referred to areas distant from the joints [15, 21, 22].

*Monarthritis of the sternoclavicular joint* without evidence of systemic disease and radiography showing erosion of the clavicular end have been reported in postmenopausal women corresponding to the dominant sternoclavicular joint and resolving within a year [5]. Such changes are usually due to degenerative changes. Consistent with this, self-limited monoarticular subacute arthritis of the sternoclavicular joint has also been reported on the dominant side in women performing strenuous physical activities [13]. It probably represents post-traumatic arthritis or erosive episodes as part of osteoarthritis. Osteoarthritis presenting as monarthritis of the sternoclavicular joint may be more common than is usually recognised (Chapter 15).

*Monarthritis of the manubriosternal joint* is rare [20, 33, 34, 36]. In the early reports it was suggested to be due to trauma [33, 34] or to repeated overexertion by hard manual work [36], which can have elicited osteoarthritis. In later studies an association with PPP, psoriasis, acne and HLA-B27 was observed [19, 20]. This indicated that MSJ monarthritis sometimes belongs to the group of seronegative arthritides. In accordance with this, MSJ arthritis may occasionally be the first manifestation of a generalised arthritis, and then for a period be monoarticular [18, 20]. However, persistent MSJ monarthritis may occur and can be associated with psoriasis vulgaris or HLA-B27 (Fig. 14.2).

The MSJ monarthritis associated with psoriasis, psoriasis in the family or HLA-B27 may be viewed as a variant of psoriatic or reactive arthritis, although triggering infection may escape detection [18, 20]. The involvement associated with PPP or acne can be regarded as a sign of a PPP- or acne-associated arthropathy (Chapter 12).

The pain of MSJ involvement often radiates to the shoulders, and sometimes also to the arms. If it is precipitated by exertion, it can simulate angina [4, 20].

*Monarthritis of the sternocostal joint* is also a rare finding. It may occur as a sign of degenerative changes or be the first manifestation of a systemic disease

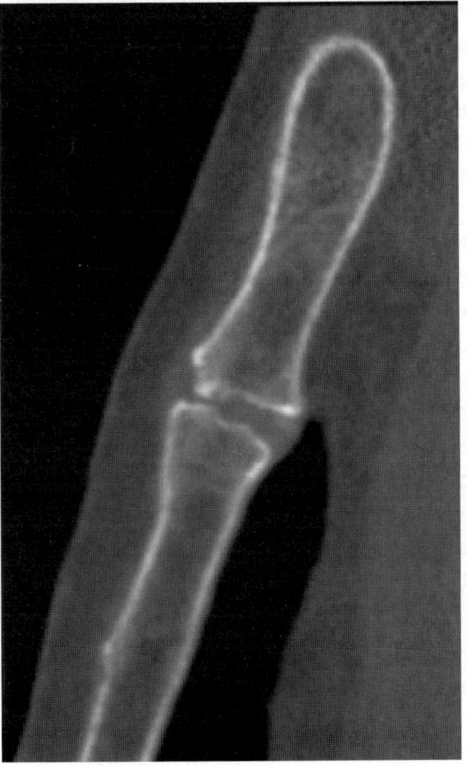

Fig. 14.2 Monarthritis of the MSJ in a 48-year-old woman with psoriasis. Sagittal CT reconstruction shows erosion of the joint facets and distension of the capsule posteriorly

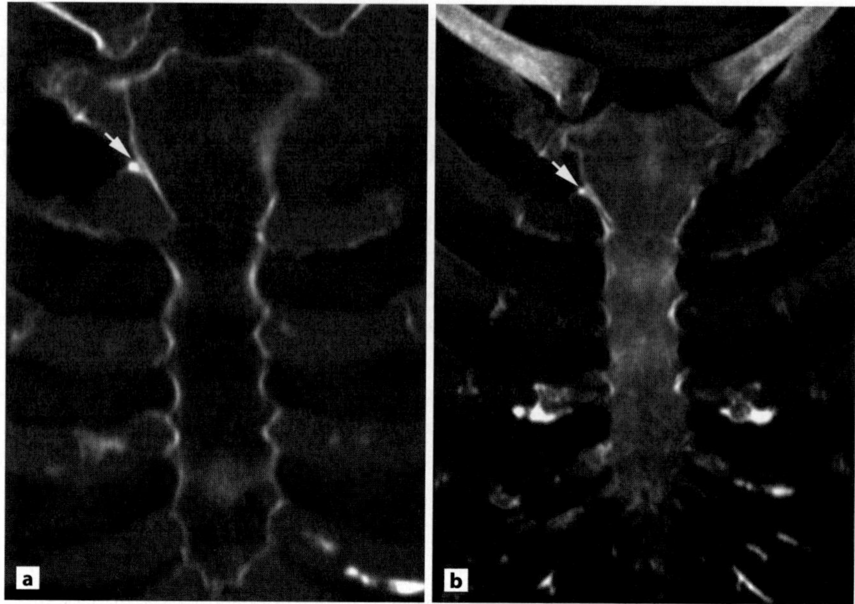

**Fig. 14.3** Osteoarthritis of the second right sternocostal joint in a 56-year-old man with synostosis of the MSJ. **a** Coronal CT reconstruction and **b** VIP view show broadening of the right second sternocostal joint with osteophyte formation (*arrow*)

(Fig. 14.3) [21]. Such changes have sometimes been termed Tietze's syndrome. This syndrome was described in 1921 as a benign self-limiting entity characterised by non-suppurative, tender, painful swelling of costal cartilage of unknown aetiology, and absence of other lesions that could establish a definite diagnosis [25, 32]. Despite the definition several disorders have been described under the term, comprising sternocostal joint swellings as part of rheumatoid [39] or seronegative arthritis [8], rheumatic fever [8] and gout [12]. Patients with idiopathic monarthritis of the sternoclavicular joint have also been included under the term Tietze's syndrome [26, 47], which should be reserved for sternocostal swellings of unknown origin and without associated disorders [23].

When looked for there are often well-defined disorders causing swelling of sternocostal joints. An analysis of 16 patients with rather similar sternocostal joint swellings disclosed different types of disorders. Nine patients had no other diseases. Five patients had concomitant PPP and/or psoriasis, one also systemic arthritic disorder, and two had HLA-B27-associated sacroiliitis. Radiographic changes with a possible bearing upon the condition occurred in seven of the nine patients with isolated sternocostal joint changes. Three patients had sternocostal joint osteoarthritis, two had persistent segmentation between the two upper segments of the sternal body, and two had ankylosis of the MSJ. Conventional tomography was normal in two patients, and a subsequent CT revealed non-specific enlargement of the involved costal cartilage adjacent to the sternum. According to the definition, the name Tietze's syndrome is to be used only in the two patients with non-specific cartilage enlargement visualised by CT. The involvement of the other seven patients with isolated sternocostal joint changes should be named in accordance with the finding of anatomical variants and/or degenerative changes.

All the patients with skin disease or HLA-B27 had radiographic changes, either erosion of the involved first sternocostal joint or erosion and/or ankylosis of the MSJ with irregularity of the adjacent second sternocostal joint. The sternocostal joint involvement in patients with systemic arthritis and/or skin disease can be regarded as a sign of seronegative arthritis, and has to be classified accordingly.

The second sternocostal joints and costal cartilages are the sites most frequently involved clinically, followed by the level of the third and fourth cartilages, equally often on the right and left side [21, 25, 32]. Involvement predominantly at the MSJ may be explained by the strain imposed on the MSJ during respiration as local strain generated during respiration can cause osteoarthrosis. One of our patients with osteoarthritis had a displaced sternal joint, and one had MSJ synostosis, conditions that alter the pattern of sternocostal mobility and can thereby cause strain on the cartilages and/or sternocostal joints during respiration (Fig. 14.3) [21]. Also the persistent sternal segmentation may alter the strain pattern [3, 21].

The SCC symptoms and clinical findings in patients with sternocostal joint swellings are rather uniform [21]. There are typically swelling and pain aggravated by deep inspiration, coughing and sneezing. The pain sometimes radiates to the shoulder [21, 25, 32] and may simulate angina [2]. The duration of symptoms varies. The pain can subside and the swelling diminish, but usually there is persistence of a hard non-tender swelling [21].

## 14.6
## Other Disorders

Other inflammatory disorders including relapsing polychondritis and Behçet's syndrome can involve the SCC region.

*Relapsing polychondritis* is considered an acquired disorder of mucopolysaccharide metabolism with a possible hypersensitivity or altered immunity component [35]. Chondritis of the ear and nose is the most common manifestation, but involvement of the costal cartilage also occurs. This causes anterior chest wall pain and the diagnosis can be suspected by increased tracer uptake at scintigraphy corresponding to the cartilages, but has to be confirmed histologically [16].

*Behçet's syndrome* is a rare clinical triad of recurrent mouth ulcers, genital ulcers and anterior uveitis. It can be associated with joint symptoms located to the SCC region [7, 48], and also clavicular hyperostosis in children [6].

## 14.7
## Conclusion

All rheumatic inflammatory disorders can involve the SCC region. SCC involvement may, however, be overlooked or misinterpreted due to the pain being referred to regions distant from the joints.

Manubriosternal joint arthritis may occasionally be the first manifestation of a generalised arthritis, and may then for a period be monoarticular. Persistent MSJ monarthritis is a rare finding, which sometimes occurs together with psoriasis or HLA-B27.

Monoarticular swelling of sternocostal joints may be due to anatomical variants, osteoarthritis and arthritic changes. Such swelling is sometimes termed Tietze's syndrome. To avoid misinterpretation this term should be used only if there is no detectable cause of the swelling at imaging or clinically.

In non-rheumatology clinics SCC pain and swelling may be regarded as signs of tumour, and the symptoms can be interpreted as signs of cardiac disease.

## References

1.  Andonopoulos AP, Meimaris N, Yiannopoulos G, Pastromas V, Dimopoulos P (2003) Large synovial cysts originating from the sternoclavicular joints in a patient with rheumatoid arthritis. Ann Rheum Dis 62:1119–1120
2.  Ausubel H, Cohen BD, Ladue JS (1959) Tietze's disease of eight years' duration. N Engl J Med 261:190
3.  Baas J, Eijsvogel M, Dijkstra P (1988) Persistent sternum synchondroses on bone scintigraphy. Eur J Nucl Med 13:572–573
4.  Bogdan A, Clark J (1950) The manubrio-sternal joint in rheumatoid arthritis. Br Med J 2:1361–1362
5.  Bremner RA (1959) Monarticular, non-infective subacute arthritis of the sterno-clavicular joint. J Bone Joint Surg Br 41-B:749–753
6.  Caravatti M, Wiesli P, Uebelhart D, Germann D, Welzl-Hinterkorner E, Schulthess G (2002) Coincidence of Behçet's disease and SAPHO syndrome. Clin Rheumatol 21:324–327

7.  Currey HL, Elson RA, Mason RM (1968) Surgical treatment of manubrio-sternal pain in Behçet's syndrome. Report of a case. J Bone Joint Surg Br 50:836–840

8.  DeHaas WHD (1952) Tietze's syndrome (in Dutch with English summary). Ned Tijdschr Geneeskd 96:254–256

9.  Dilsen N, McEwen C, Poppel M, Gersh WJ, DiTata D, Carmel P (1962) A comparative roentgenologic study of rheumatoid arthritis and rheumatoid (ankylosing) spondylitis. Arthritis Rheum 5:341–368

10.  Doube A, Clarke AK (1989) Symptomatic manubriosternal joint involvement in rheumatoid arthritis. Ann Rheum Dis 48:516–517

11.  Dura PA, Daniel TM, Frierson HF Jr, Brunner CM (1993) Chest wall mass in rheumatoid arthritis. J Rheumatol 20:910–912

12.  Frank M, De Vries A, Atsmon A (1960) Gout simulating cardiac pain. Am J Cardiol 6:929–932

13.  Glay A (1961) Destructive lesions of the clavicle. J Can Assoc Radiol 12:117–125

14.  Grosbois B, Pawlotsky Y, Chalès G, Meadeb J, Carsin M, Louboutin JY (1981) Etude clinique et radiologique de l'articulation manubrio-sternale. Comparaison entre 80 sujets témoins et 88 patients atteints de rhumatismes inflammatoires chroniques. Rev Rhum 48:495–503

15.  Hassett G, Barnsley L (2001) Pain referral from the sternoclavicular joint: a study in normal volunteers. Rheumatology (Oxford) 40:859–862

16.  Imanishi Y, Mitogawa Y, Takizawa M, Konno S, Samuta H, Ohsawa A, Kawaguchi A, Fujikawa M, Sakaida H, Shinagawa T, Yamashita H (1999) Relapsing polychondritis diagnosed by Tc-99m MDP bone scintigraphy. Clin Nucl Med 24:511–513

17.  Julkunen H (1962) Rheumatoid spondylitis. Clinical and laboratory study of 149 cases compared with 182 cases of rheumatoid arthritis. Acta Rheumatol Scand Suppl 4:1–110

18.  Jurik AG (1991) Seronegative arthritides of the anterior chest wall: a follow-up study. Skeletal Radiol 20:517–525

19.  Jurik AG (1992) Seronegative anterior chest wall syndromes. A study of the findings and course at radiography. Acta Radiol Suppl 301:1–42

20.  Jurik AG, Graudal H (1987) Monarthritis of the manubriosternal joint. A follow-up study. Rheumatol Int 7:235–241

21.  Jurik AG, Graudal H (1988) Sternocostal joint swelling: clinical Tietze's syndrome. Report of sixteen cases and review of the literature. Scand J Rheumatol 17:33–42

22.  Jurik AG, Moller BN, Jensen MK, Jensen JT, Graudal H (1986) Sclerosis and hyperostosis of the manubrium sterni. Rheumatol Int 6:171–178

23.  Jurik AG, Justesen T, Graudal H (1987) Radiographic findings in patients with clinical Tietze syndrome. Skeletal Radiol 16:517–523

24.  Kalliomaki JL, Viitanen SM, Virtama P (1968) Radiological findings of sternoclavicular joints in rheumatoid arthritis. Acta Rheumatol Scand 14:233–240

25.  Kayser HL (1956) Tietze's syndrome. A review of the literature. Am J Med 21:982–989

26.  Kennedy AC (1957) Tietze's syndrome: an unusual cause of chest wall swelling. Scott Med J 2:363–365

27. Kernodle GW, Allen NB (1986) Acute gout presenting in the manubriosternal joint. Arthritis Rheum 29:570–572

28. Khong TK, Rooney PJ (1982) Manubriosternal joint subluxation in rheumatoid arthritis. J Rheumatol 9:712–715

29. Kormano M (1970) A microradiographic and histological study of the manubrio-sternal joint in rheumatoid arthritis. Acta Rheumatol Scand 16:47–59

30. Laine VA, Vainio KJ, Pekanmaki K (1954) Shoulder affections in rheumatoid arthritis. Ann Rheum Dis 13:157–160

31. Laitinen H, Saksanen S, Suoranta H (1970) Involvement of the manubrio-sternal articulation in rheumatoid arthritis. Acta Rheum Scand 16:40–46

32. Levey GS, Calabro JJ (1962) Tietze's syndrome: report of two cases and review of the literature. Arthritis Rheum 5:261–269

33. Litchman HM, Silver CM, Simon SD, Tamura H (1969) Post-traumatic degenerative arthrosis in the manubrio-sternal joint. Clin Orthop 67:111–115

34. Lundholm G (1959) Arthritis in the manubriosternal joint after trauma. Acta Orthop Scand 29:90–97

35. McAdam LP, O'Hanlan MA, Bluestone R, Pearson CM (1976) Relapsing polychondritis: prospective study of 23 patients and a review of the literature. Medicine (Baltimore) 55:193–215

36. Reiter R (1956) Zur Kenntnis der sogenannten Chondritis und Perichondritis der oberen Synchondrose des Sternums. Z Orthop 87:436–446

37. Resnick D, Niwayama G, Goergen TG, Utsinger PD, Shapiro RF, Haselwood DH, Wiesner KB (1977) Clinical, radiographic and pathologic abnormalities in calcium pyrophosphate dihydrate deposition disease (CPPD): pseudogout. Radiology 122:1–15

38. Richman KM, Boutin RD, Vaughan LM, Haghighi P, Resnick D (1999) Tophaceous pseudogout of the sternoclavicular joint. Am J Roentgenol 172:1587–1589

39. Roberts AE (1958) Tietze's syndrome. Pa Med J 61:1497–1498

40. Sant GR, Dias E (1976) Primary gout affecting the sternoclavicular joint. Br Med J 1:262

41. Savill DL (1951) The manubrio-sternal joint in ankylosing spondylitis. J Bone Joint Surg Br 33:56–64

42. Schils JP, Resnick D, Haghighi P, Trudell D, Sartoris DJ (1989) Sternocostal joints. Anatomic, radiographic and pathologic features in adult cadavers. Invest Radiol 24:596–603

43. Schils JP, Resnick D, Haghighi PN, Trudell D, Sartoris DJ (1989) Pathogenesis of discovertebral and manubriosternal joint abnormalities in rheumatoid arthritis: a cadaveric study. J Rheumatol 16:291–297

44. Sebes JI, Salazar JE (1983) The manubriosternal joint in rheumatoid disease. Am J Roentgenol 140:117–121

45. Sokoloff F, Gleason IO (1954) The sternocostoclavicular articulation in rheumatic disease. Am J Clin Pathol 24:406–416

46. Verschuuren J, Goei The HS, Schreutelkamp I, Houben HM, Burlage F, de Korte P, Veldhuyzen VZ (1987) Radiological abnormalities of the manubriosternal joint in patients with rheumatoid arthritis and osteoarthrosis Scand J Rheumatol 16:139–142

47. Wehrmacher WH (1955) Significance of Tietze's syndrome in differential diagnosis of chest pain. J Am Med Assoc 157:505–507
48. Yamasaki O, Iwatsuki K, Kaneko F (2003) A case of SAPHO syndrome with pyoderma gangrenosum and inflammatory bowel disease masquerading as Behçet's disease. Adv Exp Med Biol 528:339–341
49. Zitnan D, Sitaj S (1976) Natural course of articular chondrocalcinosis. Arthritis Rheum 19(suppl 3):363–390

# 15 Degenerative Joint Disorders, Including Condensing Osteitis

STEPHEN P. HARDEN AND RICHARD M. BLAQUIERE

## Contents



## 15.1
## Introduction

This chapter concentrates on osteoarthritis (OA) of the sternoclavicular joint (SCJ), the archetypal degenerative joint disease and the commonest condition to affect this joint. It also covers the rather controversial topic of condensing osteitis of the clavicle. Although some authors have suggested that this condition would be better termed post-traumatic clavicular sclerosis, it is now widely accepted that it is most likely to be a degenerative process. It is still not clear whether all or any of these patients subsequently develop OA of the SCJ.

## 15.2
## Osteoarthritis of the Sternoclavicular Joint

Osteoarthritis is the most frequently identified disorder of the SCJ. Osteoarthritic changes are seen increasingly commonly with age. Kier et al. [12] performed block dissections of 55 SCJs in consecutive autopsy specimens and then performed high-resolution PA radiographs and subsequently a histological assessment to determine the severity of OA present. Some degenerative changes were identified in

50% of patients under 40 but, in comparison, were found in 97% of patients over 60. Moderately severe degenerative changes were present in only 12% of patients under 40 compared with 33% of patients over 60, while severe changes were present in no patients under 40 and 20% of those over 60. The changes were typically bilateral but often asymmetrical.

In addition to advancing years, there may be an identifiable cause of SCJ osteoarthritis. The SCJ can be involved in patients with systemic or primary OA. Arlet and Ficat [2] found clinical evidence of OA in 21 of 25 patients with generalised systemic OA. In other patients, repetitive trauma may produce a monarthritis. This may be seen in manual labourers and in those playing a lot of racket sports. There is some evidence that degenerative changes in these patients are most prominent on the side of the dominant hand [2]. Yood and Goldenberg [24] reported 18 cases of SCJ monarthritis in patients aged 20–50 years. Most of these patients were manual labourers and all of them had monarthritis on the dominant hand side. Other studies have not reliably demonstrated a strong link with dominant handedness [12]. The third group of patients with a definitive cause are those with a history of a single traumatic event, such as dislocation, subluxation or periarticular fracture [16]. Finally, there is some evidence that other conditions of the SCJ region may produce OA. These include condensing osteitis, previous joint infection and other systemic arthritides, but in all of these cases OA is not an inevitable consequence.

Patients presenting with symptomatic OA of the SCJ tend to be in or beyond the sixth decade of life. The principle symptom is local pain and this has often been present for many months or years. The pain is usually aggravated by abduction of the arm and by forward elevation of the arm above the horizontal. Swelling of the SCJ is usually present. An irregular bony prominence may be palpable and crepitus may be detected in severe cases. However, it remains surprising that patients may remain asymptomatic even with quite advanced degenerative changes. Inflammatory markers are almost invariably normal irrespective of symptoms.

The plain radiograph is usually the initial imaging investigation and this demonstrates the typical features of OA seen in most other joints. These comprise joint space narrowing, subchondral sclerosis, osteophyte formation and subchondral cysts. Kier et al. [12] found a good correlation between radiographic abnormalities and histological changes. Although sclerosis, cysts and osteophytes can be found on either side of the joint, the commonest site for these changes is the articular surface of the inferomedial clavicle [2, 12]. Osteophytes are particularly common here and are much less frequently identified at the superior clavicular surface or the sternal surface of the SCJ. There may also be partial or complete ossification of the costal cartilage of the ipsilateral first rib. However, Kier et al. [12] felt that this was more likely to represent part of the normal ageing process rather than being directly linked to OA of the SCJ as there was no significant correlation with the presence or absence of degenerative changes in the SCJ. Calcification here may be misinterpreted as a large osteophyte from the SCJ.

There are limitations to the ability of plain X-rays to demonstrate reliably SCJ pathology. Overlapping or composite shadows may obscure degenerative changes. Consequently, small subchondral cysts may be particularly difficult to define. The joint space is often difficult to assess, as the direction of the X-ray beam does not always pass perfectly through the centre of the joint. Oblique views and conventional tomography were used in the past to provide a better assessment but have been superseded by CT. Modern equipment allows the acquisition of a narrow collection of slices between 0.6 and 1.25 mm thick and these provide effectively isotropic voxels. Using a high-resolution bone algorithm and if necessary overlapping slices, reformatted images can be generated which have the same resolution in the coronal plane as they do in the axial. With an acquisition time of less than 10 s, breath-holding is not a problem.

The grading of the severity of OA is rather arbitrary but is made according to the degree to which the various radiographic features are present. So, for example, minor joint space narrowing with subtle osteophytes and small cysts represents mild disease while definite joint space narrowing with obvious osteophytes and a small number of large cysts corresponds to moderate disease. Obliteration of the joint space, large osteophytes and dense sclerosis is seen in severe cases.

These radiographic features of OA are easily identified on CT (Fig. 15.1). In particular, the joint space narrowing is much more readily identified than on plain radiographs (Fig. 15.2). CT is also able to identify degenerative changes in other nearby joints such as the acromioclavicular joint. Air may be seen within the SCJ on CT in cases of OA but this is a non-specific finding as it may be seen in normal patients with arms placed above the head. The decrease in joint pressure that this causes produces a vacuum phenomenon.

Magnetic resonance imaging (MRI) can elegantly demonstrate the changes of OA of the SCJ. Although obtaining optimal images can be difficult, we have found the most consistently useful technique is to use anterior and posterior linked coils with the patient supine and gently breathing. Small surface coils, prone examinations and respiratory gating are options. Spin echo T1 and STIR sequences are the primary weightings although spin echo T2 with or without fat saturation and proton density with fat saturation may be useful. Images should be obtained axial and coronal to the plane of the SCJ. Sagittal images are of only limited value. A slice width of 3–5 mm is usually sufficient and gadolinium is not required routinely.

Areas of subchondral sclerosis appear as low signal on both T1- and T2-weighted sequences. Subchondral cysts are usually well-defined round areas of low signal on T1 and high signal on T2 and STIR images (Fig. 15.3). The joint space loss is clearly demonstrated. Occasionally a joint effusion may be present and this

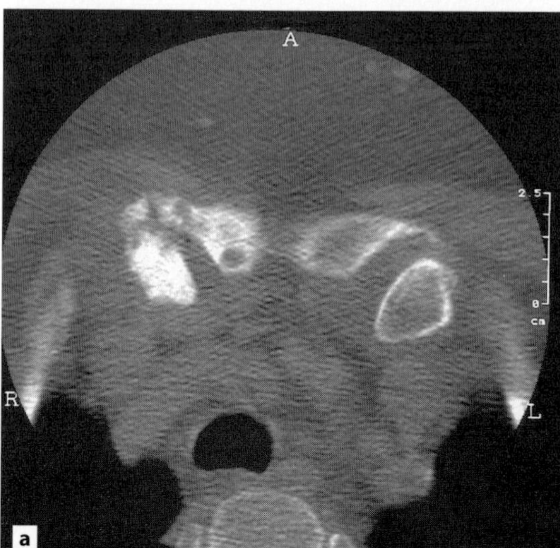

**Fig. 15.1a,b** Axial plane CT demonstrating OA of the right SCJ. Subchondral sclerosis and cysts are present and the joint space is narrowed

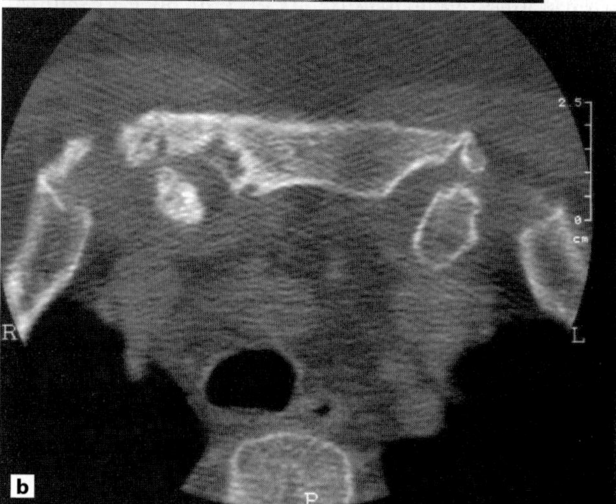

is typically of high signal on T2 and STIR images (Fig. 15.4) [7]. This may outline remnants of the degenerated intra-articular disc (Fig. 15.5). It is believed that the effusion may be due to a synovitis secondary to debris within the joint as a result of the degenerative process [20]. This may produce acute symptoms, particularly local pain, and it may be the trigger for the patient to seek medical advice. Interestingly in their series, Kier et al. [12] found no evidence of synovitis in the histological assessment of their cases, although it may be that none of their patients had symptomatic SCJ OA during life.

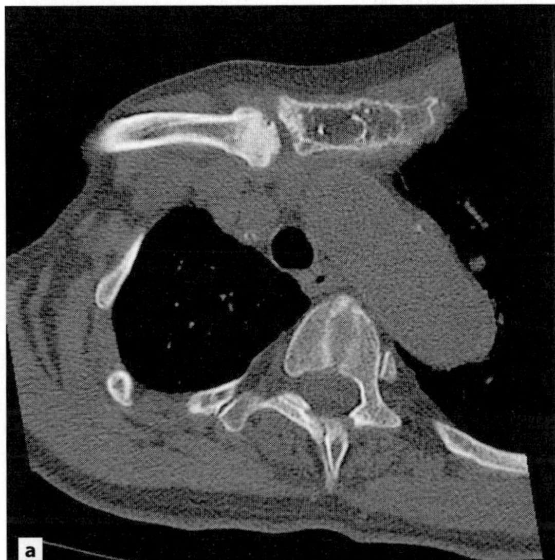

**Fig. 15.2** Computed tomography of the sternoclavicular joint with axial oblique (**a**) and coronal oblique (**b**) reconstructions. There is OA of the right SCJ with typical degenerative changes on both sides of the joint. The changes are most marked in the inferomedial aspect of the clavicle

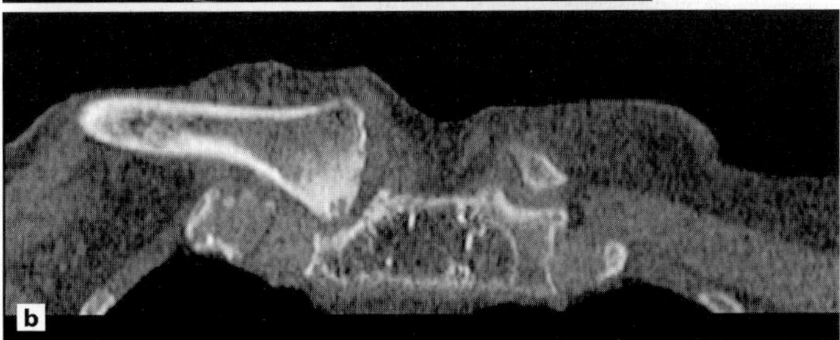

Ultrasound may be used to assess the SCJ and can demonstrate degenerative features such as osteophytes and joint space loss. The assessment of the state of the subchondral bone is less reliable.

Bone scintigraphy is rarely indicated in these patients. However, increased uptake of tracer is commonly seen around the SCJ in elderly patients and this undoubtedly corresponds to OA here. The amount of tracer uptake corresponds with osteoblastic activity in the subchondral bone.

## 15.3
## Condensing Osteitis

This is a rare and benign condition of unknown aetiology. It was first reported by Brower et al. in 1974 [3] and typically produces sclerosis of the inferomedial aspect

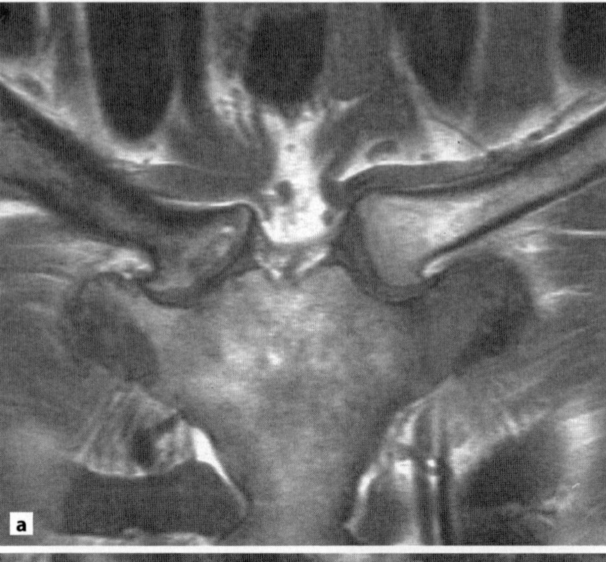

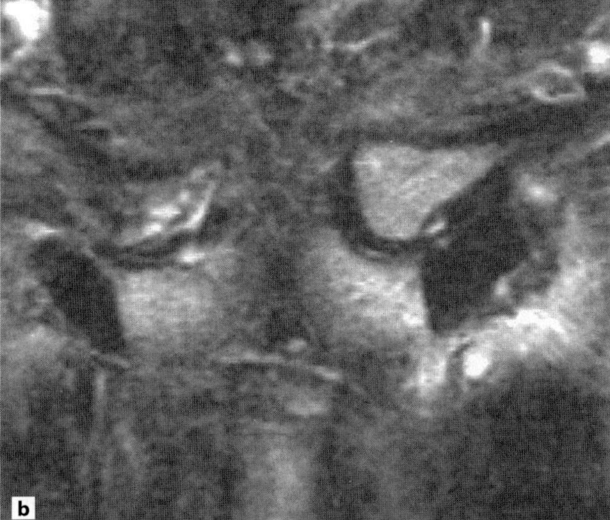

**Fig. 15.3** Magnetic resonance image of the SCJs with coronal oblique T1 (**a**) and STIR (**b**) sequences. OA of the right SCJ with subchondral cysts and some subchondral sclerosis, joint space loss and osteophyte formation

of the clavicle (Fig. 15.6). It is most commonly seen in women of mid-to-late child-bearing years but it has been reported to occur in men [6, 7].

Brower et al. [3] in their initial report suggested that this may be a degenerative process. Although the SCJ and the manubrium are normal and not involved in the disease process, the region of the clavicle involved is the same as seen in OA and there are several reports of an inferior spur with an appearance suggestive of

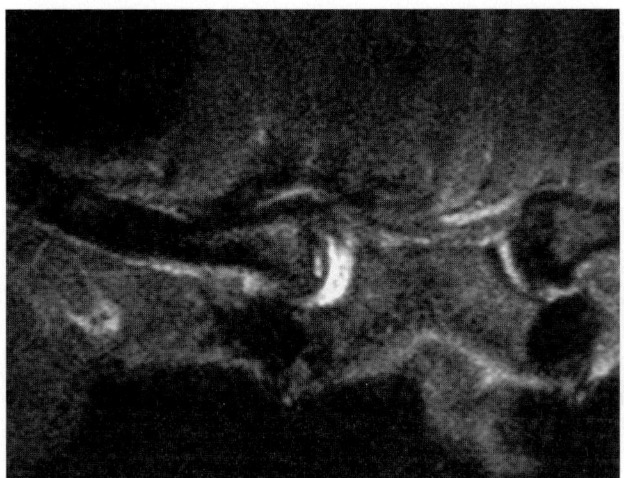

**Fig. 15.4** Coronal oblique STIR showing subchondral cysts and a joint effusion. The intra-articular disc has degenerated

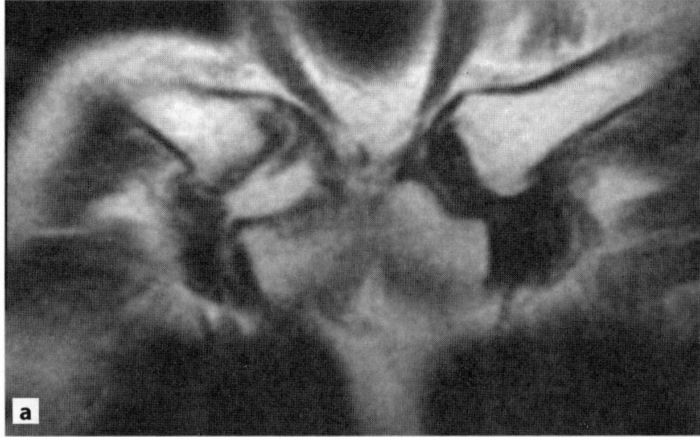

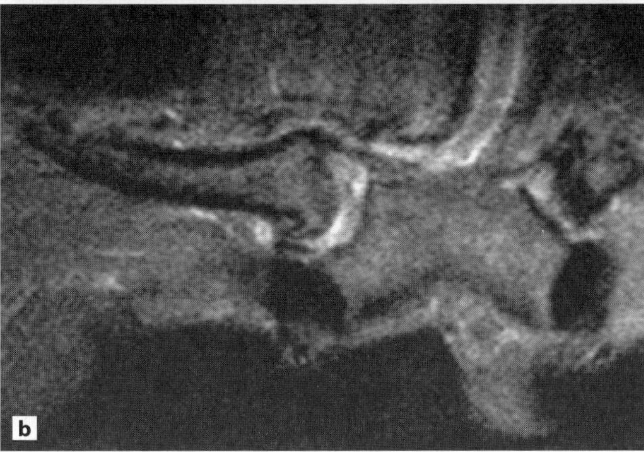

**Fig. 15.5 a** Coronal oblique T2 demonstrating right subchondral sclerosis, a joint effusion and loss of much of the intra-articular disc. **b** Coronal oblique STIR image showing a joint effusion with irregularity and disruption of the disc

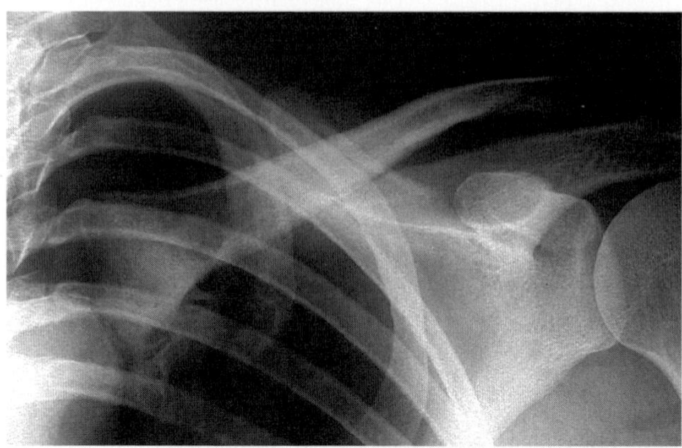

**Fig. 15.6** Radiograph of the left clavicle with sclerosis of the inferomedial clavicle. This appearance should raise a suspicion of condensing osteitis

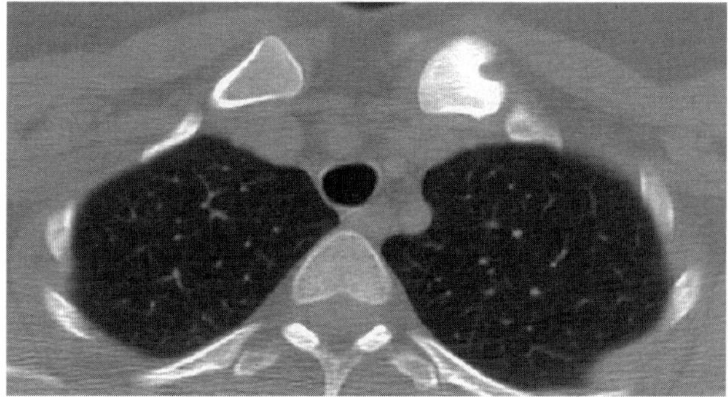

**Fig. 15.7** Axial plane CT demonstrating marked sclerosis and expansion of the inferomedial left clavicle typical of condensing osteitis. The anterior surface is deformed and protuberant although this is not strictly a true spur. The overlying soft tissues are displaced

an osteophyte (Fig. 15.7). Several studies have reported the histological features of the sclerotic process and this typically shows trabecular and cortical reinforcement with thickening of existing trabeculae [3, 13]. Much of the marrow space is obliterated. This is most likely to represent a hyperostotic response to mechanical stress [3, 4]. However, published series show a wide variation in the incidence of recognised local stress in these patients. Outwater and Oates [18] found only 2 of their 11 patients had a history of possible mechanical stress, while Jurik et al. [11] described 5 cases, 3 of whom had identifiable predisposing mechanical causes. Recorded stress mechanisms include excessive gardening, shooting, softball playing, heavy lifting and swimming [3, 11, 17]. The condition is found more commonly on the side of the dominant hand [21] but patients with bilateral condensing osteitis have been reported [11, 14].

The exact mechanism is unclear but several possibilities have been suggested. Jurik et al. [11] suggested that there may be microfractures in the medial clavicle and that these lead to a sclerotic response. Several authors have proposed a local osteonecrosis [5, 10, 11], particularly given the finding of marrow fibrosis in some cases. This had led several groups to conclude that condensing osteitis and Friedrich's disease are either the same or closely related diseases [10, 11, 18]. In fact, Friedrich's disease is a condition of children and adolescents which typically produces sclerosis of the entire medial end of the clavicle [15] and is typified histologically by necrosis and fibrosis. However, it remains the principle differential diagnosis of condensing osteitis. There may be histological evidence of marrow fibrosis in cases of condensing osteitis and this could be due to a low-grade local ischaemia, probably again related to recurrent mechanical stress. The process is strikingly similar to osteitis condensans ilii and osteitis condensans pubis. Both of these latter conditions are seen in women of mid-to-late child-bearing years and are thought to be related to mechanical stress and may represent early degenerative changes [3].

Some authors have proposed different aetiologies. Jones et al. [8] reported three cases of condensing osteitis in children. Two of the cases had positive anti-staphylolysin titres which led the authors to conclude that this disease was in fact a low-grade osteomyelitis. Other studies have performed bacteriological cultures on clavicular biopsy specimens and these have all produced no evidence of bacterial growth [13, 17]. Greenspan et al. [5] suggested that the Jones series did indeed represent low-grade osteomyelitis but that these were not cases of condensing osteitis.

Appell et al. [1] described a series of seven cases but none of these cases had typical features of condensing osteitis. At least some of the cases were believed to have a low-grade chronic osteomyelitis and four of the seven cases showed significant improvement with antibiotics. All of the cases had elevated inflammatory markers and the radiographic appearances included periosteal reactions and bone destruction. Subsequent publications have suggested that these cases also did not represent condensing osteitis [5].

Patients with condensing osteitis usually present with pain in the region of the medial clavicle although the pain can radiate to the ipsilateral supraclavicular region and the ipsilateral shoulder. Some patients describe intermittent pain while others have a more constant pain and it is not clear whether the constant pain represents a more chronic or severe form of the disease. The pain is usually mild although rarely may be intense and it has usually been present for many months prior to medical referral. Symptoms are aggravated by abduction of the arm and by forward elevation. Occasionally, patients may be asymptomatic. There is often a palpable swelling in the region of the medial clavicle and this is firm and variably tender. When tenderness is elicited it is usually mild. The overlying skin and subcutaneous tissues are invariably normal, with no signs of local inflammation. Although the range of joint movement may be reduced, it is usually normal. Inflammatory markers are always normal and alkaline phosphatase is also within normal limits.

The radiographic appearances are as originally described by Brower et al [3] with homogeneous dense sclerosis present in the inferior aspect of the medial third of the clavicle (Fig. 15.8). There may be slight expansion of the clavicle here but no bone destruction has been reported (Fig. 15.9). Several authors have identified a slight periosteal reaction histologically [3, 13] but there are no reports of periosteal reaction on plain radiographs. An inferior protuberance similar to an osteophyte has been frequently identified [4, 5]. The SCJ is normal as is the articular region of the manubrium and this is the most useful feature in excluding OA in these cases. These appearances are exquisitely demonstrated by CT which in addition identifies

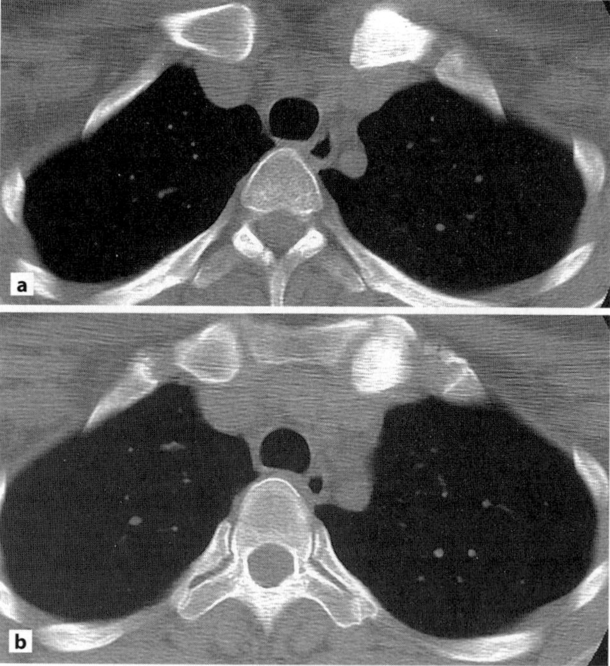

**Fig. 15.8a,b** Axial plane CT with dense sclerosis of the inferomedial left clavicle due to condensing osteitis. The manubrium and the SCJ are normal

the obliteration of the marrow space that the intense sclerosis causes. There may be minor swelling of the overlying soft tissues but this is usually absent.

There are now several reports of the MR appearances in condensing osteitis. Vierboom et al. [23] reported one case in which T1 and T2 images demonstrated low signal in the medial clavicle (Fig. 15.10). They found no high signal nidus in

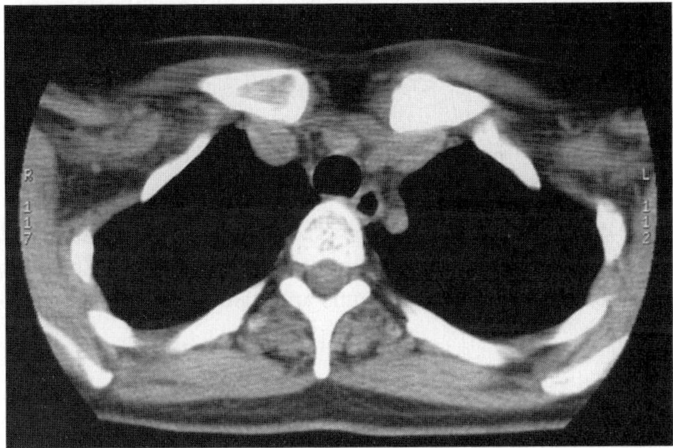

**Fig. 15.9** Sclerosis of the left medial clavicle. This is expanded slightly and the overlying soft tissues are consequently displaced but not otherwise thickened. The appearances are more in keeping with condensing osteitis than other diagnoses such as a sclerotic metastasis

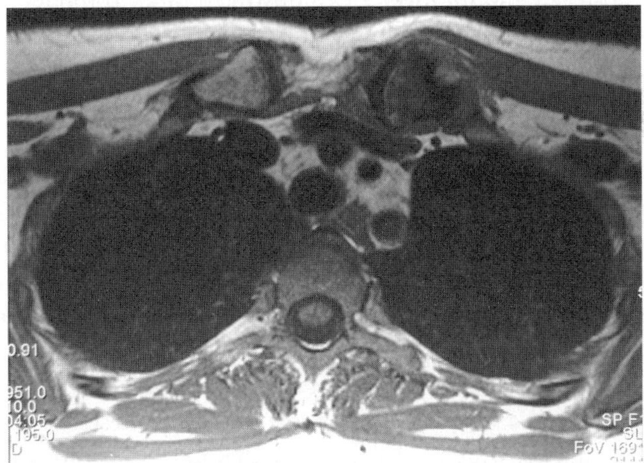

**Fig. 15.10** Axial T1-weighted MR image showing low signal in the medial left clavicle. The clavicle is expanded here. This is the MR equivalent of the typical CT appearance of condensing osteitis shown in Fig. 15.7

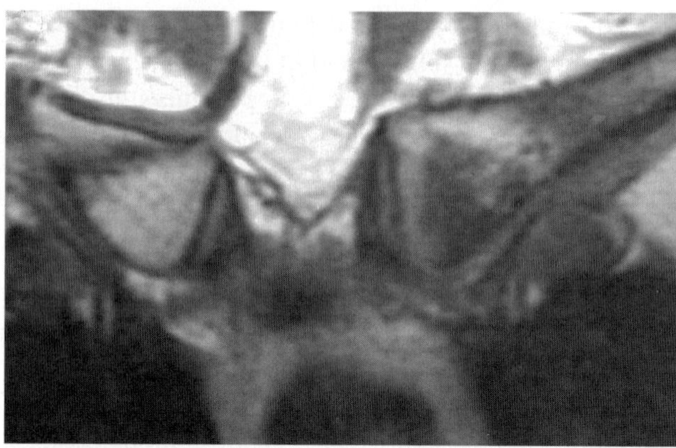

**Fig. 15.11** Oblique coronal T1 image demonstrating low signal in much of the medial left clavicle, although this is most marked in the inferomedial clavicle. These appearances together with the patient's presenting symptoms and history were indicative of condensing osteitis

the centre of the low signal abnormality and the overlying soft tissues were normal. Tait et al. [22] reported the MR findings in one patient in whom there was low signal in the medial clavicle on T1 and low to intermediate signal on T2-weighted images. Rand et al. [19] published a series of four cases and every case demonstrated low signal on T1 images (Fig. 15.11). However, T2 spin echo images showed low-to-intermediate signal, T2 gradient echo sequences showed moderate-to-high signal while T1 post-gadolinium images demonstrated mild-to-moderate intra- and periosseous enhancement. Interestingly, those patients with imaging appearances of some bone marrow oedema were those with worsening symptoms. Some reports of STIR imaging have described some evidence of increased signal in the medial clavicle (Fig. 15.12) [7].

Several studies have routinely performed bone scintigraphy on these patients and generally there is increased activity in the region of the SCJ [4, 6, 13]. There is usually no evidence of other abnormal tracer uptake in these patients. Noonan et al. [17] reported one case in which SPECT imaging was also performed and this confidently identified the abnormal activity as being solely within the medial clavicle. With current cross-sectional imaging techniques, bone scans probably have less of a role in the routine investigation of these patients.

Ultrasound also has a relatively minor role to play in these patients. It may be used to confirm that there are no degenerative changes in the joint but again it has only a limited ability to assess the subchondral bone.

The natural history of condensing osteitis remains a matter of some debate. Jurik [9] followed up 11 patients for a mean of 5 years (range 1–13 years) and found

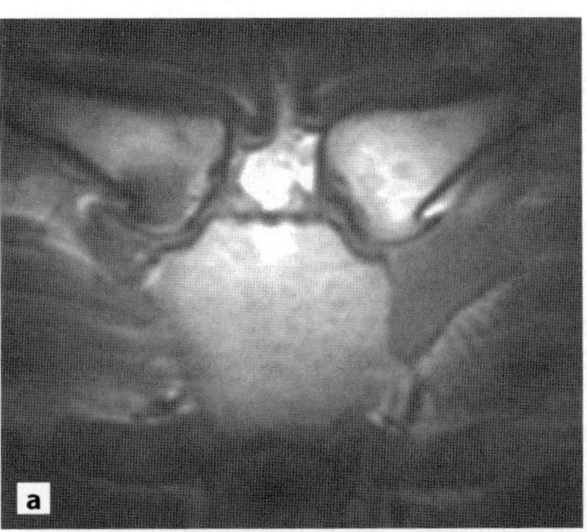
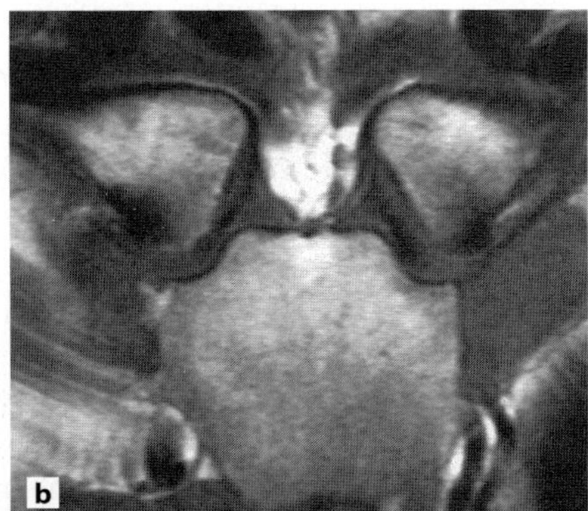
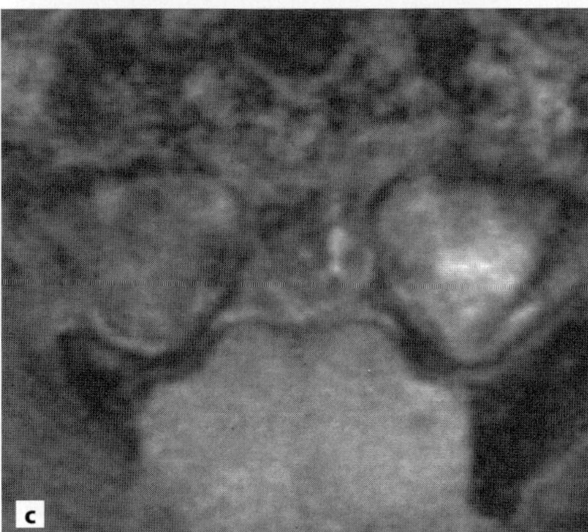

**Fig. 15.12** Coronal oblique T1-weighted MR image (**a**) in this 34-year-old woman demonstrates low signal in the inferomedial right clavicle, typical of condensing osteitis. She represented after an 8-year interval with identical symptoms on the left and at this time the coronal T1 images (**b**) show low signal in both medial clavicles. STIR images (**c**) show low signal in the right medial clavicle and intermediate to high signal on the now symptomatic left side. Note that the manubrium and the SCJs remain normal

that the degree of sclerosis regressed but that all patients developed signs of osteoarthrosis. Sng et al. [21] followed up 9 patients for a mean of 3 years and 5 of these patients had follow-up CT imaging. Of these 5 patients, 4 showed partial resolution of sclerosis compared to the previous CT but the authors acknowledged that these changes were not quantified and therefore the changes were rather subjective. The other patient showed complete resolution of sclerosis. Clearly longer term follow-up studies are required to determine the true natural history but if the improvement in sclerosis is confirmed it might indicate that this is a different disease process from OA of the SCJ.

The imaging features of condensing osteitis are quite characteristic and although OA and Friedrich's disease are the principle differential diagnoses these are usually not difficult to exclude. When this condition was first described, it was believed that it was frequently being misdiagnosed as a sclerotic bone lesion such as a metastasis, with consequent extensive investigation to search for a primary tumour. Now that it is more widely known, this occurs much less frequently.

## 15.4
## Conclusions

Degenerative disorders of the SCJ are commonly present radiographically but produce symptoms less frequently. When they do the presence of local swelling, tenderness and an abnormal radiograph can give rise to concern. In these patients MRI or CT should be used to exclude malignant or infective conditions while simultaneously differentiating the various degenerative processes.

**Acknowledgements.** We are grateful to the editor of *Clinical Radiology* for allowing us to reprint several of the images in this chapter from our recent article [7].

## References


1. Appell RG, Oppermann HC, Becker W, et al (1983) Condensing osteitis of the clavicle in childhood: a rare sclerotic bone lesion. Review of literature and report of seven patients. Pediatr Radiol 13:301–306
2. Arlet J, Ficat P (1958) Osteo-arthritis of the sternoclavicular joint. Ann Rheum Dis 17:97–100
3. Brower AC, Sweet DE, Keats TE (1974) Condensing osteitis of the clavicle: a new entity. Am J Roentgenol 121:17–21
4. Cone RO, Resnick D, Goergen TG, et al (1983) Condensing osteitis of the clavicle. Am J Roentgenol 141:387–388
5. Greenspan A, Gerscovich E, Szabo RM, et al (1991) Condensing osteitis of the clavicle: a rare but frequently misdiagnosed condition. Am J Roentgenol 156:1011–1015
6. Hamilton-Wood C, Hollingworth P, Dieppe P, et al (1985) The painful swollen sternoclavicular joint. Br J Radiol 58:941–945
7. Harden SP, Argent JD, Blaquiere RM (2004) Painful sclerosis of the medial end of the clavicle. Clin Radiol 59:992–999
8. Jones MW, Carty H, Taylor JF, et al (1990) Condensing osteitis of the clavicle: does it exist? J Bone Joint Surg Br 72-B:464–467
9. Jurik AG (1994) Non-inflammatory sclerosis of the sternal end of the clavicle: a follow-up study and review of the literature. Skeletal Radiol 23:373–378
10. Jurik AG, Moller BN (1986) Inflammatory hyperostosis and sclerosis of the clavicle. Skeletal Radiol 15:284–290
11. Jurik AG, De Carvalho A, Graudal H (1985) Sclerotic changes of the sternal end of the clavicle. Clin Radiol 36:23–25

12. Kier R, Wain SL, Apple J, et al (1986) Osteoarthritis of the sternoclavicular joint: radiographic features and pathological correlation. Invest Radiol 21:227–233
13. Kruger GD, Rock MG, Munro TG (1987) Condensing osteitis of the clavicle. J Bone Joint Surg Am 69:550–557
14. Latifi HR, Gilula LA (1992) Imaging rounds. Bilateral condensing osteitis of the clavicles. Orthop Rev 21:767–774
15. Levy M, Goldberg I, Fischel RE, et al (1981) Friedrich's disease: aseptic necrosis of the sternal end of the clavicle. J Bone Joint Surg Br 63-B:539–541
16. Noble JS (2003) Degenerative sternoclavicular arthritis and hyperostosis. Clin Sports Med 22:407–422
17. Noonan PT, Stanley MD, Sartoris DJ, et al (1998) Condensing osteitis of the clavicle in a man. Skeletal Radiol 27:291–293
18. Outwater E, Oates E (1998) Condensing osteitis of the clavicle: case report and review of the literature. J Nucl Med 29:1122–1125
19. Rand T, Schweitzer M, Rafii M, et al (1998) Condensing osteitis of the clavicle: MRI. J Comput Assist Tomogr 22:621–624
20. Resnick D, Niwayama G (1997) Degenerative disease of extraspinal locations. In: Resnick D (ed) Diagnosis of Bone and Joint Disorders. Saunders, Philadelphia
21. Sng KK, Chan BK, Chakrabarti AJ, et al (2004) Condensing osteitis of the medial clavicle: an intermediate-term follow-up. Ann Acad Med Singapore 33:499–502
22. Tait TJ, Chalmers AG, Bird HA (1994) Condensing osteitis of the clavicle: differentiation from sternocostoclavicular hyperostosis by magnetic resonance imaging. Br J Rheumatol 33:985–987
23. Vierboom MA, Steinberg JD, Mooyaart EL, et al (1992) Condensing osteitis of the clavicle: magnetic resonance imaging as an adjunct method for differential diagnosis. Ann Rheum Dis 51:539–541
24. Yood RA, Goldenberg DL (1980) Sternoclavicular joint arthritis. Arthritis Rheum 23:232–239

# 16 Infectious Disorders

ANNE GRETHE JURIK

**Contents**



## 16.1
## Introduction

Infectious lesions in the sternocostoclavicular (SCC) region are relatively rare. They mainly occur in persons with common risk factors such as intravenous drug abuse, diabetes mellitus, distant infection, steroid-treated rheumatoid arthritis, immunodeficiency including immunosuppressant therapy and alcoholism [18, 21]. Local abnormalities such as sequels of trauma or operation, the presence of a central venous catheter and definite joint disease (e.g. rheumatoid arthritis) may also play a part [12]. SCC infection in previously healthy subjects is a very rare occurrence requiring a high awareness of suspicion for the diagnostic assessment [26].

The infection may primary be located to bones or involve the joints. In the case of septic arthritis there will always be some degree of spread to bone. The micro-organisms involved are often those usually encountered in septic arthritis and osteitis [6, 13, 18], and tuberculosis also occurs [19].

## 16.2
## Pyogenic Infections

### 16.2.1
### Septic Arthritis

Septic arthritis of the sternoclavicular joint is relatively rare, but well recognised, especially among heroin users [7]. It accounts for about 1% of septic arthritis in the general population, but for 17% in intravenous drug users [18]. The increased incidence in drug users may be explained by bacteria entering the sternoclavicular joint from the adjacent subclavian vein after injection of contaminated drugs into the upper extremity, or the joint may become infected after attempted drug injection between the heads of the sternocleidomastoid muscle (Fig. 8.2) [18].

Septic arthritis of the manubriosternal joint (MSJ) is rare and mainly reported as case histories. It is important to be aware that it can occur as a complication to existing joint disorders such as rheumatoid arthritis (Fig. 16.1), reactive arthritis [24] and systemic lupus erythematosus [8], which may be associated with abnormalities of host defences and corticosteroid therapy.

It is important to diagnose septic arthritis as recovery without sequels can be obtained if it is promptly diagnosed and treated. In addition serious complications such as chest wall abscess or phlegmon and mediastinitis may occur [9, 18]. Aggressive surgical therapy is therefore often needed [15, 20].

### 16.2.1.1
### Clinical and Laboratory Findings

The symptoms and clinical findings may vary. Unlike septic arthritis of most other joints, bacterial infection of the sternoclavicular joint frequently is insidious in onset [10]. Clinical findings can consist of erythema, warmth, swelling of the joint and fever (generally low grade), and abnormal laboratory values are consistent

**❱ Fig. 16.1** Septic arthritis of the manubriosternal joint in a 68-year-old woman with steroid-treated rheumatoid arthritis and increasing swelling at the MSJ during 2 weeks. **a,b** Sagittal STIR (**a**) and axial T1-weighted (**b**) images show irregular osseous contours at the MSJ (*arrow*) with pronounced surrounding oedema both in the bones and soft tissue. **c,d** Postcontrast axial (**c**) and sagittal (**d**) T1 FS images reveal a non-enhancing multilobulated abscess (*arrows*) superficially to the bones in addition to vascularised inflammation in the surrounding soft tissue and in the bones

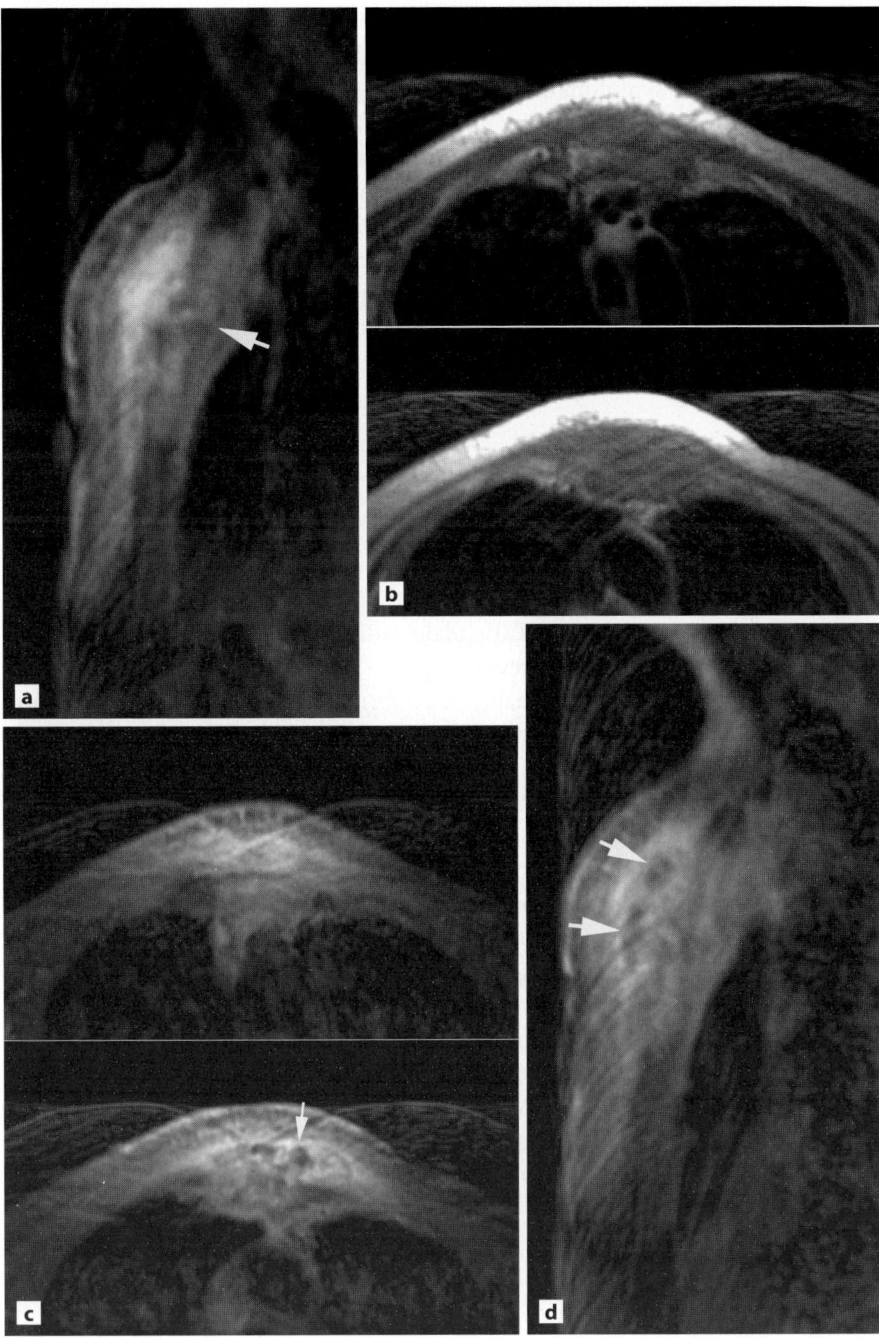

with infection [10]. However, in a recent review of 180 cases (mean age 45 years; 73% men), 78% of the patients presented with chest pain and 24% with shoulder pain after a median symptom duration of 14 days. Only 65% of the patients were febrile [18].

*Staphylococcus aureus* is the most frequent cause of septic sternoclavicular arthritis, also in intravenous drug users [18]. Certain gram-negative bacilli, particular Pseudomonas species, have a predisposition for spread to the sternoclavicular joint and were previously often the cause of septic sternoclavicular joint arthritis in intravenous drug abusers [6]. However, the frequency of Pseudomonas infection in drug users has declined with the end of an epidemic of pentazocine abuse in the 1980s [18].


## 16.2.1.2
## Imaging

The radiographic features can consist of soft tissue blurring at the superior mediastinum (Fig. 8.2). Radiographic evidence of joint space narrowing and osseous destruction gives this diagnosis. Early plain radiographs are, however, often normal, but tomography or CT may reveal erosion [10]. Cross-sectional imaging [20] in the form of CT or MRI is valuable in confirming a mass in the region of the sternoclavicular region and detecting associated osteolysis of the clavicular head and/or the manubrium (Fig. 6.2) [13]. CT or MRI should be obtained routinely to assess a possible chest wall phlegmon, retrosternal abscess or mediastinitis, which will influence the therapy (Fig. 16.2) [18]. Contrast-enhanced spiral CT scanning supplemented by multiplanar reconstruction has been found to be of value in the evaluation of suspected infection of the sternoclavicular joints. The scans obtained during the phase of high-contrast enhancement allowed definition of the extension into the soft tissue and muscle (Fig. 16.2). Bone windows demonstrated subtle cortical and periosteal abnormalities (Fig. 6.2) [21]. The sensitivity and specificity of CT for the determination of complicating mediastinal infection including abscess formation has been reported 100% [15, 16]. CT may therefore be helpful for determining surgical intervention. MRI often adds information about the extent of osseous and soft tissue involvement (Figs. 16.2 and 16.3) and early changes may be detected by MRI. Scintigraphy is valuable when suspecting multifocal disease (Fig. 9.1).

## 16.2.2
## Pyogenic Osteitis

Some degree of sternal and/or clavicular osteitis occurs in patients with septic sternoclavicular or manubriosternal arthritis (Figs. 8.2 and 16.1–16.3). Primary haematogenous sternal or clavicular osteitis is rare, and when recognised usually occurs in intravenous drug users [2], or is caused by *Staphylococcus aureus* from a local or distinct focus. However, clavicular osteomyelitis (or septic sternoclavicular arthritis) can be a complication of subclavian vein catheterisation [11], which also in rare cases may cause infection of the first costal cartilage [17]. Soft tissue infections around the puncture site occur frequently. If symptoms persist for several weeks despite topical treatment, osteomyelitis or septic sternoclavicular arthritis should be considered. Sternal osteomyelitis can also be a complication of sternotomy [22].

*Clinical Findings:* Acute osteitis is manifested by the cardinal signs of infection, but low-grade osteomyelitis with fewer symptoms also occurs.

*Imaging:* Computed tomography or MRI are valuable for achieving the diagnosis [11], if necessary supplemented by scintigraphy (Figs. 6.2, 8.2 and 16.1–3).


## 16.3
## Tuberculosis

Tuberculosis in the SCC region is rare. It may involve the sternoclavicular joints or only the bones [19]. Of 15 patients (8 men and 7 women; 16–78 years old) with tuberculosis in the SCC region, 8 had sternoclavicular joint involvement, 5 had isolated sternal involvement and 2 had isolated clavicular involvement [19].


## 16.3.1
## Tuberculous Arthritis

Tuberculous arthritis is a rare form of extrapulmonary tuberculosis and involvement of the sternoclavicular joint has been reported to account for only 1–2% of cases with tuberculous arthritis [5, 25]. Compared to other sites of skeletal tuberculosis, the SCC region has received little attention [4, 25], but some conclusions may be stated. Tuberculous infection in the sternoclavicular joint has been reported both in adults and adolescents [14], and may mimic neoplasm [5]. Patients in haemodialysis are known to develop the complication of extrapulmonary tuberculosis more frequently than the general population [5].

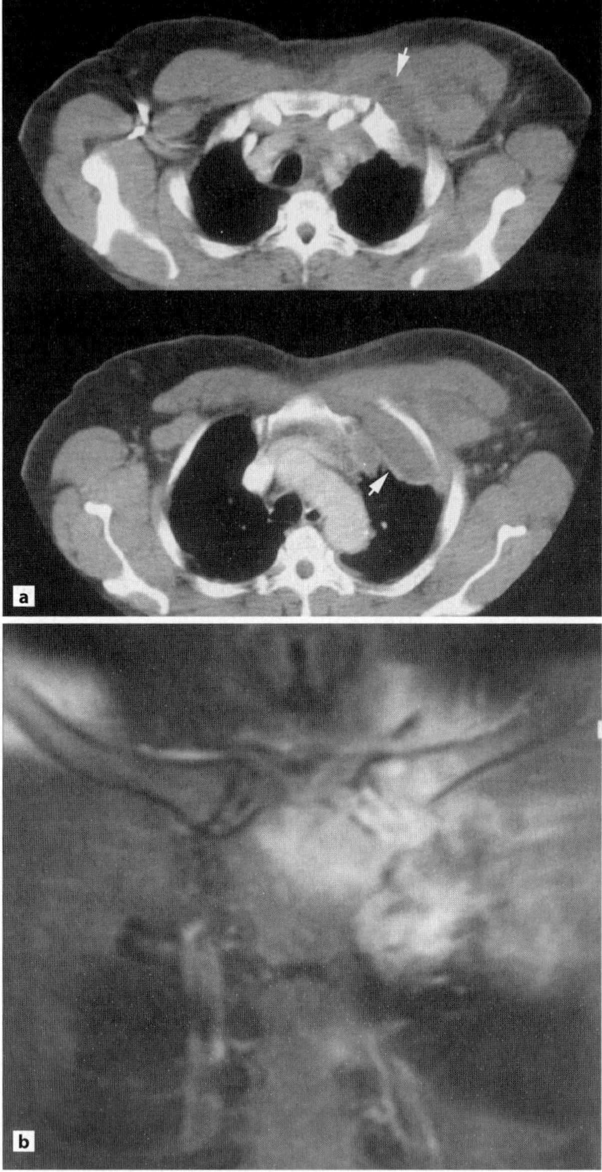

**Fig. 16.2** Septic arthritis of the sternoclavicular joint in a previously healthy 61-year-old man who, after a pneumonia, developed pain, swelling and tenderness corresponding to the left sternoclavicular joint accompanied by recurrence of fever. **a** Axial postcontrast CT slices demonstrate an avascular collection in the region of the left sternoclavicular and first sternocostal joint (*arrows*). **b** Coronal STIR shows a huge area of increased signal intensity corresponding to the left sternoclavicular joint, the surrounding bone and soft tissue

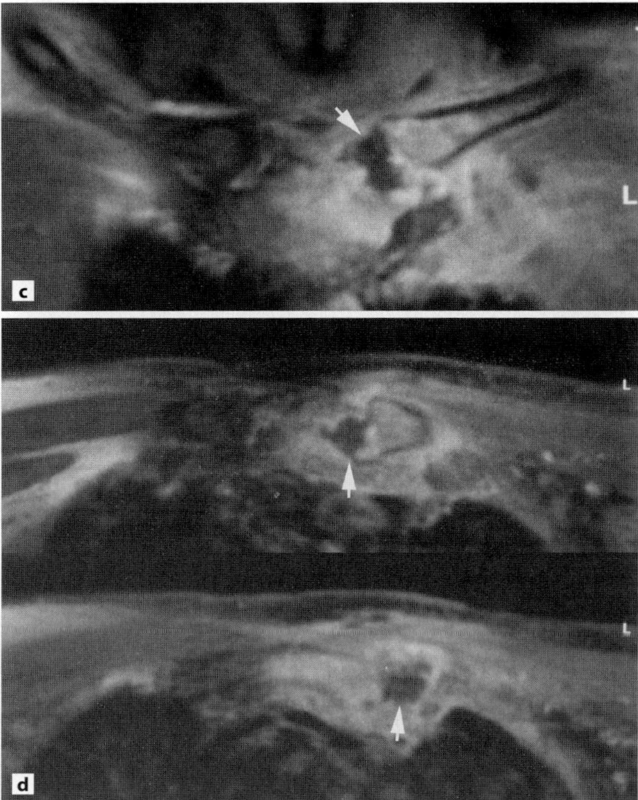

**Fig. 16.2** (*continued*) Septic arthritis of the sternoclavicular joint in a previously healthy 61-year-old man who, after a pneumonia, developed pain, swelling and tenderness corresponding to the left sternoclavicular joint accompanied by recurrence of fever. Postcontrast coronal T1 FS sequence (**c**) shows an avascular area within the joint (*arrow*) which was confirmed at axial slices (**d**)

Early diagnosis is important for a good outcome. With a worldwide occurrence of this disease, suspicion is mandatory, especially in immunocompromised patients such as AIDS patients [19] and emigrants from areas with a high frequency of tuberculosis.

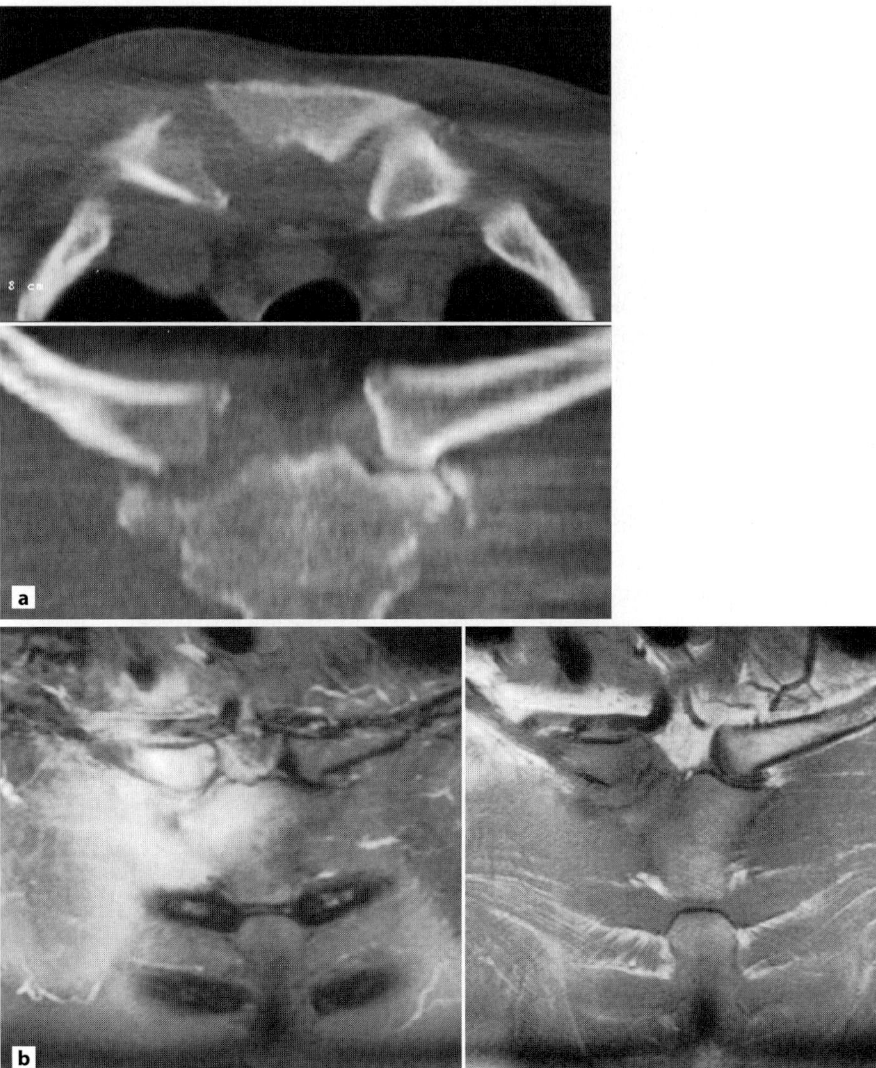

**Fig 16.3a,b** Post-traumatic sternoclavicular arthritis in a 26-year-old man who after a right-sided clavicular fracture developed pain, swelling and tenderness corresponding to the right sternoclavicular joint. Axial CT slice (*upper*) and coronal reconstruction (*lower*) show destruction of the joint facets in the right sternoclavicular joint **b** Coronal STIR (*left*) and T1-weighted image (*right*) show a huge oedema corresponding to the right sternoclavicular joint, the surrounding bone and soft tissue. The intra-articular disc is ruptured (*arrow*).

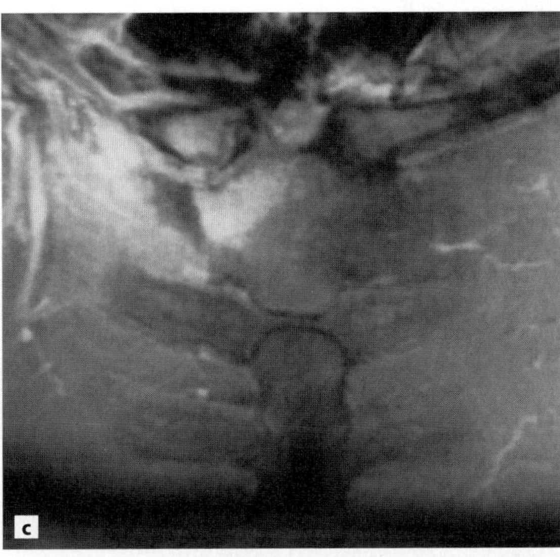

**Fig 16.3** (*continued*)Post-traumatic sternoclavicular arthritis in a 26-year-old man who after a right-sided clavicular fracture developed pain, swelling and tenderness corresponding to the right sternoclavicular joint. **c** Postcontrast T1 FS sequence did not detect any abscesses, but shows enhancement corresponding to the infected areas

## 16.3.1.1
## Clinical Findings

Clinically the symptoms may be non-specific and appear insidious. They usually consist of swelling and pain, sometimes accompanied by fever [4, 19].

## 16.3.1.2
## Imaging

Radiographs have been found diagnostic in about half of the patients only [19]. Imaging should therefore include either CT or MRI, which are helpful for defining the extent of the disease [3, 19, 25] (Fig. 16.4). MRI is particular useful in determining the extent of the lesion including marrow involvement and soft tissue extent [19, 25]. Destruction and signal intensity changes of the sternum, clavicle and adjacent cartilage and soft tissue structures may occur, representing granulation tissue or abscess formation. Displacement of the adjacent structures (vessels, trachea, etc.) and inflammatory changes in the adjacent structures in the form of cellulitis and myositis have been reported common imaging features [19].

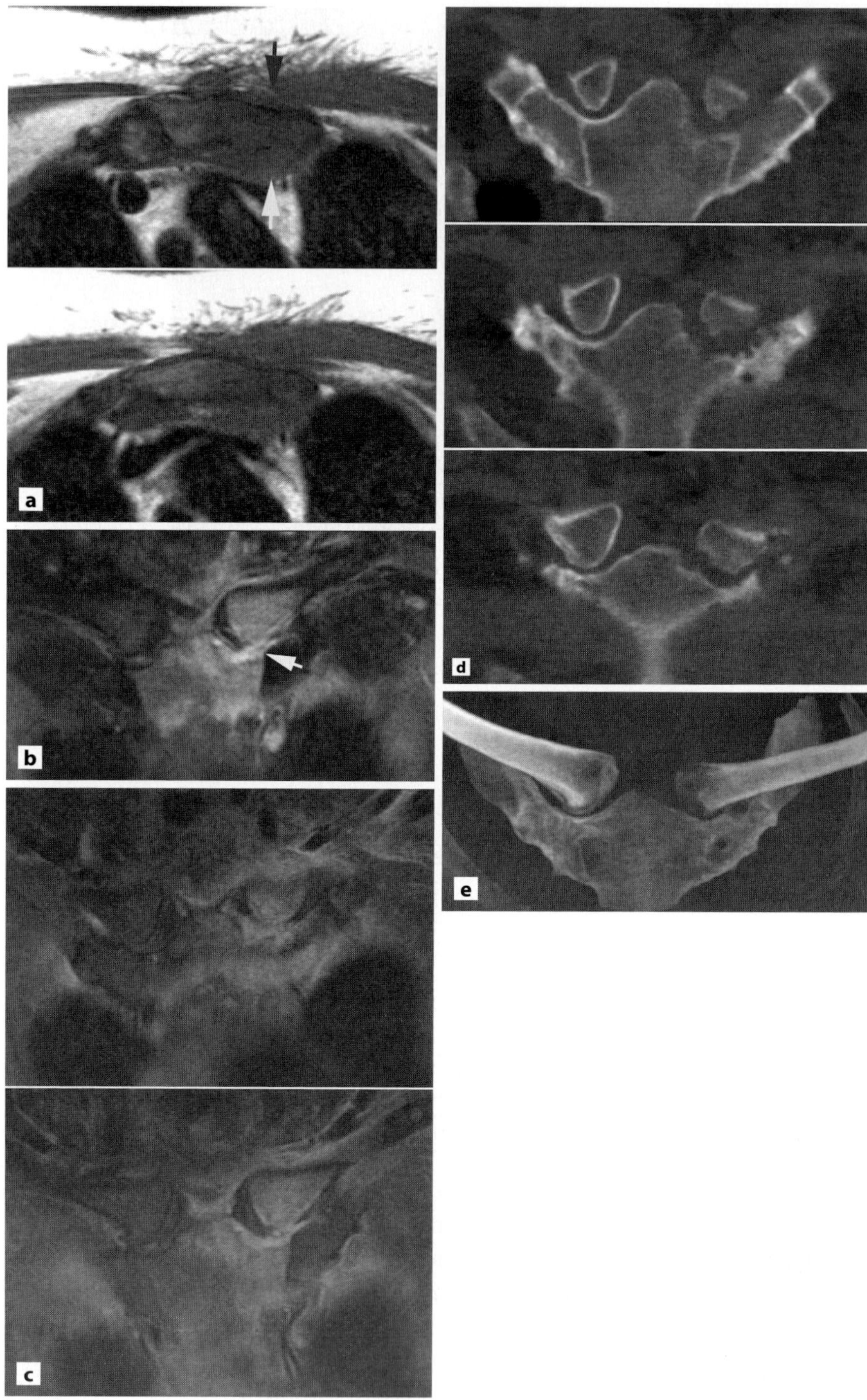

❸ **Fig 16.4** Tuberculous sternoclavicular arthritis. **a** Axial T1-weighted MR images show a mass with decreased signal intensity corresponding to the left sternoclavicular joint (*arrows*). **b** Coronal STIR shows hyperintense tissue corresponding to the joint and surrounding bone and soft tissue, most pronounced corresponding to the joint space (*arrow*). **c** Coronal postcontrast T1 FS images reveal enhancement corresponding to the abnormal tissue on STIR, but no non-enhancing areas suggesting abscess formation. **d,e** Supplementary MSCT, coronal reconstructions (**d**) and VIP (**e**) show huge osseous destruction of the joint surfaces with medial displacement of the clavicle consistent with rupture of the intra-articular disc and the costoclavicular ligament

## 16.3.2
## Tuberculous Osteitis

Primary tuberculous sternal osteitis can occur. It has been reported in a series of patients together with patients having arthritis, and also as recent case histories [19, 27]. Clavicular tuberculosis is, however, rare [23].

Plain radiography is usually not diagnostic [10] and cross-sectional imaging is needed. CT and MRI can delineate tuberculous sternal osteomyelitis [1]. CT visualises the osseous destruction and may demonstrate ring-enhancing hypodense soft tissue masses surrounding the sternum [1, 27]. At MRI the sternal bone marrow and peristernal soft tissue lesions are hypo- and hyperintense on T1-weighted images and display high signal intensity on STIR with enhancement post-gadolinium except corresponding to avascular areas. Bone scintigraphy usually shows increased tracer uptake, but there may also be areas with decreased uptake corresponding to osseous destruction [1].

## 16.4
## Differential Diagnoses

The clinical presentation of septic and tuberculous sternoclavicular arthritis and osteitis may mimic a malignancy or rheumatic arthritis, and differentiating these entities can be a challenge. However, infectious arthritis is often unilateral whereas rheumatic arthritis usually is bilateral [12].

## 16.5
## Conclusion

Infection in the SCC region is a rare finding mainly occurring in patients with decreased resistance to infection. Early diagnosis is important for a good outcome, and it is therefore important to be aware of the diagnostic possibility. Cross-sectional imaging, either CT or MRI, is important for achieving the diagnosis and delineating the extent of the disease.

## References


1.   Atasoy C, Oztekin PS, Ozdemir N, Sak SD, Erden I, Akyar S (2002) CT and MRI in tuberculous sternal osteomyelitis: a case report. Clin Imaging 26:112–115
2.   Boll KL, Jurik AG (1990) Sternal osteomyelitis in drug addicts. J Bone Joint Surg Br 72:328–329
3.   Dhillon MS, Gupta R, Rao KS, Nagi ON (2000) Bilateral sternoclavicular joint tuberculosis. Arch Orthop Trauma Surg 120:363–365
4.   Dhillon MS, Gupta RK, Bahadur R, Nagi ON (2001) Tuberculosis of the sternoclavicular joints. Acta Orthop Scand 72:514–517
5.   Fukasawa H, Suzuki H, Kato A, Yamamoto T, Fujigaki Y, Yonemura K, Hishida A (2001) Tuberculous arthritis mimicking neoplasm in a hemodialysis patient. Am J Med Sci 322:373–375
6.   Gifford DB, Patzakis M, Ivler D, Swezey RL (1975) Septic arthritis due to pseudomonas in heroin addicts. J Bone Joint Surg Am 57:631–635
7.   Goldin RH, Chow AW, Edwards JE Jr, Louie JS, Guze LB (1973) Sternoarticular septic arthritis in heroin users. N Engl J Med 289:616–618
8.   Gruber BL, Kaufman LD, Gorevic PD (1985) Septic arthritis involving the manubriosternal joint. J Rheumatol 12:803–804
9.   Haddad M, Maziak DE, Shamji FM (2002) Spontaneous sternoclavicular joint infections. Ann Thorac Surg 74:1225–1227
10.  Hermann G, Rothenberg RR, Spiera H (1983) The value of tomography in diagnosing infection of the sternoclavicular joint. Mt Sinai J Med 50:52–55
11.  Judich A, Haik J, Rosin D, Kuriansky J, Zwas ST, Ayalon A (1998) Osteomyelitis of the clavicle after subclavian vein catheterization. J Parenter Enteral Nutr 22:245–246
12.  Karten I (1969) Septic arthritis complicating rheumatoid arthritis. Ann Intern Med 70:1147–1158
13.  Kaw D, Yoon Y (2004) Pseudomonas sternoclavicular pyarthrosis. South Med J 97:705–706
14.  Khan SA, Zahid M, Asif N, Hasan AS (2002) Tuberculosis of the sternoclavicular joint. Indian J Chest Dis Allied Sci 44:271–273
15.  Novick SL, Fishman EK (2003) Anterior mediastinal extension of primary chest wall infections: role of spiral CT in detection and management. Crit Rev Comput Tomogr 44:79–93
16.  Pollack MS (1990) Staphylococcal mediastinitis due to sternoclavicular pyarthrosis: CT appearance. J Comput Assist Tomogr 14:924–927
17.  Rosenfeld LE (1985) Osteomyelitis of the first rib presenting as a cold abscess nine months after subclavian venous catheterization. Pacing Clin Electrophysiol 8:897–899

18. Ross JJ, Shamsuddin H (2004) Sternoclavicular septic arthritis: review of 180 cases. Medicine (Baltimore) 83:139–148
19. Shah J, Patkar D, Parikh B, Parmar H, Varma R, Patankar T, Prasad S (2000) Tuberculosis of the sternum and clavicle: imaging findings in 15 patients. Skeletal Radiol 29:447–453
20. Song HK, Guy TS, Kaiser LR, Shrager JB (2002) Current presentation and optimal surgical management of sternoclavicular joint infections. Ann Thorac Surg 73:427–431
21. Tecce PM, Fishman EK (1995) Spiral CT with multiplanar reconstruction in the diagnosis of sternoclavicular osteomyelitis. Skeletal Radiol 24:275–281
22. Templeton PA, Fishman EK (1992) CT evaluation of poststernotomy complications. Am J Roentgenol 159:45–50
23. Tucker GS (1990) Bilateral tuberculous osteomyelitis of the clavicle. Orthopedics 13:767–768
24. Van Linthoudt D, De Torrente A, Humair L, Ott H (1987) Septic manubriosternal arthritis in a patient with Reiter's disease. Clin Rheumatol 6:293–295
25. Yasuda T, Tamura K, Fujiwara M (1995) Tuberculous arthritis of the sternoclavicular joint. A report of three cases. J Bone Joint Surg Am 77:136–139
26. Zanelli G, Sansoni S, Migliorini L, Donati E, Cellesi C (2003) Sternoclavicular joint infection in an adult without predisposing risk factors. Infez Med 11:105–107
27. Zhao X, Chen S, Deanda A Jr, Kiev J (2006) A rare presentation of tuberculosis. Am Surg 72:96–97

# 17 Primary Bone Tumours

UKIHIDE TATEISHI, UMIO YAMAGUCHI,
MOTOTAKA MIYAKE, TETSUO MAEDA,
HIROKAZU CHUMAN AND YASUAKI ARAI

**Contents**



## 17.1 Introduction

Primary bone tumours of the sternocostoclavicular region are generally uncommon. They consist of both malignant and benign tumours of osseous and cartilaginous origin, and tumours evolving from fibrous tissue and other mesenchymal structures. Although primary bone tumours are uncommon, almost every bone tumour that occurs anywhere in the skeleton has been described in the sternocostoclavicular region [1, 2, 7, 13, 19, 25, 26, 32, 36, 37]. Tumour-like lesions such as bone cysts can also occur.

Imaging is important in the assessment of these tumours, particularly in identifying their origin and extent, response to therapy and recurrence. The imaging features of many of the lesions are non-specific, but the combination of imaging appearance, location and clinical information may suggest the diagnosis in some cases [41, 42]. Conventional chest radiography can be used to determine the location, size, rate of growth, calcification/ossification within the tumour and bone involvement. CT allows more accurate assessment of tumour morphology, composition, location and extent. When the relevant anatomy is poorly visualised on axial images, for example when the lesions parallel the ribs or are in the supraclavicular region, CT can be obtained with an angled gantry or using a thin-slice breath-hold technique with multiplanar reconstruction to clarify the anatomical relationships. MR imaging often allows tissue characterisation, accurate assessment of tumour extent and differentiation from adjacent inflammation. [18]F-fluorodeoxyglucose (FDG) positron emission tomography/computed tomography (PET/CT) may improve the localisation of regions of increased FDG uptake and the accuracy of staging of primary bone tumours of the sternocostoclavicular region.

## 17.2
## Primary Malignant Bone Tumours

This rare group of tumours mainly consists of chondrosarcoma, osteosarcoma, Ewing sarcoma or primitive neuroectodermal tumour, and pleomorphic malignant fibrous histiocytoma, which may involve both the bones and soft tissue structures.

### 17.2.1
### Chondrosarcoma

Chondrosarcomas are the most frequent primary malignant bone tumours of the chest wall, usually arising from either the costochondral arches or the sternum. Extraosseous chondrosarcomas are far less common [21, 50]. Most chondrosarcomas occur in the ribs, usually as primary lesions, but 10% arise from pre-existing benign tumours. Two peak periods of prevalence have been identified, the first before 20 years of age and the second during the sixth decade. Chest wall chondrosarcomas have a 2:1 male predilection, and most frequently occur along the upper five ribs adjacent to costal cartilage.

A permeative pattern of bone destruction, irregular contour and intratumoral mineralisation are characteristic but variable features are detected by conventional chest radiography. The degrees and types of calcification vary widely, and include calcification in the form of rings and arcs, flocculent or stippled calcification, and dense calcification.

Computed tomography is a sensitive method for delineating chondroid matrix calcifications (Fig. 17.1). The highly differentiated chondrosarcomas appear as well-defined, densely calcified masses on CT.

Magnetic resonance imaging reveals a lobulated soft tissue mass whose signal intensity is similar to that of muscle on T1-weighted MR images and equal to or

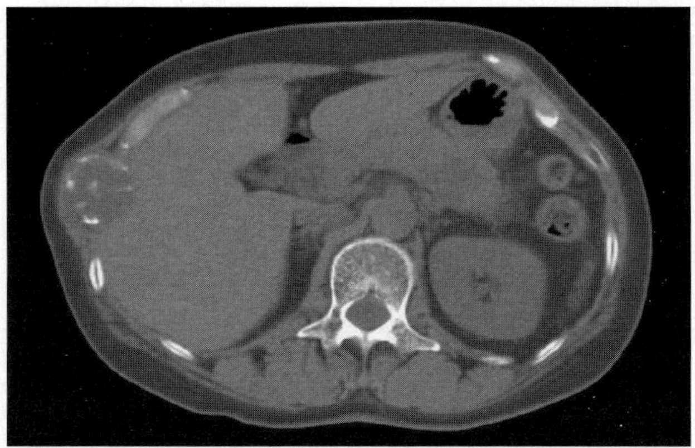

**Fig. 17.1** Chondrosarcoma in a 53-year-old woman presenting a mass arising from the right rib. Axial non-enhanced CT image demonstrates a mass with chondroid mineralisation and invasion of the overlying musculature

greater than that of fat on T2-weighted MR images. Following administration of intravenous contrast material, enhancement is typically heterogeneous, especially at the periphery (Fig. 17.2). Myxoid chondrosarcomas do not contain chondroid calcifications or exhibit bone formation, and they sometimes appear as markedly high signal intensity on T2-weighted MR images [24].

Imaging by FDG PET/CT shows significantly higher uptake in high-grade than in low-grade chondrosarcomas. Low-grade tumour often shows no radioisotope uptake on FDG PET/CT [44]. FDG PET/CT may thus be useful for predicting high-grade chondrosarcomas.

## 17.2.2
## Osteosarcoma

Osteosarcomas are malignant mesenchymal neoplasms, and they are rare in the sternocostoclavicular region. In the thoracic area they most frequently originate in the rib, scapula and clavicle and they may be accompanied by an extrapleural mass. Extraosseous osteosarcomas are less common, and the mean age of patients at presentation is 50 years in contrast to patients with its intraosseous counterpart, who usually present in their twenties or thirties. Tumours are typically manifested clinically as painful masses. Local recurrence and metastases to the lungs and lymph nodes are more frequent compared to osteosarcoma of the extremities, and they contribute to the poor survival.

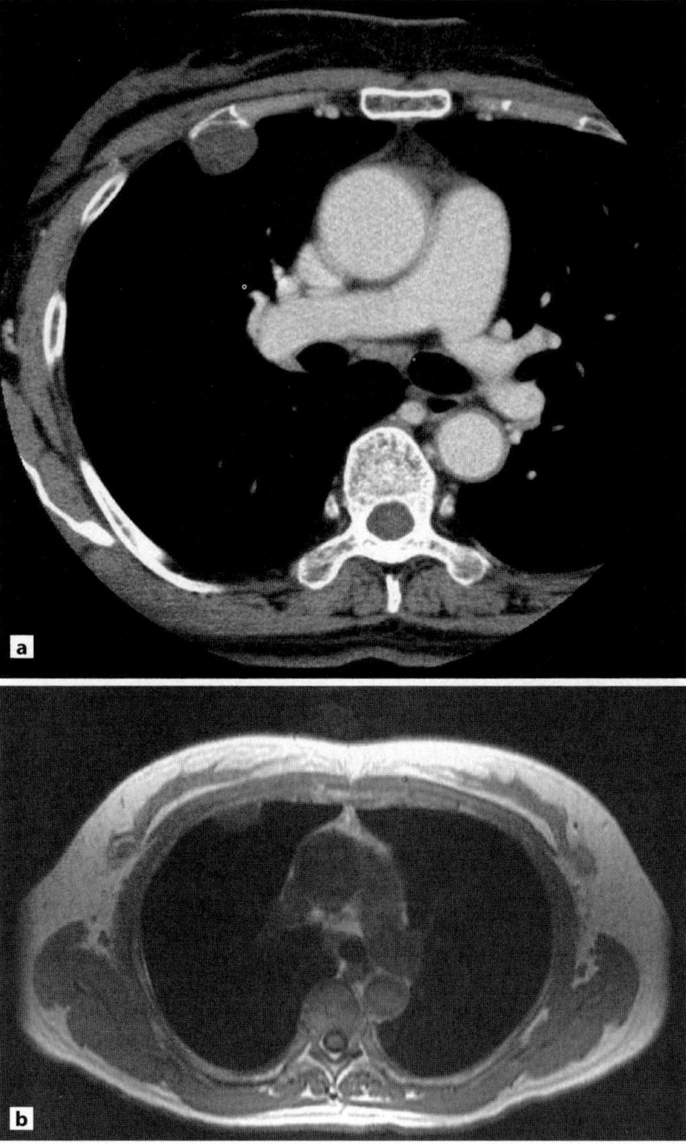

**Fig. 17.2a,b** Chondrosarcoma in a 61-year-old woman. **a** Axial contrast-enhanced CT image shows hypoattenuating mass compared to adjacent musculature. **b** Axial T1-weighted MR image shows a mass, hypointense relative to muscle

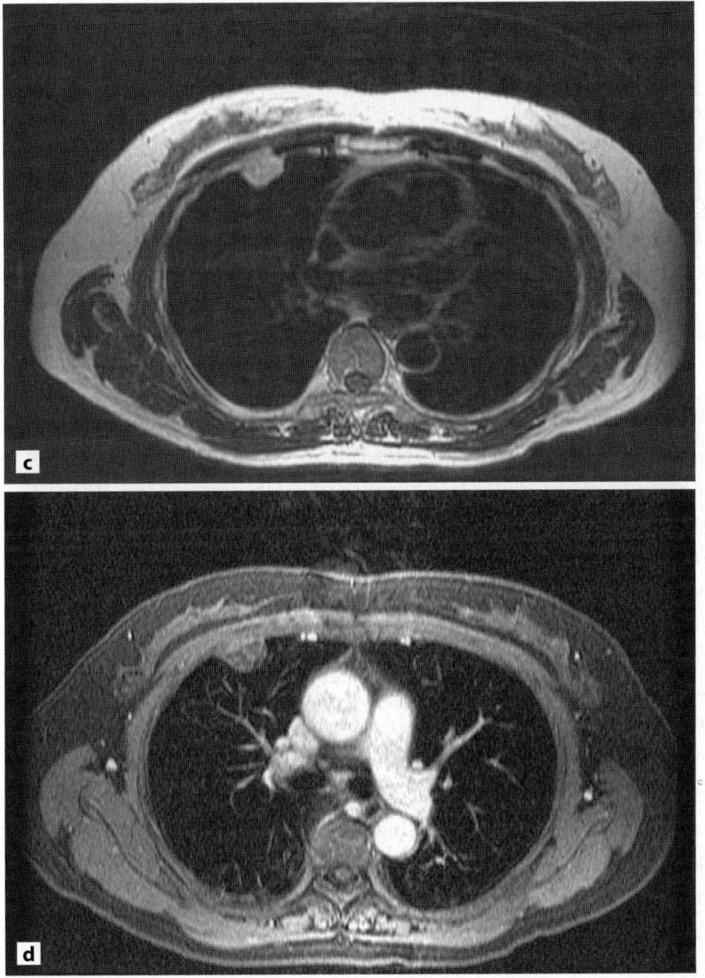

**Fig. 17.2c,d** Chondrosarcoma in a 61-year-old woman. **c** Axial T2-weighted MR image shows a homogeneous mass with long T2, suggestive of the chondroid matrix. **d** Axial contrast-enhanced fat saturated T1-weighted MR image shows slight peripheral and heterogeneous enhancement

Radiographs show calcification or osteoid bone matrix within a mass that may be lytic or sclerotic. An important feature of the mineralisation on CT is its spatial distribution, which is greatest at the centre of the lesion and least at the periphery.

Magnetic resonance imaging shows a multilobulated mass that may be heterogeneously hypo- to isointense relative to muscle on T1-weighted MR images. Mixed but predominantly high signal intensity is observed on T2-weighted MR

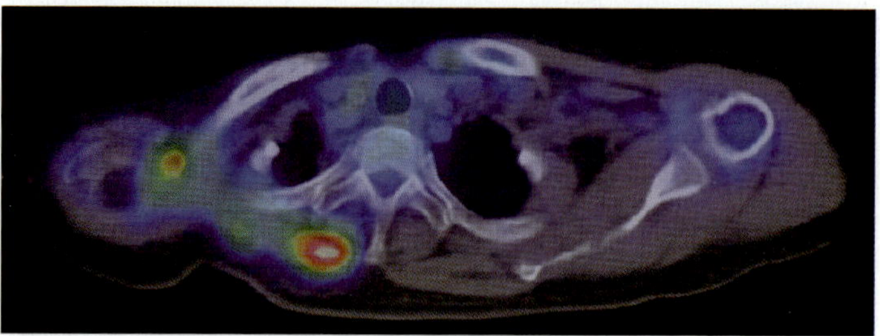

**Fig. 17.3** Osteosarcoma in a 58-year-old woman. Axial FDG PET/CT image shows abnormal accumulation in the rib and scapular region

images. The tumour shows heterogeneous enhancement after administration of intravenous contrast media [39]. FDG PET provides a precise tool for non-invasive evaluation of the therapeutic response of osteosarcoma [34, 43]. The decreases in FDG uptake by osteosarcomas correlate well with the amount of tumour necrosis. Patients whose lesions show a marked decrease of FDG uptake after therapy have a more favourable prognosis (Fig. 17.3).

## 17.2.3
## Ewing Sarcoma/Primitive Neuroectodermal Tumour

Askin first described a clinicopathological entity characterised by malignant small cell tumours in 20 children and adolescents, which appeared to originate in the soft tissues of the chest wall [4]. The tumour, known as primitive neuroectodermal tumour (PNET), is now recognised as a more aggressive type of Ewing sarcoma (ES). Both of these tumours probably develop from embryonal neural crest cells, and they contain several balanced reciprocal translocations. The translocation points have been cloned, and they have been found to be identical in all the tumours. ES/PNET develops either as a solitary mass or multiple masses with an eccentric growth pattern [10]. The sarcoma usually arises in the ribs, scapula, clavicle or sternum, but occasionally is of extraskeletal origin. Expansion of chest wall tumours may cause the lung to collapse, or the neoplasm may invade the lung. It tends to displace adjacent soft tissue structures rather than to invade or encase them. Larger tumours show direct infiltration of the surrounding structures.

At CT, the tumours are visualised as large, ill-defined masses having an inhomogeneous appearance due to extensive haemorrhage or cystic degeneration [52]. They may be seen to contain calcification.

At MRI, tumours generally have signal intensity equal to or greater than that of muscle on T1-weighted MR images (Fig. 17.4). Larger tumours appear as heteroge-

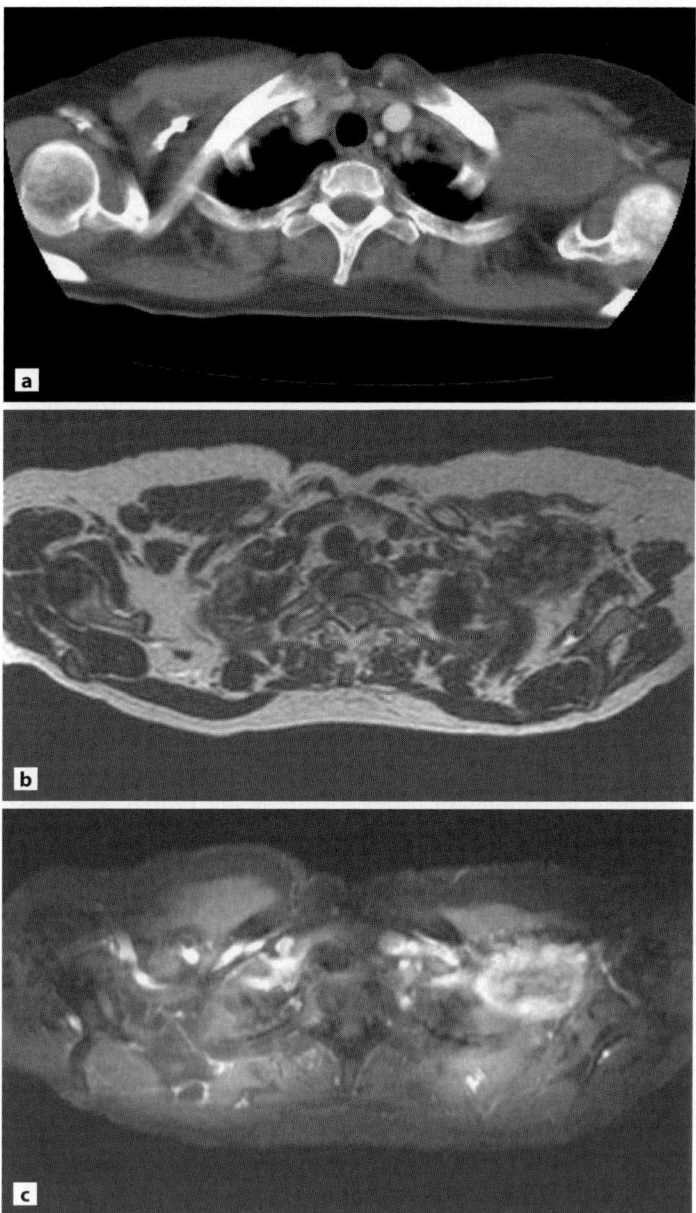

**Fig. 17.4** Ewing sarcoma/primitive neuroectodermal tumour (ES/PNET) in a 57-year-old woman. **a** Axial contrast-enhanced CT scan shows an ill-defined mass arising from the left supraclavicular region. **b** Axial T2-weighted MR image shows isointense signal relative to muscle. **c** Axial contrast-enhanced fat-saturated T1-weighted MR image shows heterogeneous enhancement extending into the surrounding soft tissues

neous masses, frequently with evidence of haemorrhage or necrosis, while smaller ones tend to be more homogeneous. On T2-weighted images, the tumours tend to manifest as inhomogeneous high signal intensity [52]. Tumours show marked enhancement after intravenous administration of contrast material (Fig. 17.4).

The appearance of ES/PNET on FDG PET imaging correlates with their histological response to neoadjuvant chemotherapy [16]. A peripheral rim of FDG accumulation has been found to correlate pathologically with the formation of a fibrous pseudocapsule. The pretreatment maximal standard uptake values (SUV) after neoadjuvant chemotherapy independently identify patients at high risk of recurrence.

## 17.2.4
## Pleomorphic Malignant Fibrous Histiocytoma/ Undifferentiated High-grade Pleomorphic Sarcoma

Pleomorphic malignant fibrous histiocytoma (PMFH) is the most common soft tissue sarcoma of late adult life, but it rarely occurs in the chest wall. The tumours arise in deep fascia or skeletal muscle, and rarely in bone, although involvement of adjacent bone is common. PMFH was initially described as having a histiocytic origin, although the histogenesis of the tumour is still uncertain [12]. PMFH are the most common form, accounting for over two thirds of all cases.

Pleomorphic malignant fibrous histiocytoma appears on CT as a non-specific, heterogeneously enhancing mass arising along muscle and fascial planes (Fig. 17.5). At MRI, PMFH may be either homogeneous or heterogeneous on both T1-weighted and T2-weighted MR images. Most tumours have signal intensity equal to that of muscle on T1-weighted MR images and show iso- or hyperintensity relative to fat on T2-weighted MR images [40]. FDG PET shows intense accumulation in PMFH. Maximal SUV correlates well with tumour grade [45].

## 17.3
## Primary Benign Tumours

## 17.3.1
## Osteochondroma

Osteochondromas are relatively common skeletal lesions, and are regarded as neoplasms or aberration of normal tissue growth. In the ribs, they are particularly frequent at the costochondral junction. The tumours are characteristically pedunculated osseous protuberances arising from the surface of the parent bone.

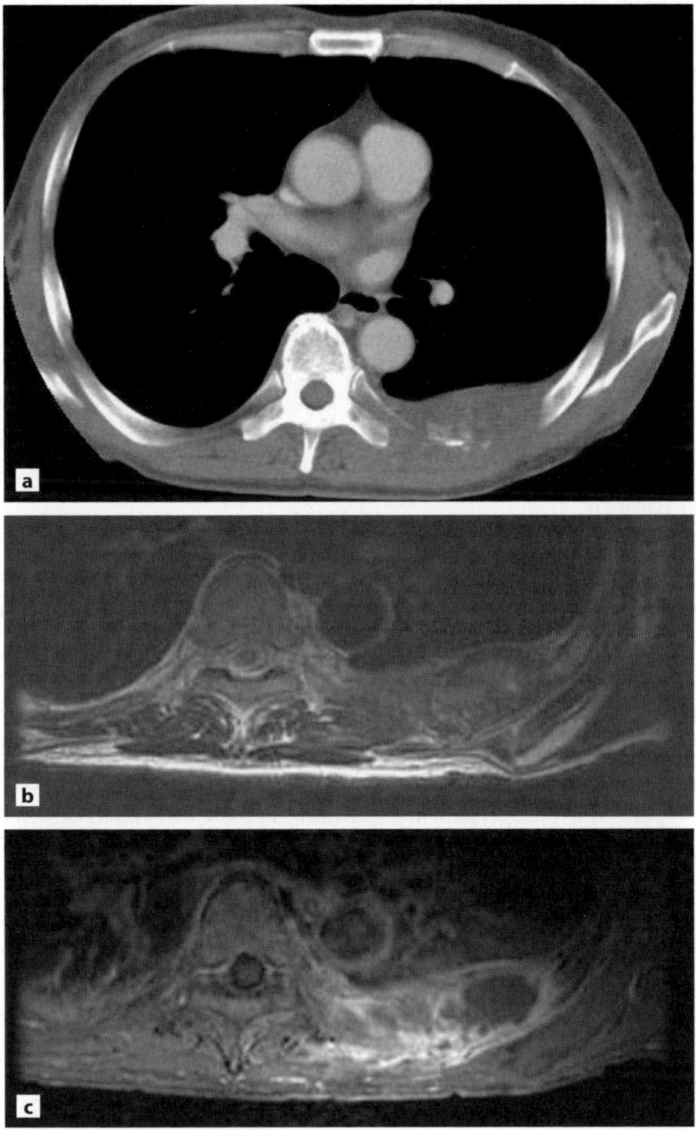

**Fig. 17.5** Pleomorphic malignant fibrous histiocytoma (PMFH) in a 65-year-old man. **a** Axial contrast-enhanced CT scan shows a destructive mass originating in the left rib and extending into the surrounding soft tissues. **b** Axial T2-weighted MR image shows heterogeneous signal intensity within the tumour **c** Axial contrast-enhanced fat-saturated T1-weighted MR image shows heterogeneous enhancement

Conventional radiography may show a "cap" composed of hyaline cartilage that can be calcified and is then optimally visualised on CT. The cartilaginous tissue in the cap appears as high signal intensity on T2-weighted MR images. Continuity between cortical and medullary bone in the extremities can be detected by CT or MRI studies, but it is seldom present in the ribs (Fig. 17.6). Several complications are associated with this tumour, including fractures, osseous deformity, vascular injury, neural compression, bursa formation and malignant transformation [28]. Bone destruction, irregular calcification, thickening of the cartilage cap or the development of pain at the lesion site suggests malignant transformation. Although FDG PET imaging of osteochondromas does not show significant accumulation, tumours that have undergone malignant transformation may show abnormal uptake of FDG.

### 17.3.2
### Giant Cell Tumour

Giant cell tumours (GCTs) are relatively common benign skeletal tumours of uncertain origin that contain abundant giant cells mixed with spindle stromal cells and vascular sinuses filled or lined by tumour cells. Tumours are typically solitary, although in rare cases multicentric GCTs occur simultaneously or metachronously. GCTs typically present in the fourth or fifth decades of life after closure of the epiphyses. Thoracic GCTs are rare, usually arising in the subchondral regions in the flat or tubular bones of the chest wall, including the sternum, clavicle and ribs.

On conventional radiographs, the tumours appear as eccentric, osteolytic lesions causing cortical thinning and expansion. CT allows evaluation of tumour extent and its relationship to surrounding structures. At MRI, the tumour typically manifests as low signal intensity on T1-weighted and relative high signal intensity on T2-weighted MR images [8, 9]. Fluid-fluid levels within the tumour are less common than in aneurysmal bone cysts [23, 29]. FDG PET imaging of GCTs shows abnormal uptake reflecting tracer trapping in giant cells, foamy cells and lymphocytes within the lesion. Enhanced FDG uptake is attributable to enhanced vascular angiogenesis and increased FDG transport [38].

### 17.3.3
### Chondromyxoid Fibroma

Chondromyxoid fibromas are the least common benign cartilaginous neoplasms, composed of varying proportions of chondroid, myxomatous and fibrous

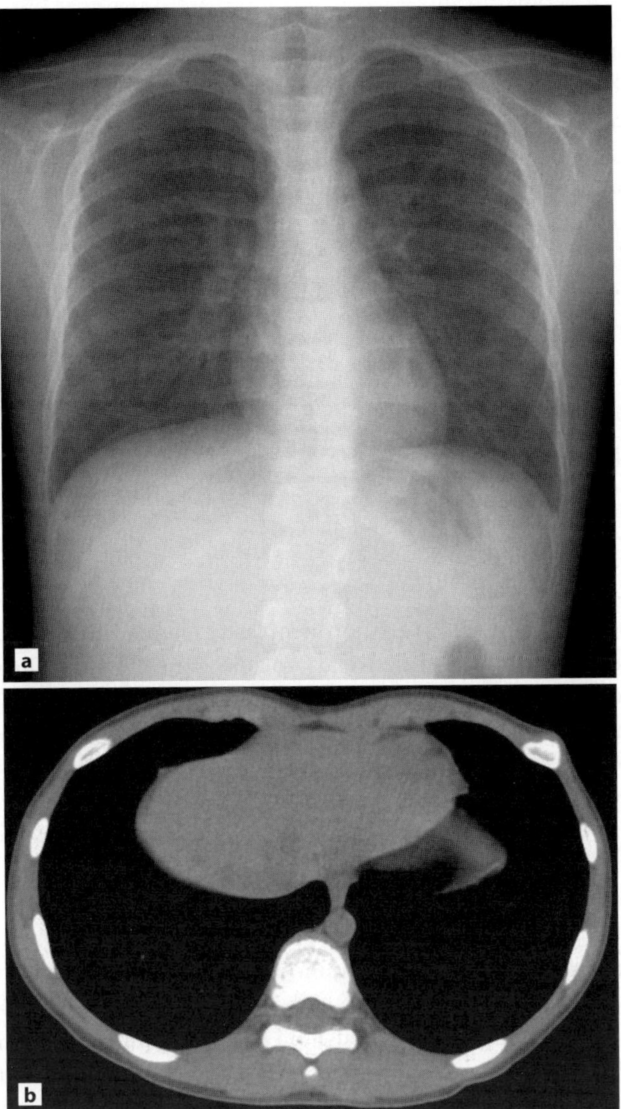

**Fig. 17.6 Osteochondroma** in a 6-year-old boy. **a** Chest radiograph shows dense calcification in the left rib. **b** Axial non-enhanced CT image shows a tumour with pronounced calcification projecting slightly

components arranged in lobules separated by vascular sclerotic bands. Chondro-myxoid fibromas typically occur in patients under 30 years of age. The tumour is rare in the chest wall, but occasionally occurs in the ribs, spine or scapula.

On conventional radiographs, chondromyxoid fibromas usually appear as well-demarcated masses with scalloped, sclerotic borders and no internal calcification [11]. Cortical expansion, exuberant endosteal sclerosis and overlapping areas of cortical scalloping, which may give the impression of coarse trabeculation, are present [51]. At MRI, the tumours show heterogeneous signal intensity on T2-weighted and diffuse enhancement on T1-weighted MR images after intravenous administration of contrast media.

## 17.4
## Tumour-like Lesions

### 17.4.1
### Aneurysmal Bone Cyst

Aneurysmal bone cysts (ABCs) are non-neoplastic masses with potential for rapid growth, bone destruction and extension into adjacent soft tissue. The masses contain a meshwork of multiple blood-filled cysts lined by fibroblasts and multinucleated osteoclast-type giant cells. Although a sclerotic margin around the lesion may indicate its benign nature, soft tissue extension can make it difficult to differentiate an ABC from a sarcoma. Most ABCs occur in patients under the age of 30 years. The most common site of involvement in the thoracic region is the posterior elements of the spine.

Conventional radiography shows an expanding lesion with a well-defined inner margin. CT is useful in delineating the size and location of the intraosseous and extraosseous components of the tumour (Fig. 17.7). MRI typically shows an expanding, lobulated or septated mass with a thin, well-defined rim of low signal intensity [5, 53]. The presence of a fluid-fluid level within the tumour indicates the haemorrhagic nature of the cyst contents; however, fluid-fluid levels may also be found in other osseous lesions, including GCTs, simple bone cysts and chondro-blastomas [17, 18].

### 17.4.2
### Fibrous Dysplasia

Fibrous dysplasia is a skeletal developmental anomaly of bone-forming mesen-chyme in which osteoblasts fail to undergo normal morphological differentiation

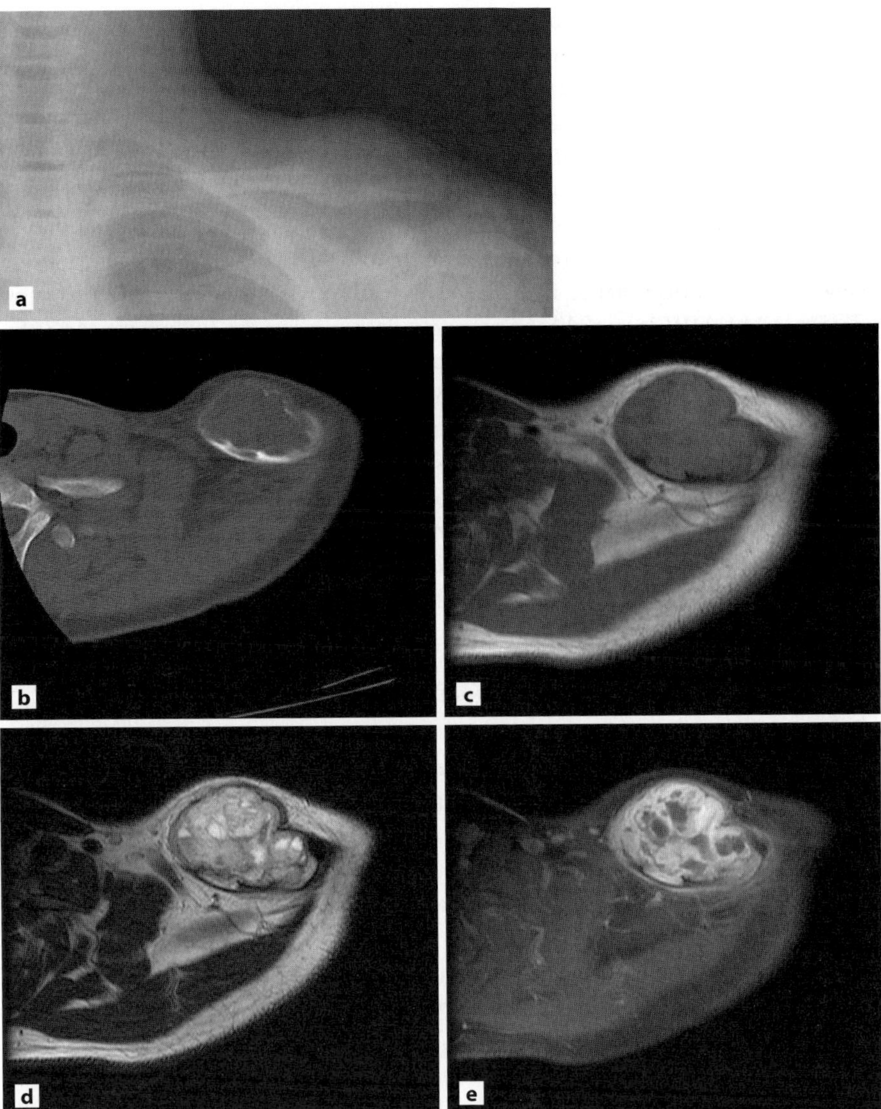

**Fig. 17.7** Aneurysmal bone cyst in a 13-year-old boy. **a** Radiograph of the left clavicle shows an expansive mass. **b** Axial non-enhanced CT image through the clavicle shows a lytic mass with poorly delineated septations. **c** Axial T1-weighted MR image shows a mass, slightly hyperintense relative to muscle. **d** Axial T2-weighted MR image shows a heterogeneous mass with signal hyperintense to fat and containing a fluid-fluid level with multiple septations of hypointense signal. **e** Axial contrast-enhanced fat saturated T1-weighted (600/15) MR image shows heterogeneous enhancement

and maturation. Approximately 70–80% of cases are monostotic, and the other 20–30% are polyostotic. The age of patients with monostotic disease ranges from 10 to 70 years, but recognition is most frequent between 20 and 30 years of age. Patients are usually asymptomatic, although complication by pathological fracture is sometimes manifested clinically as pain. The ribs are commonly affected, whereas the clavicle is only occasionally involved.

Conventional radiography characteristically shows unilateral, fusiform enlargement and deformity with cortical thickening and increased trabeculation of one or more ribs. Amorphous or irregular calcification is often seen in the lesion on CT (Fig. 17.8). MRI is useful for accurately determining the full extent of the lesion (Fig. 17.8). The signal intensity characteristics are various, although the areas of involvement typically display low signal intensity on T1-weighted MR images and low, intermediate or high signal intensity on T2-weighted MR images [20, 22, 49]. Monostotic involvement does not usually convert to polyostotic disease and, in most patients, the size and number of lesions do not increase at the time of the initial radiological evaluation. Malignant transformation is rare, although osteosarcoma and fibrosarcoma may develop after radiation to the involved bones. FDG PET imaging of fibrous dysplasia shows abnormal uptake similar to that of malignant bone tumours [35].

## 17.5
## Management of Primary Bone Tumours of the Sternocostoclavicular Region

Tumours involving the sternocostoclavicular region are rare and a heterogeneous group that ranges from benign lesions to highly aggressive lesions. The clinical management of these tumours therefore differs substantially from the wait-and-see policy or local marginal surgery to cases that need a multimodality approach, including systemic chemotherapy, radiotherapy and surgical intervention. Surgical resection of the tumour is the only acceptable goal of treatment for most of these tumours. For low-grade tumours, such as chondrosarcomas, the preferred treatment is complete resection, because no effective chemotherapy or radiotherapy is available for these tumours. Osteosarcoma and ES/PNET respond to chemotherapy, and ES/PNET responds to radiotherapy. Perioperative chemotherapy or/and radiotherapy of these tumours result in improved local control, fewer metastases and better postoperative survival than in patients who do not receive perioperative treatment. Surgical resection of tumours involving the sternocostoclavicular region, however, often presents a challenge, because the presence of the thoracic cage and adjacent neurovascular structures make dissection with tumour-free margins difficult.

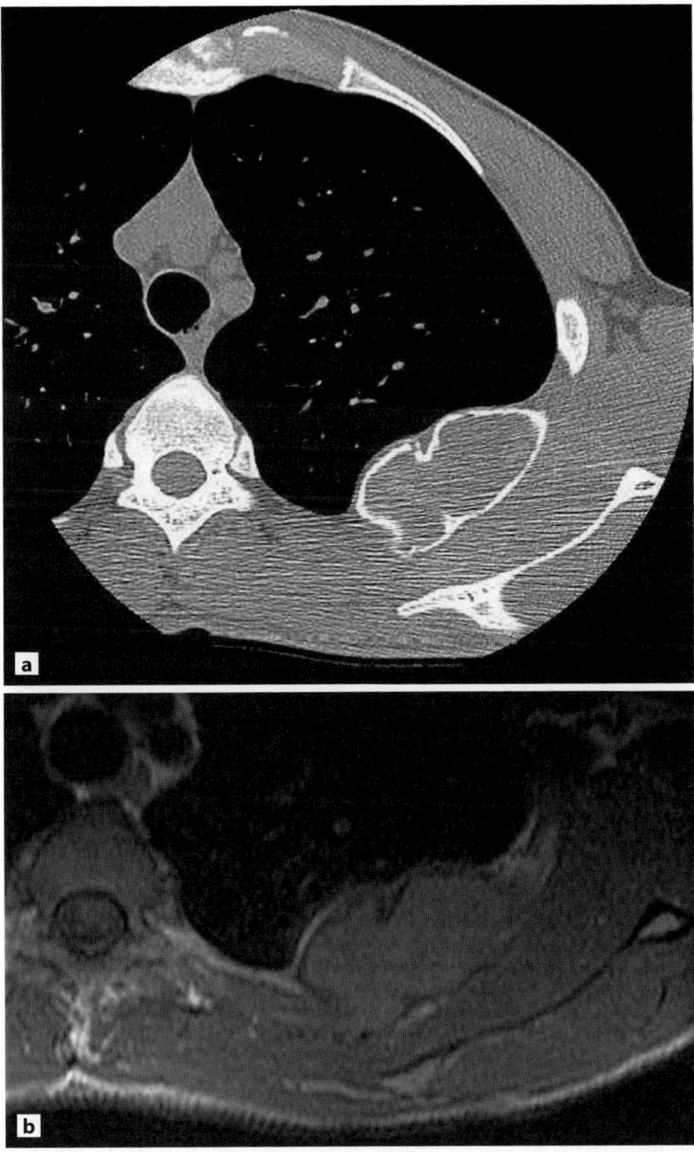

**Fig. 17.8** Fibrous dysplasia in a 34-year-old man. **a** Axial non-enhanced CT scan shows an expansive mass with ground-glass mineralisation. **b** Axial T1-weighted MR image shows a mass with signal isointense to muscle. **c,d** *see page 222*

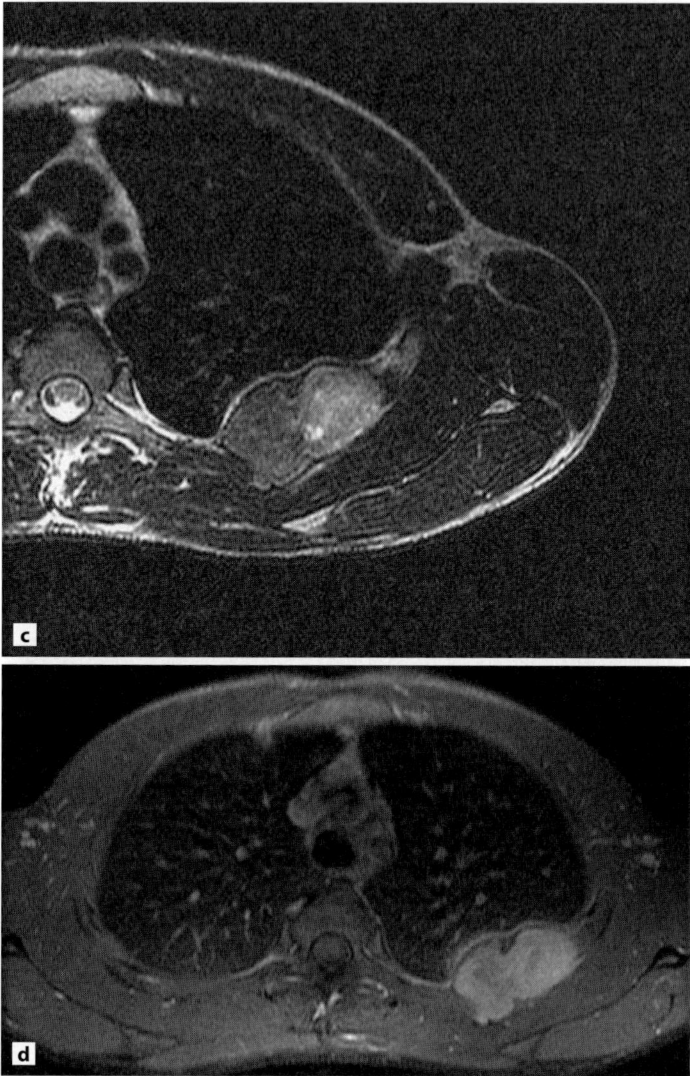

**Fig. 17.8** (*continued*) **c,d** Fibrous dysplasia in a 34-year-old man. **c** Axial T2-weighted MR image shows heterogeneous signal intensity within the tumour. **d** Axial contrast-enhanced fat-saturated T1-weighted MR image shows heterogeneous enhancement

## 17.5.1
## Surgical Management of Primary Tumours of the Sternum

Surgery for sternal tumours has long been considered a challenge because the anatomical aspects make full-thickness resections difficult without compromising the stability and reconstruction of the thoracic wall [7, 19, 25, 26]. For these reasons, the aggressiveness, size and location of the tumour determine the extent of resection. Preoperative imaging allows precise location of the tumour and detection of possible invasion of the lung, pericardium, brachiocephalic vein and superior vena cava. The use of musculocutaneous flaps and prosthetic materials allowing simultaneous reconstruction of defects in the chest wall make wide full-thickness resection of the sternum recommended [33, 46]. Ensuring a tumour-free margin defines the extent of resection. Tumours of the upper third of the sternum require resection of the manubrium, most of the sternal body, the proximal ends of the clavicles and the adjacent sternocostal cartilages. Tumours of the middle third of the sternum require resection of the sternal body but not of the manubrium or xiphoid process. In the deep aspect of the tumour, adherent pleura or pericardium should be resected. To restore the ventilatory mechanics and protect the intrathoracic organs, many prosthetic materials with various degrees of flexibility are available to reconstruct the defects after removal of the sternum (Fig. 17.9).

## 17.5.2
## Surgical Management of Primary Tumours of the Clavicle

Surgical management of primary clavicle tumours includes partial or total resection. Total resection of the clavicle is only performed if needed to obtain tumour-free margins as it may influence the function of the shoulder. Fortunately it is rarely needed. For partial resection of the clavicle, preservation of the coracoclavicular ligament is important when resecting the lateral end of the clavicle because the stump of the clavicle loses its stability without it and presses upwards against the soft tissues in the supraclavicular region, resulting in pain and disability. If the coracoclavicular ligament cannot be preserved or repaired, the lateral two thirds of the clavicle must be resected [1, 46]. Resection of the middle third of the clavicle is acceptable and there is no functional disability [1]. When the medial end of the clavicle is resected, the costoclavicular ligament should be preserved or the inner third of the clavicle should be resected for the same reasons as in resection of the lateral part of the clavicle [1]. If the tumour is near the sternoclavicular joint, it may be necessary to perform an en bloc resection of the sternoclavicular joint with a portion of the sternum. When the tumour has a soft tissue component, the deep

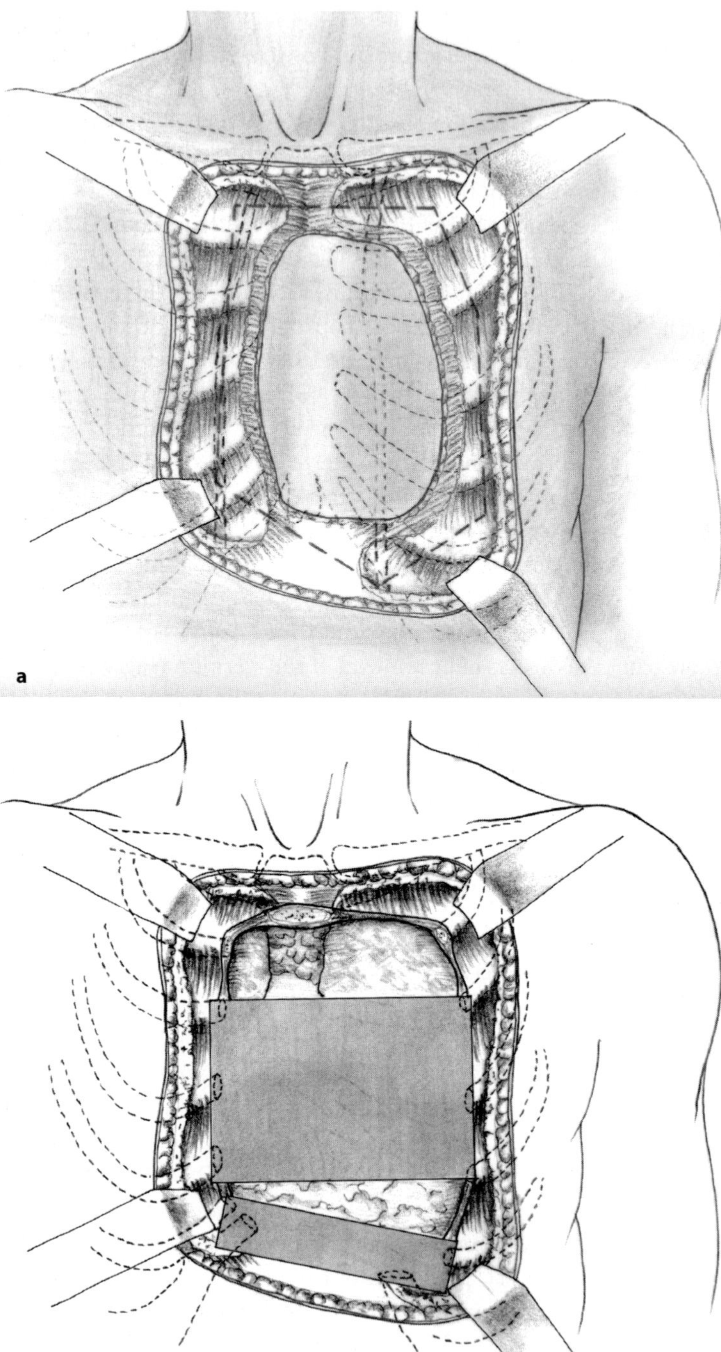

◁ **Fig. 17.9 a** Drawing showing the skin and muscle excision to be incorporated with resection of the sternum. **b** Titanium mesh is used to reconstruct the defect of the anterior chest wall

anatomical aspect of the clavicle sometimes makes it difficult to obtain a tumour-free margin. The subclavian vessels and the brachial plexus lie beneath the clavicle as they pass from the root of the neck to the axilla. When the tumour is very near these vital vessels, it is important to remove the myofascial layer covering the vessels with the tumour when the clavicle is resected en bloc.

### 17.5.3
### Surgical Management of Primary Tumours of the Ribs

The distribution of rib tumours depends on whether they are benign or malignant [3, 14, 15, 31, 33, 47, 48]. It is generally agreed that all primary rib tumours should be treated by complete en bloc resection. Even when large segments of the chest wall are resected, it is well tolerated and usually results in little functional impairment [6]. Careful evaluation of clinical and radiological findings is important to determine whether it is a benign or malignant tumour prior to surgery. There should be no hesitation to perform radical wide resection if the tumour is malignant to prevent local recurrences and dissemination of tumour cells in the thoracic cavity. The resection must include the involved rib and a wide surgical margin including the corresponding costochondral arches, and several partial ribs above and below the tumour [14, 31, 33, 47]. If there is infiltration of the soft tissue, pleura, lung parenchyma or diaphragm, the involved parts should also be resected. If the tumour is near the sternum, combined sternal resection should be performed. When there is a large defect in the chest wall, reconstruction of the bony thorax is necessary to maintain sufficient chest wall fixation and adequate respiratory function. Materials used to repair the bony defect include autologous tissue, such as periosteum or ribs, or prosthetic materials [3, 27, 30]. In some situations, musculocutaneous flaps may be necessary to cover soft tissue defects.

### 17.6
### Conclusion

Primary bone tumours of the sternocostoclavicular region include a diverse group of lesions of osseous and cartilaginous origin. Radiological assessment is an essential component of the management of these tumours. Evaluation usually includes conventional chest radiography to detect and localise the lesion, cross-sectional imaging (CT or MRI) to further characterise and define tumour extent, and anato-metabolic correlations with FDG PET/CT. Several of the primary bone tumours of the sternocostoclavicular region have characteristic features that allow confident identification. However, many tumours have non-specific imaging features and biopsy is frequently required for diagnosis. Despite this, imaging remains important to patient management and is frequently used to facilitate biopsy, assess postprocedural complications, monitor tumours that are not excised and assess significant prognostic imaging characteristics.

**Acknowledgements.** The authors acknowledge the help of Dr. Akira Kawai, Dr. Fumihiko Nakatani and Dr. Yasuo Beppu for their contribution to the study. This work was funded by BMS Freedom to Discovery Grant and was supported in part by grants for Scientific Research Expenses for Health and Welfare Programs, number 17–12.

# References


1.  Abbott LC, Lucas DB (1954) The function of the clavicle: its surgical significance. Ann Surg 140:583–599
2.  Anderson HS (1931) Lesions of clavicle. Radiology 16:181–186
3.  Arnold PG, Pairolero PC (1981) Chest wall reconstruction. Ann Thorac Surg 32:325–326
4.  Askin FB, Rosai J, Sibley RK, Dehner LP, McAlister WH (1979) Malignant small cell tumor of the thoracopulmonary region in childhood: a distinctive clinicopathologic entity of uncertain histogenesis. Cancer 43:2438–2451
5.  Beltran J, Simon DC, Levy M, et al (1986) Aneurysmal bone cysts: MR imaging at 1.5 T. Radiology 158:689–690
6.  Campbell DA (1950) Reconstruction of the anterior thoracic wall. J Thorac Surg 19:456–461
7.  Chapelier AR, Missana MC, Couturaud B, et al (2004) Sternal resection and reconstruction for primary malignant tumors. Ann Thorac Surg 77:1001–1007
8.  Cooper KL, Beabout JW, Dahlin DC (1984) Giant cell tumor: ossification in soft-tissue implants. Radiology 153:597–602
9.  Dahlin DC (1985) Caldwell Lecture. Giant cell tumor of bone: highlights of 407 cases. AJR 144:955–960
10. Dehner LP (1993) Primitive neuroectodermal tumor and Ewing's sarcoma. Am J Surg Pathol 17:1–13
11. Feldman F, Hecht HL, Johnston AD (1970) Chondromyxoid fibroma of bone. Radiology 94:249–260
12. Fletcher CD, Gustafson P, Rydholm A, Willen H, Akerman M (2001) Clinicopathologic re-evaluation of 100 malignant fibrous histiocytomas: prognostic relevance of subclassification. J Clin Oncol 19:3045–3050

13. Glay A (1961) Destructive lesions of clavicle. J Can Assoc Radiol 12:117–125

14. Graeber GM, Snyder RJ, Fleming AW, et al (1982) Initial and long term results in the management of primary chest wall neoplasms. Ann Thorac Surg 34:664–673

15. Graham J, Usher FC, Perry SL (1960) Marlex mesh as a prosthesis in the repair of thoracic wall defects. Ann Surg 151:469–479

16. Hawkins DS, Schuetze SM, Butrynski JE, et al (2005) [18F]Fluorodeoxyglucose positron emission tomography predicts outcome for Ewing sarcoma family of tumors. J Clin Oncol 23:8828–8834

17. Hudson TM (1984) Fluid levels in aneurysmal bone cysts: a CT feature. AJR 142:1001–1004

18. Hudson TM, Hamlin DJ, Fitzsimmons JR (1985) Magnetic resonance imaging of fluid levels in an aneurysmal bone cyst and in anticoagulated human blood. Skeletal Radiol 13:267–270

19. Incarbone M, Nava M, Lequaglie C, et al (1997) Sternal resection for primary or secondary tumors. J Thorac Cardiovasc Surg 114:93–99

20. Jee WH, Choi KH, Choe BY, Park JM, Shinn KS (1996) Fibrous dysplasia: MR imaging characteristics with radiopathologic correlation. AJR 167:1523–1527

21. Kransdorf MJ, Meis JM (1993) From the archives of the AFIP. Extraskeletal osseous and cartilaginous tumors of the extremities. Radiographics 13:853–884

22. Kransdorf MJ, Moser RP Jr, Gilkey FW (1990) Fibrous dysplasia. Radiographics 10:519–537

23. Lee MJ, Sallomi DF, Munk PL, et al (1998) Pictorial review: giant cell tumours of bone. Clin Radiol 53:481–489

24. Lee FY, Yu J, Chang SS, et al (2004) Diagnostic value and limitations of fluorine-18 fluorodeoxyglucose positron emission tomography for cartilaginous tumors of bone. J Bone Joint Surg Am 86:2677–2685

25. Lequaglie C, Massone PB, Giudice G, et al (2002) Gold standard for sternectomies and plastic reconstructions after resections for primary or secondary sternal neoplasms. Ann Surg Oncol 9:472–479

26. Martini N, Huvos AG, Smith J, Beattie EJ Jr (1974) Primary malignant tumors of the sternum. Surg Gynecol Obstet 138:391–395

27. McCormack P, Bains M, Beattie ED Jr, et al (1981) New trends in skeletal reconstruction after resection. Ann Thorac Surg 31:45–52

28. Murphey MD, Choi JJ, Kransdorf MJ, et al (2000) Imaging of osteochondroma: variants and complications with radiologic-pathologic correlation. Radiographics 20:1407–1434

29. Murphey MD, Nomikos GC, Flemming DJ, Gannon FH, Temple HT, Kransdorf MJ (2001) From the archives of AFIP. Imaging of giant cell tumor and giant cell reparative granuloma of bone: radiologic-pathologic correlation. Radiographics 21:1283–1309

30. Pairolero PC, Arnold PG (1985) Chest wall tumors: experience with 100 consecutive patients. J Thorac Cardiovasc Surg 90:367–372

31. Pascuzzi CA, Dahlin DC, Clagett OT (1957) Primary tumors of the ribs and sternum. Surg Gynecol Obstet 104:390–400

32. Pratt GF, Dahlin DC, Ghormley RK (1958) Tumors of scapula and clavicle. Surg Gynecol Obstet 106:536–544

33. Schmidt FE, Trummer MJ (1972) Primary tumours of the ribs. Ann Thorac Surg 13:251–257
34. Schulte M, Brecht-Krauss D, Werner M, et al (1999) Evaluation of neoadjuvant therapy response of osteogenic sarcoma using FDG PET. J Nucl Med 40:1637–1643
35. Shigesawa T, Sugawara Y, Shinohara I, et al (2005) Bone metastasis detected by FDG PET in a patient with breast cancer and fibrous dysplasia. Clin Nucl Med 30:571–573
36. Smith J, McLachlan D, Huvos AG, et al (1975) Primary bone tumors of the clavicle and scapula. AJR 124:113–123
37. Smith J, Yuppa F, Watson RC (1988) Primary tumors and tumor-like lesions of the clavicle. Skeletal Radiol 17:235–246
38. Strauss LG, Dimitrakopoulou-Strauss A, Koczan D, et al (2004) 18F-FDG kinetics and gene expression in giant cell tumors. J Nucl Med 45:1528–1535
39. Sundaram M, McGuire MH, Herbold DR (1987) Magnetic resonance imaging of osteosarcoma. Skeletal Radiol 16:23–29
40. Tateishi U, Kusumoto M, Nishihara H, et al (2002) Primary malignant fibrous histiocytoma of the chest wall: CT and MR appearance. J Comput Assist Tomogr 26:558–563
41. Tateishi U, Gladish GW, Kusumoto M, et al (2003) Chest wall tumors: radiologic findings and pathologic correlation: part 1. Benign tumors. Radiographics 23:1477–1490
42. Tateishi U, Gladish GW, Kusumoto M, et al (2003) Chest wall tumors: radiologic findings and pathologic correlation: part 2. Malignant tumors. Radiographics 23:1491–1508
43. Tateishi U, Yamaguchi U, Terauchi T, et al (2005) Extraskeletal osteosarcoma: extensive tumor thrombus on fused PET-CT images. Ann Nucl Med 19:729–732
44. Tateishi U, Hasegawa T, Nojima T, et al (2006) MRI features of extraskeletal myxoid chondrosarcoma. Skeletal Radiol 35:27–33
45. Tateishi U, Yamaguchi U, Seki K, et al (2006) Glut-1 expression and enhanced glucose metabolism are associated with tumor grade in bone and soft tissue sarcomas: a prospective evaluation by [F-18]-fluorodeoxyglucose positron emission tomography. Eur J Nucl Med Mol Imaging 33:683–691
46. Teitelbaum SL (1969) Tumours of the chest wall. Surg Gynecol Obstet 129:1059–1073
47. Teitelbaum SL (1972) Twenty years experience with intrinsic tumors of the bony thorax at a large institution. J Thorac Cardiovasc Surg 63:776–782
48. Threlkel JB, Adkins RB (1971) Primary chest wall tumors. Ann Thorac Surg 11:450–459
49. Utz JA, Kransdorf MJ, Jelinek JS, Moser RP Jr, Berrey BH (1989) MR appearance of fibrous dysplasia. J Comput Assist Tomogr 13:845–851
50. Varma DG, Ayala AG, Carrasco CH, et al (1992) Chondrosarcoma: MR imaging with pathologic correlation. Radiographics 12:687–704
51. Wilson AJ, Kyriakos M, Ackerman LV (1991) Chondromyxoid fibroma: radiographic appearance in 38 cases and in a review of the literature. Radiology 179:513–518
52. Winer-Muram HT, Kauffman WM, Gronemeyer SA, Jennings SG (1993) Primitive neuroectodermal tumors of the chest wall (Askin tumors): CT and MR findings. AJR 161:265–268
53. Zimmer WD, Berquist TH, Sim FH, et al (1984) Magnetic resonance imaging of aneurysmal bone cyst. Mayo Clin Proc 59:633–636

# 18 Other Malignant Disorders

UKIHIDE TATEISHI, UMIO YAMAGUCHI,
MOTOTAKA MIYAKE, TETSUO MAEDA,
HIROKAZU CHUMAN AND YASUAKI ARAI

**Contents**



## 18.1
## Introduction

Malignant disorders of the sternocostoclavicular region include a diverse group of lesions having a wide variety of histological lineages. The region can be involved in all forms of malignancies, but those usually encountered are metastases (Fig. 7.3), primary bone tumours (Chapter 17), soft tissue tumours and myeloproliferative disorders.

Although radiographs are useful for detecting cortical destruction, they do not allow comprehensive assessment of chest wall tumours [1]. CT and MR imaging often provide additional information regarding local extent and focal tumour invasion as well as tissue characterisation. $^{18}$F-fluorodeoxyglucose (FDG) positron emission tomography combined with CT (PET/CT) can reveal the localisation of target lesions and increase the accuracy in staging and grading of malignant disorders of the sternocostoclavicular region.

This chapter reviews the clinical and imaging features of malignant disorders of the sternocostoclavicular region except primary bone tumours (Chapter 17).

## 18.2
## Malignant Soft Tissue Tumours and Allied Disorders

Malignant soft tissue tumours are more frequent than primary bone tumours. The most frequent tumour types are aggressive fibromatosis, liposarcoma (Fig. 7.2) and malignant fibrous histiocytoma (sometimes involving the bones; Chapter 17), but a large variety of other tumour types are seen as described in the following.

### 18.2.1
### Aggressive Fibromatosis

Aggressive fibromatosis or desmoid tumour is a common tumour. It accounts for 54% of low-grade sarcomas of the chest wall. The chest wall has been reported as the site of origin in 10–28% of patients with shoulder involvement being most common. Aggressive fibromatosis is generally regarded as a neoplasm having intermediate behaviour and tends to occur in adolescents and young adults. The lesions do not metastasise, but usually infiltrate locally although spontaneous regression has been observed. The exact pathogenesis is unknown; however, trauma, endocrine and genetic factors representing chromosomal abnormalities of +8, +20, and 5q- may be implicated. Aggressive fibromatosis may occur as a feature of Gardner's syndrome, but this association is strongest for abdominal fibromatosis.

Computed tomography shows variable attenuation and enhancement due to variations in tumour composition. An infiltrative pattern is common in young patients, whereas a nodular pattern is frequent in adults. The tumour is usually confined to the musculature and adjacent fascia, but encasement of adjacent nerves and vessels sometimes occurs (Fig. 18.1). Infiltration of overlying subcutaneous tissue is uncommon. The lesion may cause pressure erosion of adjacent bones, but bone invasion is unusual.

At MRI, the tumours show hypo- or isointense signal areas compared to muscle on T1-weighted images, while on T2-weighted images, they are mostly intermediate, although very low and extremely high signal intensities are occasionally seen [8]. Low signal intensity areas on T2-weighted images are thought to be attributable to an increased amount of collagen [1]. Differences in signal intensity between different tumour components, between asynchronous multicentric tumours and between primary and recurrent lesions represent combinations of variations in cellular content, amount of collagen, water content of the extracellular space and vascularity [5]. FDG PET imaging of aggressive fibromatosis shows abnormal uptake similar to that of malignant bone tumour [18].

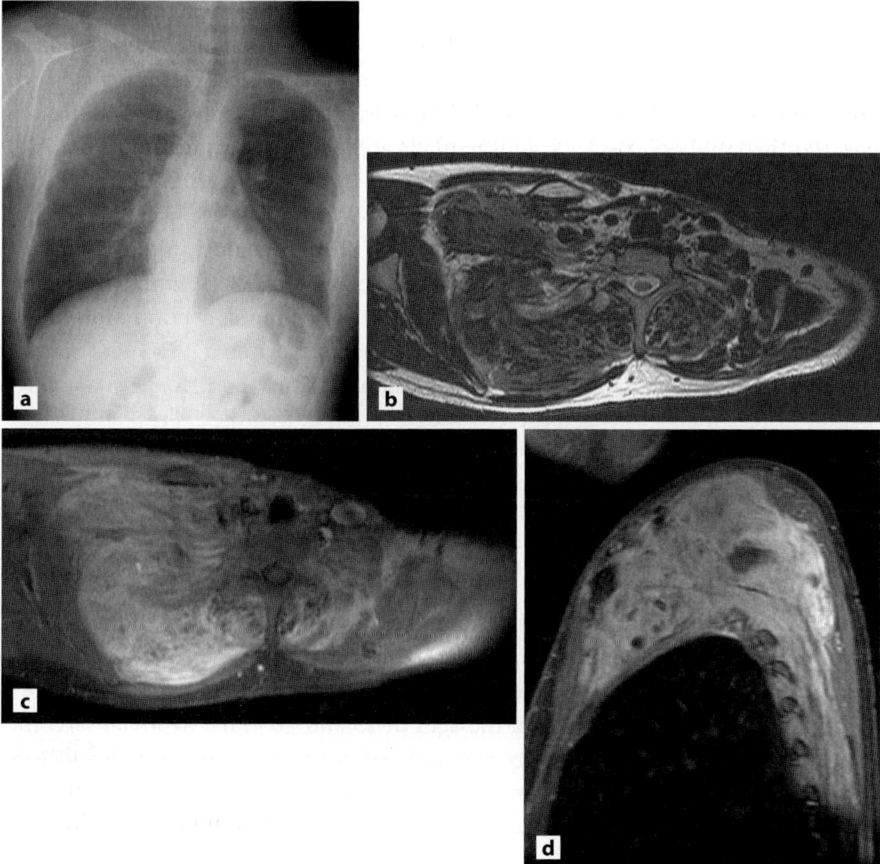

**Fig. 18.1** Aggressive fibromatosis in a 42-year-old man. **a** Chest radiograph shows increased attenuation of soft tissue mass in the right clavicular region. **b** Axial T2-weighted MR image shows infiltrative mass isointense relative to muscle. **c** Axial contrast-enhanced fat saturated T1-weighted MR image shows marked enhancement with invasion of the musculature. **d** Sagittal contrast-enhanced fat saturated T1-weighted MR image shows invasion of adjacent vascular structures

## 18.2.2
## Angiosarcoma

Angiosarcomas are malignant endothelial neoplasms characterised by vasoformative architecture. Patients with angiosarcoma frequently present with an enlarging, painful mass that is occasionally associated with haemorrhage, anaemia or coagulopathy [17]. Chronic lymphoedema is the most widely recognised predisposing factor to angiosarcoma, but the tumour is also associated with radiation therapy and chemical exposure. Tumours arising in the deep soft tissues show a predilection for the lower extremities, whereas the cutaneous forms are often found in the head and neck. Angiosarcomas are thus rare in the sternocostoclavicular region.

Magnetic resonance imaging shows a heterogeneous mass, which becomes sharply delineated with intravenous gadolinium administration [6]. Feeding vessels are usually seen in the periphery of the tumour (Fig. 18.2). Fibrous thickening, soft tissue nodules, increased fat attenuation and fluid collection around the muscles characterise the tumours associated with lymphoedema. FDG PET reveals intense accumulation in angiosarcomatous lesions and may contribute to the diagnosis of distant metastases and thereby the selection of treatment [15].

### 18.2.3
### Synovial Sarcoma

Synovial sarcomas are rare, malignant mesenchymal neoplasms that mostly occur in the para-articular regions, usually close to joint capsules, bursae and tendon sheaths of the extremities. Synovial sarcoma in the chest wall is extremely rare and usually occurs in patients between the ages of 15 and 40 years. Synovial sarcoma is a clinically and morphologically well-defined entity that has been extensively described, but its biological features remain a matter of controversy. A definitive diagnosis is made by identifying a t(x;18)(p11; q11) translocation in the tumour cells.

Computed tomography shows a soft tissue mass of slightly higher density than muscle which may infiltrate adjacent structures. Cortical bone erosion or invasion is well depicted on CT, as are intratumoral calcifications, which are noted in 20–30% of cases.

At MRI, most tumours show heterogeneous signal intensity that is predominately isointense relative to muscle on T1-weighted images [10]. Small foci of high signal on T1-weighted images suggest haemorrhage and are noted in 45% of cases. Fluid-fluid levels can be a striking finding, and they are seen in 15–25% of patients. Haemorrhage with fluid-fluid levels or high signal intensity on all pulse sequences may be associated with a poorer prognosis, because such tumours are usually large with extensive tissue invasion. On T2-weighted images, marked heterogeneity is the rule, and various degrees of internal septation may be noted (Fig. 18.3). This finding is especially true for larger tumours, which show a heterogeneous signal pattern in more than 85% of the cases. A triple signal pattern on T2-weighted im-

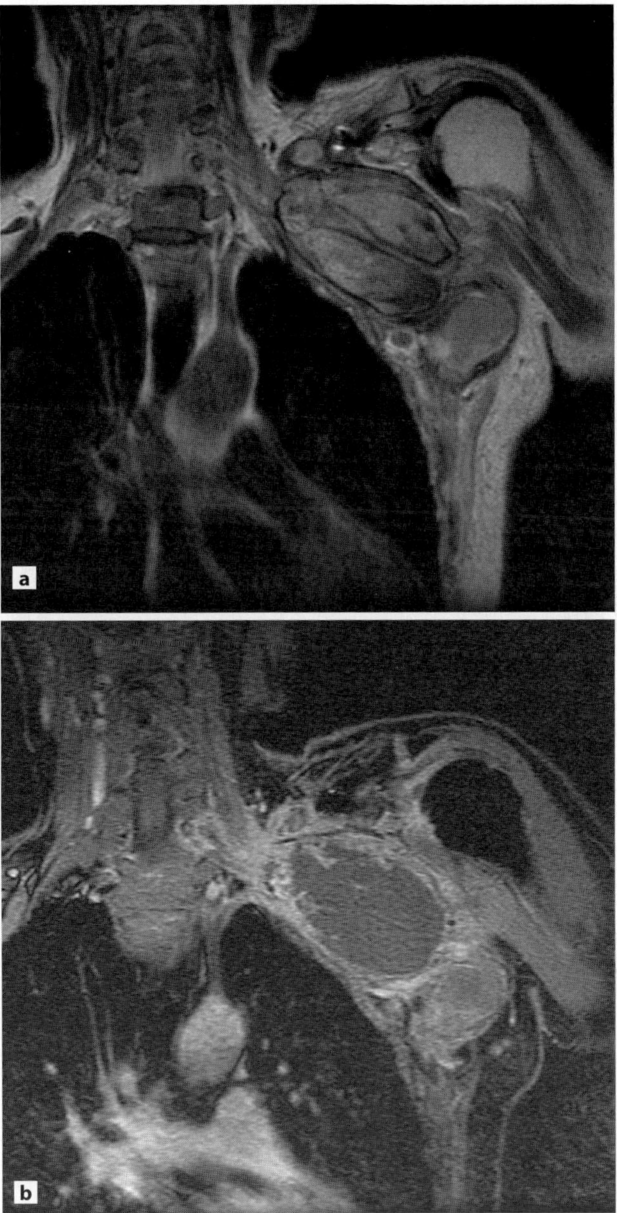

**Fig. 18.2** Angiosarcoma in a 77-year-old man presenting with a large mass arising from the subclavicular region. **a** Tumour infiltrates from the subclavicular region to the axilla. Coronal T2-weighted MR image shows a multiloculated heterogeneous mass. **b** Tumour shows heterogeneous and peripheral enhancement suggestive of necrosis

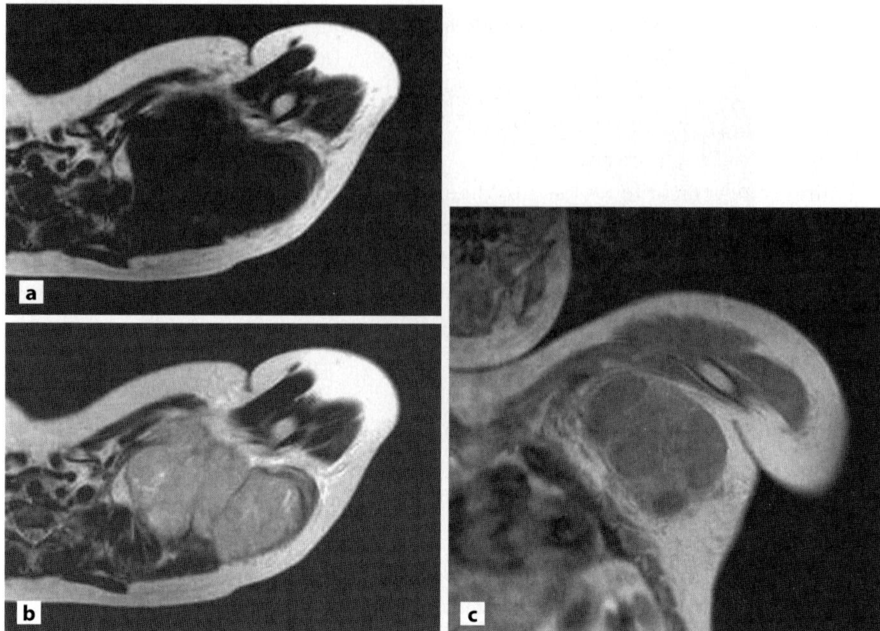

**Fig. 18.3** Synovial sarcoma in a 13-year-old boy. **a** Axial T1-weighted MR image shows soft tissue mass isointense relative to muscle. **b** Axial T2-weighted MR image shows heterogeneous signal intensity and internal septations. **c** Coronal contrast-enhanced T1-weighted MR image shows heterogeneous enhancement

ages is noted in 33% of cases, which consists of a high signal similar to that of fluid, an intermediate signal intensity iso- or hyperintense relative to fat, and low signal intensity closer to that of fibrous tissue. This triple signal pattern on T2-weighted images together with the small high signal foci on T1-weighted images, the presence of calcifications and proximity to a joint suggest the diagnosis [20, 21].

## 18.2.4
## Malignant Peripheral Nerve Sheath Tumour

Malignant peripheral nerve sheath tumours (MPNST) are malignant neoplasms of nerve sheath origin that can locally infiltrate and metastasise. They represent approximately 6% of all malignant soft tissue tumours. Although up to 50% of MPNSTs are associated with type 1 neurofibromatosis (NF-1), only about 5% of patients with NF-1 develop MPNST. MPNSTs have a predilection for the proximal portions of the limbs and the trunk followed by the head and neck. A slow-growing mass and pain are the most common symptoms. However, the onset of pain and sudden enlargement of a pre-existing neurofibroma indicate malignant transformation. Necrosis, haemorrhage and calcification are common features and cause heterogeneity of the tumour.

Plain radiographs can be used to detect calcification or osseous change within the area of a pre-existing neurofibroma and, when observed, the possibility of malignant transformation to MPNST should be considered.

Precontrast CT usually shows a large heterogeneous mass with or without intralesional calcification, bone erosion and bone destruction. Contrast-enhanced CT shows heterogeneous, predominantly peripheral, enhancement.

Magnetic resonance imaging can show an invasive mass located along the course of a nerve [13]. MPNST shows isointensity or slightly high intensity compared to muscle on T1-weighted images and markedly high intensity on T2-weighted images. On contrast-enhanced T1-weighted images they appear as areas of heterogeneous enhancement (Fig. 18.4). These findings reflect the heterogeneity of the tumour. Ill-defined margins, invasion of surrounding fatty tissue or adjacent

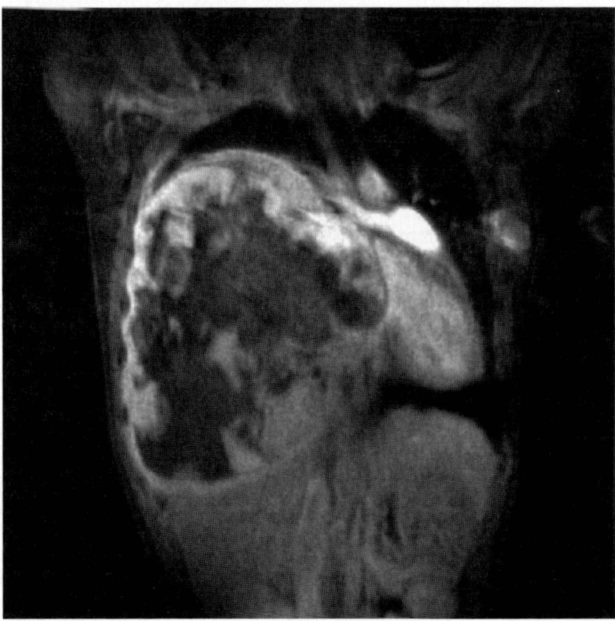

**Fig. 18.4** Malignant peripheral nerve sheath tumour. MRI, coronal contrast enhanced image show a large inhomogeneous tumour with compression of the chest wall, mediastinal viscera, liver and the right lower lobe of the lung

structures, perilesional oedema, irregular bone destruction, involvement of lymph nodes and pleural effusion can be helpful in establishing the diagnosis of MPNST. Malignant transformation of neurofibromas may result in loss of the target-like appearance of the benign lesions (a peripheral area of high signal intensity with a central area of low signal intensity) on T2-weighted images.

Abnormal [67]Ga-citrate uptake in patients with NF-1 suggests malignant transformation and indicates the need for further evaluation by other imaging methods. FDG PET has become the predominant non-invasive technique for biological tumour evaluation. Several studies have reported the usefulness of FDG PET in differentiating high-grade soft tissue sarcomas from low-grade or benign soft tissue tumours. MPNSTs yield higher standard uptake values (SUV) than benign tumours, but there is an overlap between the SUVs of malignant and benign tumours. FDG PET has been reported capable of identifying sarcomatous change within neurofibromatosis.

## 18.2.5
## Low-grade Fibromyxoid Sarcoma

Low-grade fibromyxoid sarcoma (LGFMS) is a spindle cell tumour with mixed histological features. The tumour is grossly well circumscribed, but there is often extensive microscopic infiltration of the surrounding soft tissue. Histopathologically, the tumour shows intermingled fibrous and myxoid zones with abrupt abutting or gradual transition. Paradoxically LGFMS often has an aggressive behaviour. LGFMS can be a serious disease with a recurrence rate of 68%, a metastasis rate of 41% and a mortality rate of 18%. However, in a recent study ascertained prospectively, the rates of recurrence, metastasis and death were 9%, 6% and 2%, respectively [9]. LGFMS typically affects young adults. The median age at presentation is 15–34 years, and there is no sex difference. It presents as a slow-growing, non-tender and firm tumour. Up to 19% of cases occur in patients younger than 18 years old. Most lesions arise from the deep soft tissue at the lower limbs or thoracic wall, followed by the groin, buttock, axilla and retroperitoneum. Superficial lesions occur in less than 10–20% of cases.

Only a few reports have described the imaging features of LGFMS. Plain radiographs reveal well-delineated soft tissue mass. Precontrast CT sometimes demonstrates a homogeneously isodense mass displaying heterogeneous contrast enhancement. To our knowledge, there has been only one report in the English literature describing the MRI features (Fig. 18.5). Koh et al. have reported MRI features of two cases with LGFMS [11]. The first patient had a large and ovoid mass within the thigh, including some intralesional nodules within the tumour showing a target-like appearance. The second patient had a dumbbell-shaped lesion with invasive features. There have been no reports of the scintigraphy or FDG-PET findings in LGFMS.

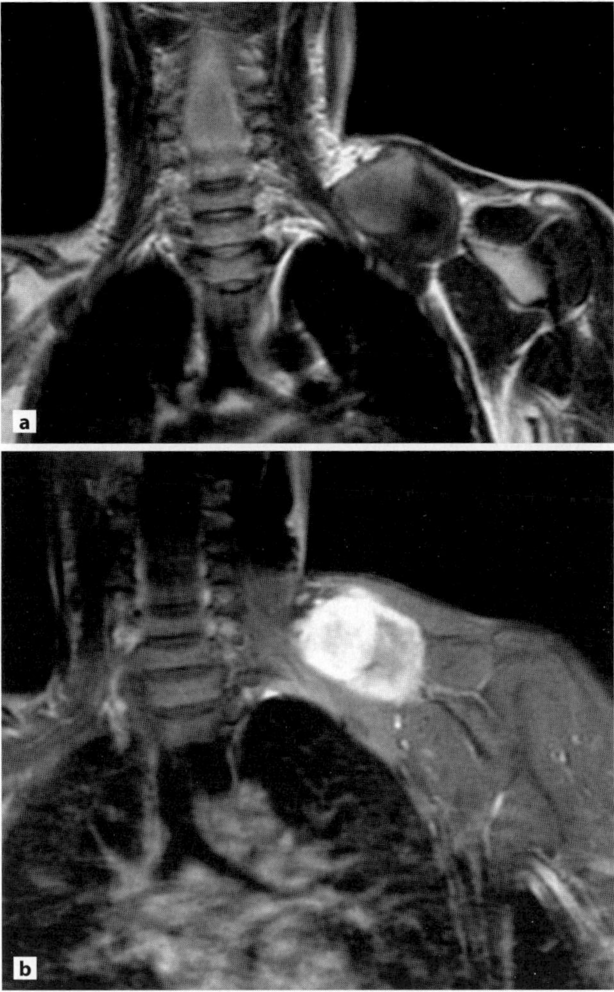

**Fig. 18.5** Low-grade fibromyxoid sarcoma in the left supraclavicular region of a 10-year-old boy. **a** On coronal T2-weighted MR images, the tumour showed heterogeneously low to high signal intensity. **b** The tumour enhanced heterogeneously on coronal contrast-enhanced T1-weighted MR images. The area of lower signal intensity on T2-weighted MR image enhances less than areas of higher signal intensity on T2-weighted MR image; the former represents the area of increased cellularity and the latter the myxoid area

### 18.2.6
### Ossifying Fibromyxoid Tumour of Soft Parts

Ossifying fibromyxoid tumour of soft parts is a rare histologically benign or low-grade malignant tumour of uncertain origin [7]. It affects men more frequently (64%) than women, and occurs from 14 to 79 years of age with a median of 50 years. Approximately 70% of the lesions arise in the extremities and the second most common site is the chest wall. Most patients present with a small, painless, well-defined, subcutaneous mass, typically covered by a thick fibrous pseudocapsule with or without a shell of bone. Approximately 80% of the lesions are surrounded by an incomplete shell of metaplastic lamellar bone, and the other 20% completely lack a shell of bone (non-ossifying variant). Fatty marrow spaces can be seen between the metaplastic bone trabeculae. The atypical or malignant type of this tumour is characterised by hypercellularity and/or increased numbers of mitotic figures, and they tend to have a much less complete shell of bone than benign examples.

Plain radiographs reveal a well-circumscribed, lobulated mass containing irregular calcifications and surrounded by an incomplete ring of calcification [19]. Erosion or destruction of underlying bone and a periosteal reaction simulating a parosteal osteosarcoma has been reported. CT is capable of demonstrating the typical lamellar bone formation. Contrast-enhanced CT may reveal significant enhancement of the soft tissue because of high vascularity. At MRI, a high intensity area on T1-weighted images reflects fatty marrow spaces, and a high intensity area on T2-weighted images corresponds to myxoid material. Contrast-enhanced T1-weighted images show heterogeneous enhancement (Fig. 18.6). At bone scintigraphy, the localised increase in uptake correlates with the mature bone formation in the tumour, although this is not a specific finding.

## 18.3
## Myeloproliferative and Allied Disorders

### 18.3.1
### Malignant Lymphoma

Extranodal diffuse B-cell lymphoma is the most frequent primary chest wall lymphoma and presents a multinodal or diffuse infiltrative pattern. Malignant lymphoma mainly occurs in the sixth decade of life. An increased incidence has been described in patients who have undergone orthopaedic surgery using metallic

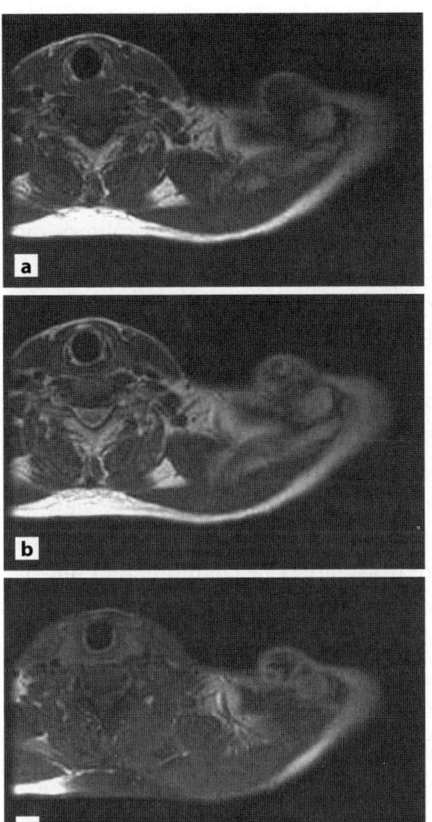

**Fig. 18.6** Ossifying fibromyxoid tumour in a 59-year-old man. **a** On axial T1-weighted MR image, tumour shows homogeneous isointensity compared to that of muscle. **b** Focal myxoid components show high intensity on axial T2-weighted MR image. **c** On axial contrast-enhanced T1-weighted MR image, the tumour shows heterogeneous enhancement

implants, in patients with AIDS or those receiving immunosuppressive therapy, for example after organ transplantation.

Computed tomography shows attenuation similar to that of muscle, and poor, diffuse enhancement after intravenous injection of contrast material [12, 16]. At MRI, lymphomas appear as large masses with signal intensity comparable to or slightly lower than adjacent muscle on T1-weighted images, and hyperintense on T2-weighted or STIR images (Fig. 7.4). Infiltration along the neurovascular bundle and extension through the subcutaneous tissues is common. FDG PET has been reported to detect viable tumours in malignant lymphomas, and can be used to improve staging at the initial diagnosis by detecting active lesions. FDG PET may also be used in patients with residual masses, and can be used to differentiate between active lymphoma and inactive fibrotic tissue.

### 18.3.2
### Solitary and Multiple Myeloma

Solitary and multiple myeloma are plasma cell tumours that occur in the form of a single mass or as diffuse marrow involvement. Solitary myelomas occur in a younger age group (mean age about 50 years) than multiple myeloma that has a peak age of presentation at 65–70 years. Many cases of apparently solitary myeloma progress over time to multiple myeloma.

Solitary myeloma of bone manifests radiologically as a multicystic expansive mass or purely osteolytic focus without expansion. The less common extraosseous solitary myeloma, which presents as a non-specific soft tissue mass, progresses to multiple myeloma less frequently [3]. In multiple myeloma, the abnormal accumulation of plasma cells in bone marrow is associated with multiple areas of osteolysis because the plasma cells produce an osteoclastic stimulating factor.

Multiple osteolytic lesions with discrete margins are typically detected radiographically in the vertebral column, ribs and clavicles. Sclerosis in the lesions generally develops after a pathological fracture, irradiation or chemotherapy for osteolytic lesions, although it is occasionally seen in untreated lesions.

Tumours are detected as low signal intensity on T1-weighted images and high signal intensity on T2-weighted images. Contrast-enhanced MR images may be an effective means of monitoring the response to therapy [14]. Bone scintigraphy may be false-negative, but FDG PET is highly accurate for detecting the extent of multiple active lesions [4]. FDG PET may also contribute to the initial staging of solitary myelomas.

### 18.3.3
### Granulocytic Sarcoma

Granulocytic sarcoma, also called extramedullary myeloblastoma, is an uncommon malignant tumour that rarely involves the chest wall. It is essentially a solid tumour that contains precursor cells. This tumour can occur as a complication during the course of chronic myeloid leukaemia or other myeloproliferative disorders. Tumour manifests as an infiltrative mass in the periosteal regions, soft tissues of the neck or trunk, central nervous system and skin.

▶ **Fig. 18.7** Granulocytic sarcoma in a 47-year-old man. **a** Axial T2-weighted MR image shows a mass with heterogeneous increased signal intensity relative to muscle in the sternal region. **b** Axial contrast-enhanced fat saturated T1-weighted (600/15) MR image shows pronounced and heterogeneous enhancement of tumour. **c** Axial FDG PET/CT image shows abnormal uptake within the tumour

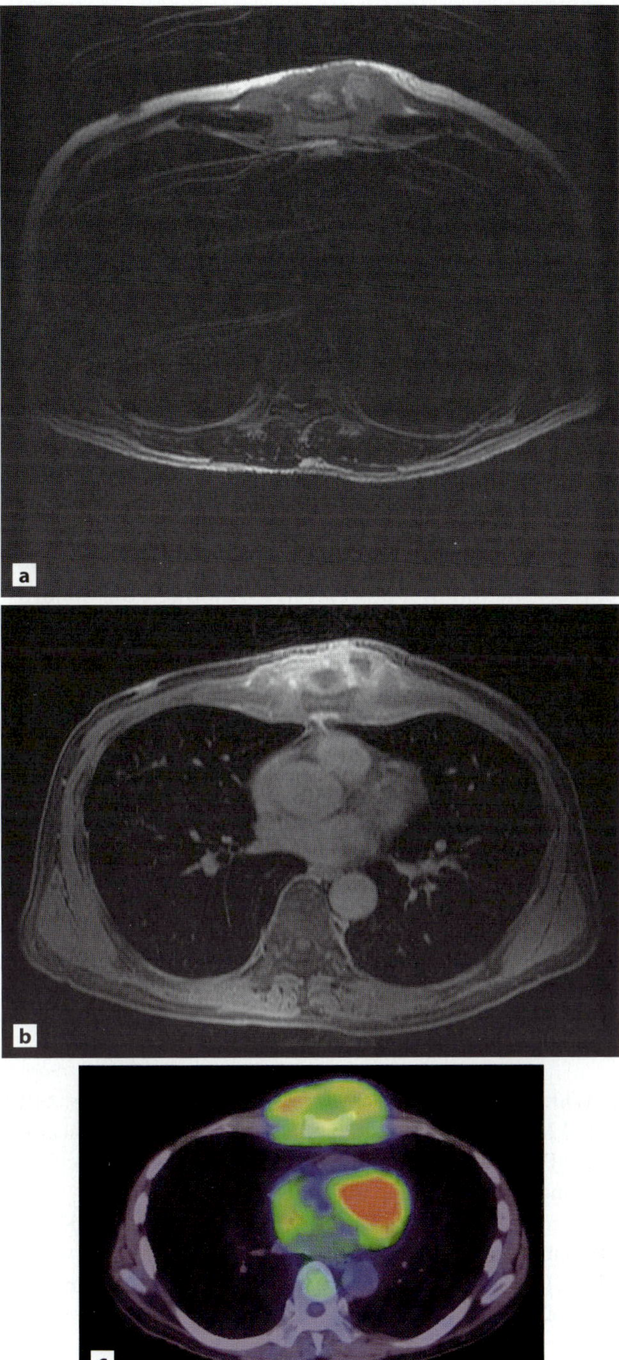

Computed tomography shows non-calcified, irregular masses with poorly defined margins. At MRI, tumours appear as irregular and homogeneous masses with signal intensity comparable to or slightly lower than that of adjacent muscles on T1-weighted images and hyperintense on T2-weighted images [2]. Contrast-enhanced MR images reveal homogeneous enhancement and may be an effective means of detecting and monitoring the response to therapy. FDG PET reveals hypermetabolic masses and may also be useful for detecting active lesions (Fig. 18.7).

## 18.4
## Conclusion

Malignant disorders of the sternocostoclavicular region include a diverse group of lesions with a wide variety of histological lineages. Evaluation of tumours usually includes conventional chest radiography to detect and localise the lesions, CT or MRI to further characterise the tumour and define its extent, and investigation of anato-metabolic correlation by FDG PET/CT. Although the majority of these tumours have a non-specific appearance, in some patients, the combination of clinical and imaging findings may suggest the diagnosis. Despite their non-specific appearances, imaging is important for the staging, grading, therapeutic planning and follow-up of malignant disorders of the sternocostoclavicular region.

**Acknowledgements.** The authors acknowledge the help of Dr. Akira Kawai, Dr. Fumihiko Nakatani and Dr. Yasuo Beppu for their contribution to the study. This work was funded by BMS Freedom to Discovery Grant and was supported in part by grants for Scientific Research Expenses for Health and Welfare Programs, number 17–12.

## References

1.   Ackman JB, Whitman GJ, Chew FS (1994) Aggressive fibromatosis. AJR 163:544
2.   Arthur S (2000) Myeloblastoma (chloroma) in leukemia. J Clin Oncol 18:3993–3997
3.   Bataille R, Sany J (1981) Solitary myeloma: clinical and prognostic features of a review of 114 cases. Cancer 48:845–851
4.   Bredella MA, Steinbach L, Caputo G, et al (2005) Value of FDG PET in the assessment of patients with multiple myeloma. AJR 184:1199–1024
5.   Casillas J, Sais GJ, Greve JL, Iparraguirre MC, Morillo G (1991) Imaging of intra- and extraabdominal desmoid tumors. Radiographics 11:959–968

6.  Coldwell DM, Baron RL, Charnsangavej C (1989) Angiosarcoma. Diagnosis and clinical course. Acta Radiol 30:627–631

7.  Enzinger FM, Weiss SW, Liang CY (1989) Ossifying fibromyxoid tumor of soft parts. A clinicopathological analysis of 59 cases. Am J Surg Pathol 13:817–827

8.  Feld R, Burk DL Jr, McCue P, Mitchell DG, Lackman R, Rifkin MD (1990) MRI of aggressive fibromatosis: frequent appearance of high signal intensity on T2-weighted images. Magn Reson Imaging 8:583–588

9.  Folpe AL, Lane KL, Paull G, et al (2000) Low-grade fibromyxoid sarcoma and hyalinizung spindle cell tumor with giant rosettes: a clinicopathologic study of 73 cases supporting their identity and assessing the impact of high-grade areas. Am J Surg Pathol 24:1353–1360

10.  Jones BC, Sundaram M, Kransdorf MJ (1993) Synovial sarcoma: MRI findings in 34 patients. AJR 161:827–830

11.  Koh SH, Choe HS, Lee IJ, et al (2005) Low-grade fibromyxoid sarcoma: ultrasound and magnetic resonance findings in two cases. Skeletal Radiol 34:550–554

12.  Lee VS, Martinez S, Coleman RE (1997) Primary muscle lymphoma: clinical and imaging findings. Radiology 203:237–244

13.  Levine E, Huntrakoon M, Wetzel LH (1987) Malignant nerve-sheath neoplasms in neurofibromatosis: distinction from benign tumors by using imaging techniques. AJR 149:1059–1064

14.  Libshitz HI, Malthouse SR, Cunningham D, MacVicar AD, Husband JE (1992) Multiple myeloma: appearance at MRI. Radiology 182:833–837

15.  Maeda T, Tateishi U, Hasegawa T, et al (2006) Primary hepatic angiosarcoma on co-registered FDG-PET and CT images. AJR (in press)

16.  Malloy PC, Fishman EK, Magid D (1992) Lymphoma of bone, muscle, and skin: CT findings. AJR 159:805–809

17.  Meis-Kindblom JM, Kindblom LG (1998) Angiosarcoma of soft tissue: a study of 80 cases. Am J Surg Pathol 22:683–697

18.  Meller J, Lehmann K, Altenvoerde G, et al (2000) F-18-FDG PET for the detection of aggressive fibromatosis. Nuklearmedizin 39:115–117

19.  Schaffler G, Raith J, Ranner G, Weybora W, Jeserschek R (1997) Radiographic appearance of an ossifying fibromyxoid tumor of soft parts. Skeletal Radiol 26:615–618

20.  Tateishi U, Gladish GW, Kusumoto M, et al (2003) Chest wall tumors: radiologic findings and pathologic correlation: part 2. malignant tumors. Radiographics 23:1491–1508

21.  Tateishi U, Hasegawa T, Beppu Y, et al (2004) Synovial sarcoma of the soft tissues: prognostic significance of imaging features. J Comput Assist Tomogr 28:140–148

# 19   Miscellaneous Disorders

ANNE GRETHE JURIK

**Contents**



## 19.1
## Introduction

The sternocostoclavicular (SCC) region can be involved by all kinds of musculo-skeletal disorders. Apart from the disorders dealt with in Chapters 10–18 the following disorders have been observed.

## 19.2
## Metabolic Disorders

Osteoarthropathy in primary and secondary *hyperparathyroidism* can involve the sternoclavicular region. Subperiosteal bone resorption and sclerosis, particularly along the inferior margin of the clavicle, result in widening and irregularity of the sternoclavicular joint. The changes are related predominantly to trabecular destruction beneath cartilage surfaces, substitutive fibrosis and new bone formation

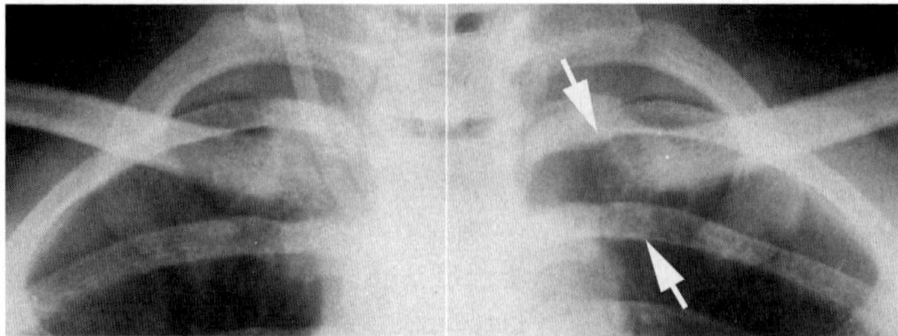

**Fig. 19.1** Hyperparathyroidism. AP radiograph of the sternoclavicular joints in a 25-year-old woman with secondary hyperparathyroidism. There are irregular joint facets with manifest osseous resorption in the medial part of the clavicles (*arrows*). The joint space thereby looks widened

(Fig. 19.1) [8]. Careful analysis of the sternoclavicular region on frontal chest film will usually disclose manifest changes. A radiographic diagnosis of hyperparathyroidism can thus be obtained from an otherwise negative chest study [13]. Also tumour-like calcific deposition may occur in the SCC region as part of hyperparathyroidism [7].

## 19.3
## Amyloidosis

Amyloid deposition is an important complication of long-term haemodialysis. It may be deposited in and around synovia, ligaments, tendons and bones, and may involve the sternoclavicular region [2]. The main radiographic features are periarticular soft tissue swelling, subchondral cysts and articular erosion. This appearance may simulate arthritis or infection [2]. Bone scintigraphy can sometimes be used to differentiate amyloidosis from infection because joint destruction due to amyloid deposition may fail to take up tracer.

## 19.4
## Synovial Osteochondromatosis

Synovial osteochondromatosis is a disorder characterised by hyperplastic proliferation of connective tissue in the synovial membrane with formation of metaplastic cartilage. It occurs mainly as a monarticular involvement of large joints, but can occur corresponding to the sternoclavicular joint even in children [14].

## 19.5
## Postoperative Disorders

Sternotomy for heart and vessel surgery may imply several postoperative changes or complications. *Postoperative infection* can be a serious complication with abscess formation and fistula. In a later stage *pseudoarthrosis* may be seen due to inadequate healing with widening of the sternotomy cleft and smoothing of the bone surface [12]. Occasionally broken cerclage wires cause pain and can be seen at radiography [11]. Osseous resorption around fixation material can also occur due to metalosis.

## 19.6
## Spontaneous Atraumatic Subluxation

Spontaneous atraumatic subluxation of the sternoclavicular joint is a relatively rare problem, occurring most commonly in teenagers and young adults who have general laxity. The subluxation occurs either during routine overhead activities or during overhead sports activities [9]. Spontaneous subluxation can also occur as part of a degenerative process or non-infectious subacute arthritis (Fig. 19.2) [10].

## 19.7
## Other Disorders

*Pagets' disease* occurs rarely in the SCC region. Polyostotic Pagets' disease may involve the manubrium and sternal body [3], and monostotic lesions can be seen in the clavicle. It presents as an enlarged and irregular dense osseous lesion. The definite diagnosis is usually based on typical histological features of active osteoclast resorption and osteoblast production.

*Osteopetrosis*, also named Albers Schoenberg disease, and other disorders involving the bone marrow may involve the SCC region (Fig. 19.3). Osteopetrosis represents a heterogeneous group of disorders characterised by an increase in bone density due to a defect in osteoclastic bone resorption [1].

*Avascular necrosis* or aseptic necrosis of the clavicular head (Friedrich's disease) has been reported [5] and may also occur corresponding to the sternum in disorders disposing to necrosis, such as sickle cell disease [6]. Also *Langerhans' cell histiocytosis* has been reported in the sternum [4].

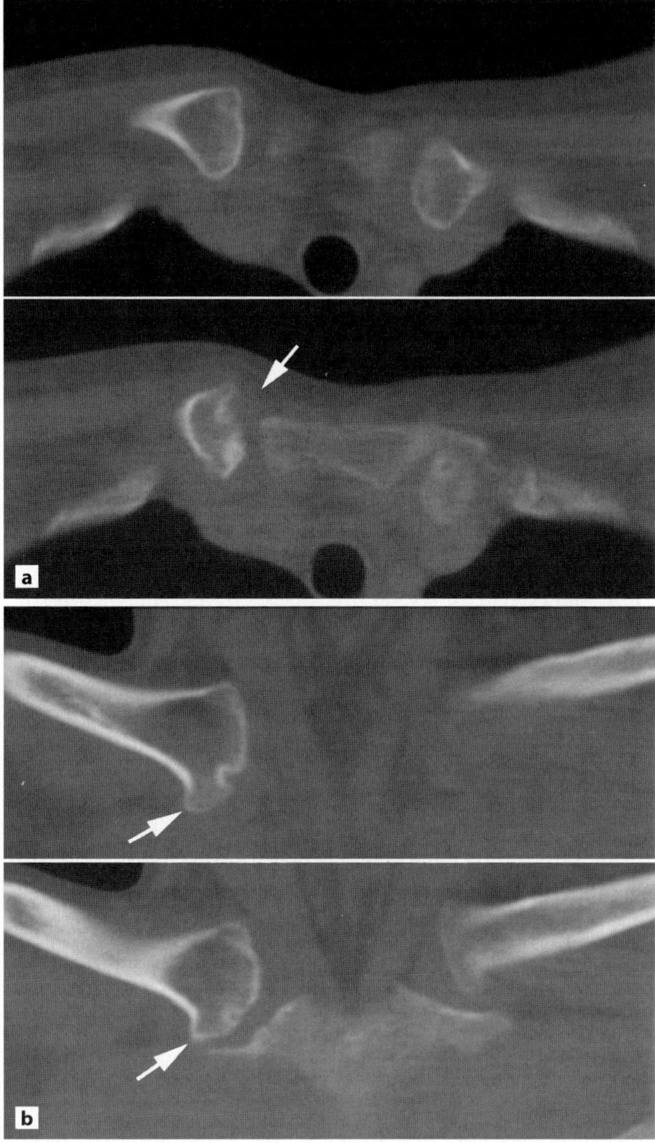

**Fig. 19.2** Spontaneous atraumatic subluxation of the sternoclavicular joint in a 62-year-old woman with a sudden swelling at the right sternoclavicular joint. **a** Axial CT slices show the clavicular joint facet displaced anteriorly (*arrow*) in relation to the sternum. **b** Coronal reconstruction shows definite signs of osteoarthritis in the form of osteophytes (*arrows*) and subchondral cysts

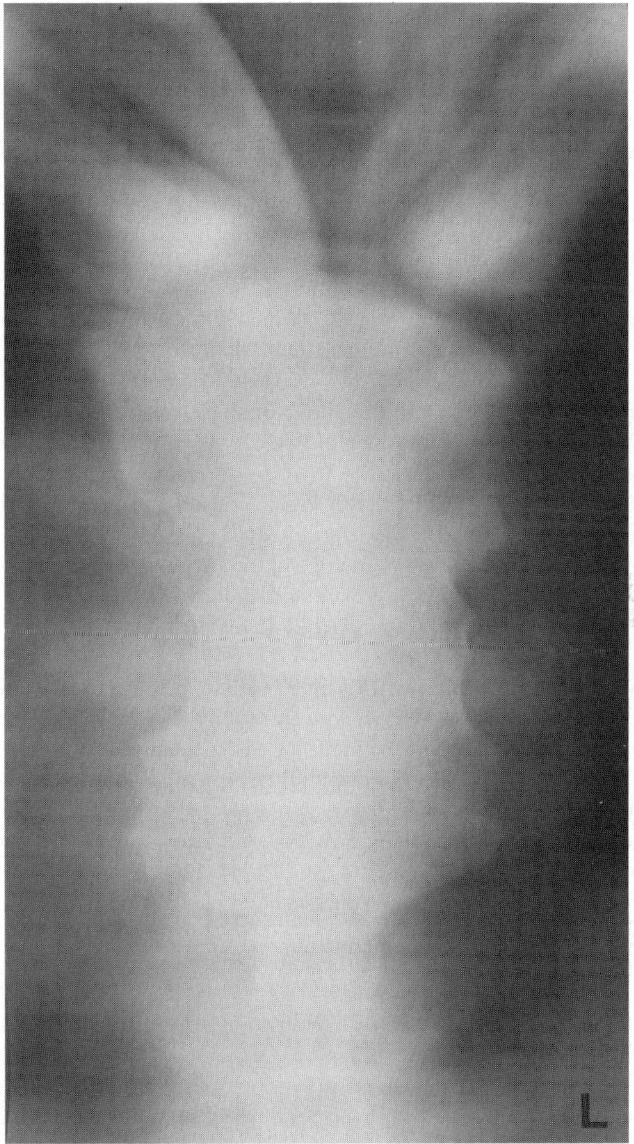

**Fig. 19.3** Osteopetrosis. Frontal tomography of a 20-year-old woman with inherent osteopetrosis. There is a homogeneous increased osseous density of the sternum and the medial part of the clavicles

## 19.8
## Conclusions

Many different disorders may involve the SCC region and have to be taken into consideration in patients with SCC symptoms or abnormal radiological findings.

## References


1.  Balemans W, Van Wesenbeeck L, Van Hul W (2005) A clinical and molecular overview of the human osteopetroses. Calcif Tissue Int 77:263–274
2.  Cameron EW, Resnik CS, Light PD, Sun CC (1997) Hemodialysis-related amyloidosis of the sternoclavicular joint. Skeletal Radiol 26:428–430
3.  Dowling K, Hutto RL, Dowling EA (1991) Sternal mass in a patient with Paget's disease. Invest Radiol 26:615–619
4.  Fazio N, Spaggiari L, Pelosi G, Presicci F, Preda L (2005) Langerhans' cell histiocytosis. Lancet 365:598
5.  Jurik AG (1994) Noninflammatory sclerosis of the sternal end of the clavicle: a follow-up study and review of the literature. Skeletal Radiol 23:373–378
6.  Knight-Madden JM, Sang MM, Ramphel PS (2005) Trap-door sternum in sickle cell disease. J Pediatr 146:845
7.  O'Malley BM, Haller JO, Twersky J, Tejani AH (1989) CT appearance of large sternoclavicular calcific masses in a teenager with chronic renal disease and secondary hyperparathyroidism, on hemodialysis maintenance. Pediatr Radiol 19:339–340
8.  Resnick D, Niwayama G (1976) Subchondral resorption of bone in renal osteodystrophy. Radiology 118:315–321
9.  Rockwood CA Jr, Odor JM (1989) Spontaneous atraumatic anterior subluxation of the sternoclavicular joint. J Bone Joint Surg Am 71:1280–1288
10. Sadr B, Swann M (1979) Spontaneous dislocation of the sterno-clavicular joint. Acta Orthop Scand 50:269–274
11. Shih CM, Su YY, Lin SJ, Shih CC (2005) Failure analysis of explanted sternal wires. Biomaterials 26:2053–2059
12. Templeton PA, Fishman EK (1992) CT evaluation of poststernotomy complications. Am J Roentgenol 159:45–50
13. Teplick JG, Eftekhari F, Haskin ME (1974) Erosion of the sternal ends of the clavicles. A new sign of primary and secondary hyperparathyroidism. Radiology 113:323–326
14. Vrdoljak J, Irha E (2000) Synovial osteochondromatosis of the sternoclavicular joint. Pediatr Radiol 30:181–183

# Subject Index

Printing: Krips bv, Meppel
Binding: Stürtz, Würzburg